ACLS
Review

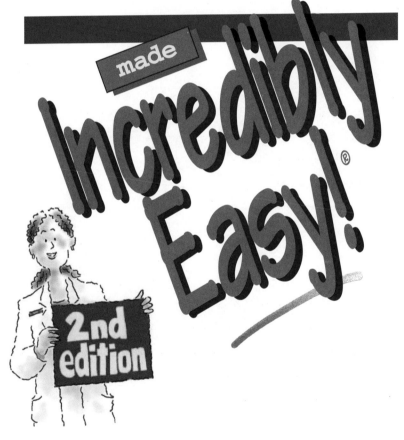

made
Incredibly
Easy!®

2nd
edition

ACLS Review

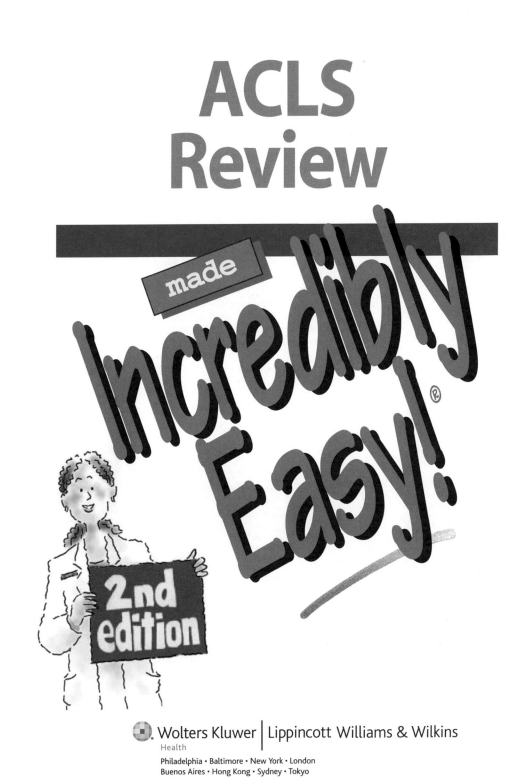

made

Incredibly

Easy!®

2nd edition

Wolters Kluwer | Lippincott Williams & Wilkins
Health

Philadelphia · Baltimore · New York · London
Buenos Aires · Hong Kong · Sydney · Tokyo

Staff

Clinical Director
Joan M. Robinson, RN, MSN

Clinical Project Manager
Lorraine Hallowell, RN, BSN, RVS

Clinical Editor
Kate Stout, RN, MSN

Product Director
David Moreau

Product Manager
Rosanne Hallowell

Editor
Karen C. Comerford

Copy Editor
Jerry Altobelli

Editorial Assistants
Karen J. Kirk, Jeri O'Shea, Linda K. Ruhf

Art Director
Elaine Kasmer

Designer
Joseph John Clark

Illustrator
Bot Roda

Vendor Manager
Karyn Crislip

Manufacturing Manager
Beth J. Welsh

Production and Indexing Services
SPi Global

Printed in China.

ACLSMIE2E010112

Library of Congress Cataloging-in-Publication Data

ACLS review made incredibly easy!—2nd ed.
   p. ; cm.
   Includes bibliographical references and index.
   ISBN 978-1-60831-288-7
   I. Lippincott Williams & Wilkins.
   [DNLM: 1. Advanced Cardiac Life Support—methods—Problems and Exercises. 2. Arrhythmias, Cardiac—therapy—Problems and Exercises. 3. Certification—methods—Problems and Exercises. WG 18.2]

LC classification not assigned
616.1'230250076—dc23

2011032644

Contents

Appendices and index

Contributors and consultants

Linda Cason, MSN, RN-BC, NE-BC, CNRN
Manager Employee Education &
 Development Department
Deaconess Hospital
Evansville, IN

Wendeline J. Grbach, RN, MSN, CCRN,
 CLNC
Curriculum Developer for Simulation
 Education
UPMC Shadyside School of Nursing
Pittsburgh, PA

Molly Groban, RN, MS, MAEd, CEN, CCRN,
 SANE, MICN, LNC
Director of Education
JFK Memorial Hospital
Indio, CA

Elizabeth E. Hand, RN, MS
ECC Instructor
Hillcrest Medical Center
Tulsa, OK

Kathleen M. Hill, RN, MSN, CCNS-CSC
Clinical Nurse Specialist, Surgical
 Intensive Care Unit
Cleveland Clinic
Cleveland, OH

Cynthia Holt, RN, MN, CCRN, CCNS, APN
Cardiovascular Clinical Nurse
 Specialist
Morristown Memorial Hospital
Morristown, NJ

Jared Kutzin, RN, DNP, MPH
Director of Nursing & Clinical
 Simulation
Institute for Medical Simulation &
 Advanced Learning
Bronx, NY

Brenda Lammert, RN, BSN
Staff Development Specialist
Good Samaritan Hospital
Vincennes, IN

Margaret McAtee, RN, MN, ACNP-BC,
 CCRN
Cardiovascular Nurse Practitioner
Baylor All Saints Medical Center
Fort Worth, TX

Kathryn Moore, RN, DNP, CCRN, CEN,
 ACNP-BC, ANP-BC
Assistant Professor
University of Kentucky College of
 Nursing
Lexington

Cheryl Schmitz, RN, MS, CNS-BC, CEN
Clinical Specialist for Emergency
 Services
Inova Loudoun Hospital
Leesburg, VA

Not another boring foreword

If you're like me, you're too busy to wade through a foreword that uses pretentious terms and umpteen dull paragraphs to get to the point. So let's cut right to the chase! Here's why *ACLS Review Made Incredibly Easy*, 2nd edition, is so terrific:

It will teach you the important things you need to know about advanced cardiac life support. (And it will leave out all the fluff that wastes your time.)

It will help you remember what you've learned.

It will make you smile as it enhances your knowledge and skills.

Don't believe me? Try these recurring logos on for size:

Peak technique—provides tips for performing procedures

Go with the flow—presents need-to-know algorithms

Now I get it!—explains complex processes in an easy-to-understand way

Memory jogger—reinforces learning through acronyms and other tools that aid recall

See? I told you! And that's not all. Look for me and my friends in the margins throughout this book. We'll be there to explain key concepts, provide important care reminders, and offer reassurance. Oh, and if you don't mind, we'll be spicing up the pages with a bit of humor along the way, to teach and entertain in a way that no other resource can.

I hope you find this book helpful. Best of luck throughout your career!

Joy

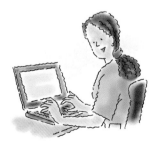

ACLS essentials

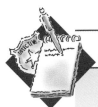

Just the facts

In this chapter, you'll learn:

♦ core concepts of advanced cardiac life support (ACLS)

♦ basic components of the ACLS course

♦ study strategies to help you prepare for the ACLS examination.

What is ACLS?

Advanced cardiac life support (ACLS) is a systematic approach to resuscitation efforts. ACLS training gives rescuers a coordinated way to approach critically ill patients, regardless of response team size. (See *ACLS core concepts*, page 2.)

Health care workers seeking ACLS training include physicians, registered nurses (RNs), advanced emergency medical services (EMS) personnel, and dental and surgical care professionals.

> Don't sweat ACLS training! Six to eight hours of coursework will prepare you for the written and practical examination.

ACLS training

The foundation of ACLS is high-quality basic life support (BLS). A current BLS card is required of ACLS training participants.

The ACLS card is granted after a person successfully finishes an initial 2-day course or an 8-hour recertification course. The course involves lectures on ACLS concepts and hands-on practice using simulated ACLS situations, followed by a written and practical examination. Certification cards are issued only to active healthcare providers with the appropriate skills and knowledge to participate in ACLS.

Keep in mind that the completion card, which verifies that you've successfully completed the course, isn't a license

ACLS core concepts

Here are the core concepts and skills you'll need for advanced cardiac life support (ACLS) training.

General skills

For all devices and procedures, you should know:

- indications
- precautions
- proper use.

For every medication, you should know:

- why to use it
- when to use it
- how to administer it
- what to watch for.

Airway management

You should know how to perform and assist with endotracheal intubation. You should also know alternative ventilation techniques, such as how to use a bag-valve mask device and laryngeal mask airway.

Early management

You should know how to manage the first 30 minutes of emergencies that result from such causes as:

- acute coronary syndrome
- cardiac arrest associated with trauma
- cardiac arrest involving a pregnant patient
- cardiac tamponade
- drowning and near-drowning
- electrocution and lightning strike

- hypothermia
- pneumothorax
- possible drug overdose
- stroke
- thrombosis.

Electrical therapy

You should know how to safely use electrical devices, such as an automated external defibrillator, conventional defibrillator, and pacemakers.

Emergency conditions

You should be able to identify indications for ACLS, such as asystole, pulseless electrical activity, supraventricular tachycardias, ventricular tachycardia, and ventricular fibrillation. You should also be able to institute proper treatment for the identified indication quickly.

I.V. and invasive techniques

You should be familiar with I.V. and invasive therapeutic techniques, such as peripheral and central I.V. line insertion and intraosseous cannulation.

Pharmacology

You should know the action, indication, dosages, and precautions for the major drugs used during ACLS, such as adenosine, amiodarone, and epinephrine.

to perform techniques discussed or reviewed in the course (such as endotracheal intubation or I.V. catheterization). Instead, each person's scope of practice and state license determines her ability to perform these techniques. ACLS renewal is required every 2 years.

Online possibilities

Electronic courses may be available to provide part of the initial and recertification education online but they can't be used exclusively to assess a participant's competence. Hands-on performance assessment of individual rescuers and teams is essential.

Born to teach

After completing your course, if you show exemplary understanding of the core concepts and you're interested in teaching an ACLS course, you can follow the formal process to become an ACLS instructor.

ACLS examination

The ACLS examination includes a written or online section and a practical section. The written section, issued by the AHA, contains 30 to 50 multiple-choice questions, depending on the version used. The test takes about 1 hour.

To pass the written section of the examination, you must answer 84% of the questions correctly. If you don't pass the written section, you may take it a second time at a later date.

"Mega" practice

The practical section of the examination follows the written section and must be completed with an authorized instructor at a training center. During this section, you'll have the opportunity to participate in established case scenarios called a Megacode. A Megacode is a recreation of an emergency situation in which a team approach is used to give appropriate treatment. Every team member will have a chance to enact each role, including the team leader, person in charge of the airway, medication provider, and cardiopulmonary resuscitation provider. You'll be expected to precisely and thoroughly carry out all the necessary steps of each role, which may take 5 to 10 minutes, depending on the case scenario.

Study strategies

The ACLS examination calls for thorough preparation. The test assesses both knowledge of ACLS concepts and the ability to apply those concepts during high-pressure emergency situations. Still, as a trained health care professional, you should view the ACLS examination as just another step in your professional development. If you study and prepare effectively, you'll feel confident about the examination.

You can choose from several study strategies. Not all strategies are appropriate for every student. A combination of strategies will help you learn ACLS concepts and be enthusiastic about the material.

> **Key points**
>
> **Taking the examination**
> • The examination consists of written and practical sections.
> • The passing grade is 84%.
> • Participation in established case scenarios is required.
> • A team approach is used for the Megacode.

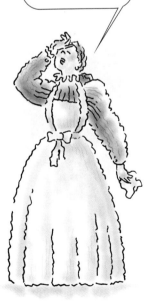

I'm ready for my role. Oh, this is the Megacode audition? Well, then, I think I might be a bit overdressed...

Determining your strengths and weaknesses

ACLS training focuses on a broad range of skills, from airway management to pharmacology to leadership during emergency situations. Chances are, you feel more familiar with some areas than with others.

Make a list and check it twice

One good way to begin your study preparation is to look at the list of ACLS core concepts provided in this chapter. On a sheet of paper, create two columns. Title one column "know well." Title the other "need review." Now go through the list of ACLS core concepts and place each one in either the "know well" or "need review" column, depending on how confident you feel about the material. Don't worry if one column is longer than the other. This will provide an initial guide to how much time you should allot for each topic.

Remember, you'll still study topics listed in the "know well" column; you just won't spend as much time on those topics as you'll spend on topics in the "need review" column.

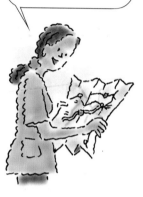

Putting ACLS concepts into "know well" and "need review" columns will help you map out how much time you need to spend studying each topic.

Setting your schedule

Most people can identify a period in the day when they feel most alert. For example, if you feel more energized in the morning, set aside some time in the morning for topics that need more review. Then you can use time in the afternoon or evening, when you feel less alert, for topics that need less review. If the opposite is true, plan your schedule accordingly.

Eight days a week

Now you're ready to set up a basic study schedule. Using a calendar or organizer, determine how many days you have before the ACLS examination. Fill in those dates with specific times and topics to study. For example, you might schedule I.V. techniques for a Wednesday afternoon and electrical therapy for a Friday morning.

Keep in mind that you shouldn't study all day. Set aside time for regular activities. Also, know your own study capabilities and set realistic goals. You'll feel better about yourself—and your chances of passing the ACLS examination—when you regularly meet your goals. (See *Creating an effective study space.*)

Get creative

Even the most determined student needs an occasional change of pace to stay motivated. Consider studying with a group or using audiovisual or other devices to make your study time more effective.

> ### Key points
>
> **Study tips**
> • Use a combination of study strategies to help you learn.
> • Create a guide of "know well" and "needs review."
> • Devise a study schedule.
> • Use additional materials to maintain motivation.

Creating an effective study space

When preparing for the advanced cardiac life support examination, it's important to use your time and space effectively. Time is wasted when you study in places where it's hard to concentrate. Look for a study space that:
- is quiet, convenient, and away from traffic
- has soft lighting that allows you to see clearly without straining your eyes
- has a temperature between 65° and 70° F (18.3° and 21.1° C)
- contains a solid chair that aids good posture
- contains flowers, green plants, or familiar photos, paintings, or other elements that give you a sense of comfort.

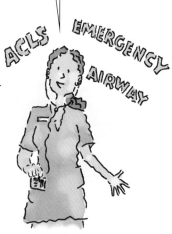

Using a recording device is a portable and effective way to enhance your memorization of core concepts.

Study buddies

Studying with a partner or group can be an excellent way to energize yourself. Working with a partner allows you to test one another and encourage and motivate each other. When choosing a partner, select someone with similar goals, motivation, and knowledge; otherwise, you may waste valuable time chatting or needlessly reviewing basic material.

Visualize success

Audiovisual tools can also enhance your study routine. Flash cards, flowcharts, drawings, and diagrams all provide images that may improve your retention. Even the process of creating these materials will help you learn. (See *Virtual studying*.)

Do you hear what I hear?

If you understand and retain information more effectively by hearing rather than seeing, consider using a handheld recording

Virtual studying

Many internet sites offer study materials to help you prepare for the advanced cardiac life support (ACLS) examination. For example, several sites offer ACLS simulators that allow you to practice your ACLS skills on virtual patients and offer immediate feedback as well as a fun approach to studying. Remember, ACLS information and recommendations may change, so check to see when a site was last updated before relying on it too heavily.

In addition, many professional sites (such as the American Medical Association, the American Heart Association [AHA], and various other nursing and medical sites) offer materials to help you research and understand specific concepts and provide up-to-date information on the changing field of health care.

When you do your research, beware of online ACLS courses that may not be approved by the AHA. Your health care facility may not find them to be acceptable courses.

device (such as a tape recorder or even an electronic organizer or cell phone) to record key ideas. Like flash cards, a recording is portable and perfect for short study periods during the day.

Quick quiz

1. What's advanced cardiac life support?
   A. Systematic approach to life support
   B. Life support with use of a ventilator
   C. A 2-day course with 6 to 8 hours of lecture
   D. A written and practical examination

Answer: A. ACLS is a systematic approach to resuscitation that provides rescuers with memory aids for the treatment of critically ill patients.

2. To prepare for the ACLS examination, you should:
   A. study all day, the day prior to the examination.
   B. determine a study strategy that works for you.
   C. not study at all.
   D. study for several weeks prior to the examination.

Answer: B. Not all study strategies are appropriate for every student. Determine a study strategy that works for you to adequately prepare for the ACLS examination.

3. An ACLS card should be obtained by which professionals?
   A. RNs, physicians, and advanced EMS personnel
   B. Physicians, licensed practical nurses (LPNs), and nursing students
   C. Dental care professionals, nursing students, and RNs
   D. LPNs, physician's assistants, and surgical care professionals

Answer: A. Health care workers seeking ACLS training include physicians, RNs, and advanced EMS personnel. Dental and surgical care professionals also seek ACLS training.

Scoring

✩✩✩ If you answered all three questions correctly, way to go! You really know your essentials.

✩✩ If you answered two questions correctly, keep up the good work! You're "essentially" on the right track.

✩ If you answered fewer than two questions correctly, nice try! Next time, you're sure to get an "A" on ACLS.

ACLS in practice

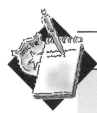

Just the facts

In this chapter, you'll learn:

♦ American Heart Association's "chain of survival"

♦ CABD surveys that form the basis of advanced cardiac life support

♦ phased-response approach to emergency response team management

♦ purpose of treatment algorithms.

The chain of survival

The chain of survival describes a chain of events—each interdependent—that plays a crucial role in helping a patient survive cardiac arrest. This series of events is called a "chain" because each link must be strong for the process to work. If one link is weak or missing, poor survival rates will result even if the rest of the emergency cardiac care system is excellent.

The five links in the adult chain of survival are:

immediate recognition and activation of the emergency response system

early cardiopulmonary resuscitation (CPR) with high-quality chest compressions

rapid defibrillation

effective advanced cardiac life support (ACLS)

integrated post–cardiac arrest care.

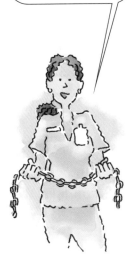

The chain of survival describes a chain of events that plays a crucial role in helping a patient survive cardiac arrest.

The first link: Immediate recognition and activation

Immediate recognition and activation consists of the events that occur between the patient's collapse, recognition of the cardiac arrest and activation of the emergency response system, and the arrival of emergency medical services (EMS) personnel. The faster the EMS team arrives, the greater the patient's chance for survival. Immediate recognition and activation aims to bring EMS personnel to the scene as quickly as possible.

Follow the five steps

Immediate recognition and activation involves these steps:
- Someone quickly recognizes the patient's collapse and need for the emergency response system.
- Someone rapidly activates an EMS response team, usually by telephone. (In the United States, dialing 911 is the typical method. In a hospital setting, a specific "code" is established to activate the facility's emergency team.)
- Dispatchers quickly recognize an emergency situation and guide an EMS response team to the patient, providing as much information about the type of emergency as possible.
- EMS personnel arrive quickly with emergency equipment, including a defibrillator, oxygen, airway management devices, and medication.
- EMS personnel correctly identify the type of emergency and begin appropriate treatment.

The second link: Early CPR

Early, effective CPR bridges the gap between the patient's collapse and the arrival of EMS personnel with emergency equipment. Even with an effective emergency response system, a delay between the patient's collapse and the arrival of EMS personnel may be unavoidable.

Many studies confirm the value of bystander CPR (an attempt to provide CPR by a person who isn't part of the organized emergency response system) and show that CPR is most effective when started immediately after a person collapses. Bystander CPR seems to have the greatest impact on the survival rates of infants and children.

Skill builders

New approaches to teaching CPR have helped to improve skill retention. These include simplified teaching materials, practice-while-watching and practice-after-watching videos, and emphasis on regular practice. The growing use of computer software and the internet to practice skills may also help to improve the quality and frequency of bystander CPR.

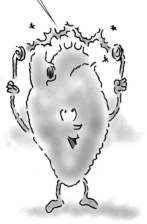

Wow! I got a real charge out of that! I feel so much better now.

The third link: Rapid defibrillation

When performed correctly, rapid defibrillation is the most effective way to improve the patient's chance for survival. Because early defibrillation is so important, any action that safely shortens the time between collapse and defibrillation can have a significant impact. Typically, EMS personnel equipped with automated external defibrillators (AEDs) perform defibrillation.

Eye on AEDs

Because AEDs have evolved into user-friendly devices, large numbers of people can be trained to use them. Programs that equip firefighters, police, and airplane personnel with AEDs and train them in AED use show positive results. Instruction courses on public access defibrillation are widely available, especially as airports and public buildings, such as hotels, office buildings, and malls, obtain AEDs.

The fourth link: Effective ACLS

After defibrillation, effective ACLS performed by trained personnel, including advanced airway management and the administration of rhythm-appropriate I.V. medications, is the next step in patient care.

EMS systems should provide a minimum of two responders trained in ACLS for all emergencies. Studies show that an ideal response team consists of two members trained in ACLS supported by two members trained in basic life support (BLS).

The fifth link: Integrated post–cardiac arrest care

Following return of spontaneous circulation (ROSC), integrated post–cardiac arrest care emphasizes the importance of comprehensive, multidisciplinary care, including interventions to optimize hemodynamic, neurologic, and metabolic function and possibly the use of therapeutic hypothermia. (See *Post–cardiac arrest care*, pages 329, 330.)

BLS vs. ACLS

A thorough understanding of BLS principles will prepare you to learn more advanced ACLS skills. BLS involves CPR and airway management and includes such skills as closed-chest compressions and the abdominal thrust. Any trained person who reaches a patient before ACLS-trained personnel arrive can perform BLS interventions. These interventions, such as performing CPR with effective chest compressions and administering ventilations, form an important bridge between the patient's collapse and the start of ACLS.

ACLS is an advanced version of BLS that adds more complex interventions, such as intubating the patient, initiating I.V. access, and giving medications. However, both BLS and ACLS emphasize the same elements: circulation, airway, and breathing.

Remember…an emergency calls for CAB—circulation, airway, breathing.

Initial CABD steps

Although mastering individual skills (such as providing airway management and establishing I.V. access) is important for performing ACLS, only by understanding its systematic approach will you be able to use those skills effectively in a cardiac emergency.

ACLS uses a two-pronged approach: Initial CABD steps followed by progressive CABD steps. You should use this approach with all potential cardiac arrest patients and at all major decision points during a difficult resuscitation effort.

Initial CABD steps focus on basic CPR and defibrillation. They include:
- Circulation—Perform chest compressions.
- Airway—Open the airway.
- Breathing—Ventilate the patient.
- Defibrillation—Defibrillate ventricular fibrillation (VF) and pulseless ventricular tachycardia (VT).

Circulation

After you assess the patient and determine unresponsiveness, call for help; then place the patient in the supine position on a hard, flat surface. Pulse detection is unreliable, even when performed by trained rescuers, so attempt a pulse check over 5–10 seconds, and then proceed to performing chest compressions if you are unable to detect a pulse or are uncertain of a pulse.

Key points

Initial CABD steps
- Assess the patient—call for help.
- **C**—Assist circulation, chest compressions.
- **A**—Establish a patent airway.
- **B**—Ensure breathing.
- **D**—Deliver shocks as soon as possible.

BLS to the rescue

If the patient is unresponsive and not breathing normally and a pulse is not detected, perform closed-chest compressions using BLS techniques:

- Kneel with your knees apart for a wide base of support.
- Place the heel of one hand over the lower half of the patient's sternum (center of the chest) at the nipple line and then place your other hand on top of the first with your hands overlapped.
- Lock your elbows and keep your shoulders directly over the patient. Your body will now act as a fulcrum as you apply chest compressions.
- Give chest compressions hard and fast. Compress at least 2″ (5 cm) for an adult at a rate of at least 100/minute. Remember to allow the chest to completely recoil after each compression. Minimize interruptions in compressions, but if multiple rescuers are available, rotate the task of compressions every 2 minutes (five cycles of CPR).
- Give 30 compressions and 2 breaths for both one- and two-person CPR until an advanced airway is in place. For two-person CPR, one team member performs compressions while the other performs rescue breathing. Deliver ventilations at 8 to 10 breaths/minute.
- After an advanced airway is in place, deliver compressions at a rate of at least 100/minute continuously without interruptions for ventilations. The team member providing ventilations gives 8 to 10 breaths/minute.

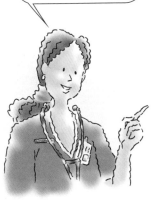

After you assess the patient and determine unresponsiveness, call for help.

Airway

To open the patient's airway, open his mouth using the basic CPR head-tilt, chin-lift maneuver. As a health care provider, if you suspect neck injury, use the jaw-thrust maneuver. If the jaw-thrust maneuver doesn't effectively open the airway, use the head-tilt, chin-lift maneuver.

Breathing

Once you have opened the patient's airway, begin ventilations with a pocket face mask or bag-valve mask device. Provide two rescue ventilations with each breath delivered in 1 second. If his chest doesn't rise with rescue ventilations, reposition the airway and reattempt ventilation. If you're still unsuccessful, follow the American Heart Association's (AHA) steps for obstructed airway.

Defibrillation

The CAB (circulation, airway, breathing) approach to emergency care is familiar to many health care workers; however, the initial CABD steps of ACLS adds an important step—defibrillation. Defibrillation must occur as soon as possible. For example, a person in VF has almost no chance of survival if defibrillation doesn't occur within 10 minutes of collapse. That means you must move swiftly and efficiently through the CAB portion of the survey in order to proceed quickly to defibrillation.

The AED advantage

Current ACLS training emphasizes the use of AEDs for defibrillation. AEDs are computerized, low-maintenance defibrillators that analyze the patient's heart rhythm to determine if a shockable rhythm is present. If the AED detects a shockable rhythm, it charges and then prompts the rescuer to press a button to deliver the shock.

All AEDs operate using four steps:

Power—Turn the AED on.

Attachment—Attach the pads to the patient.

Analysis—Place the AED into analyze mode to detect a shockable rhythm.

Shock—Press the shock button when indicated.

Repeat these steps with effective CPR until VF or VT is no longer present. If an AED isn't available, follow steps for using a manual defibrillator.

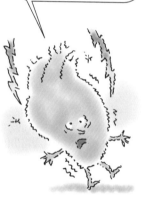

The ACLS primary survey adds defibrillation to the CAB approach to emergency care. Thanks, I needed that!

Progressive CABD steps

After completing the initial CABD steps, move immediately to progressive CABD steps, using the same basic concepts but with more in-depth interventions and assessments. It includes:
• Circulation—Gain I.V. access, determine the heart rhythm, and give medications appropriate to that rhythm.
• Airway—Insert an advanced airway.
• Breathing—Assess bilateral chest movement and ventilation.
• Differential diagnosis—Search for, find, and treat reversible causes of the arrest.

Circulation

The circulation component of the secondary CABD survey involves several interventions ultimately designed to identify arrhythmias and determine and deliver appropriate medication to the patient. As one person obtains I.V. access, another attaches cardiac monitor leads, identifies the heart rhythm, and measures blood pressure.

After you obtain I.V. access and identify the heart rhythm, decide which medication to administer to help restore heart rate and rhythm. Then determine the need for other treatments, such as cardioversion (restoring normal heart rhythm using shock) or defibrillation.

Airway

Reassess the airway to make sure that it's still open. If a bag-valve mask device is providing adequate airway management, you may defer insertion of an endotracheal (ET) tube until after return of spontaneous circulation, or after CPR and defibrillation have been provided. An ET tube should be inserted as quickly as possible.

Breathing

After insertion of an ET tube, confirm oxygenation and monitor ventilation with an end-tidal carbon dioxide detector and an oxygen saturation monitor. Also assess for equal chest movement during ventilation. Auscultate for bilateral breath sounds using a five-point technique (left and right anterior chest, left and right midaxillary points, and over the stomach). Make any necessary adjustments to ensure that the patient is breathing adequately, including removing the tube, if necessary, and starting over.

When you're confident that the ET tube is in place, secure it to prevent dislodgment. Confirm its placement using waveform capnography or an exhaled esophageal detector device. A chest X-ray and arterial blood gas levels help to accurately evaluate adequate ventilation.

Differential diagnosis

You need to consider potentially reversible causes of the cardiopulmonary emergency, such as hypovolemia, hypoxia, acidosis,

Key points

Progressive CABD steps
- **C**—Perform interventions to deliver medications, identify heart rhythm, and monitor blood pressure.
- **A**—Reassess the airway; intubate as soon as possible.
- **B**—Check for breath sounds; confirm tube placement.
- **D**—Determine what caused the event.

Keep in mind that an ET tube should be inserted as quickly as possible!

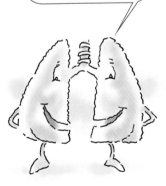

hyperkalemia, hypokalemia, hypothermia, drug overdose, cardiac tamponade, tension pneumothorax, coronary thrombosis, or pulmonary thrombosis. Even if you succeed in establishing a perfusing rhythm, cardiac arrest can recur if the underlying cause isn't identified and appropriately treated.

Organized team approach

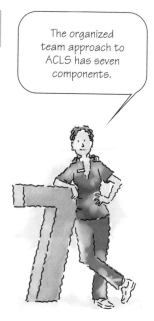

The organized team approach to ACLS has seven components.

The CABD steps provide an overall structure for patient care before, during, and after a cardiopulmonary emergency. Similarly, an organized team approach provides an overall structure for managing the emergency response team and guides the team through all phases of an emergency, from preparation to post-emergency evaluation.

An organized team approach has components that may slightly overlap in an actual emergency:

- anticipation
- entry
- resuscitation
- maintenance
- family notification
- transfer
- debriefing.

Anticipation

The anticipation component involves the rescuers' preparations as they move to the scene of a possible cardiac arrest or wait for the arrival of a patient with possible cardiac arrest. Steps in this component include gathering the team, agreeing on a leader, delineating duties, preparing and checking equipment, and positioning the rescuers.

Entry

In the entry component, the team makes first contact with the patient. Steps to perform during this component include obtaining entry vital signs, transferring the patient in an orderly manner from BLS personnel to the ACLS team (if applicable), gathering a concise history, and repeating vital sign assessment.

Resuscitation

During the resuscitation component, the team leader needs to keep the team focused on the basics of circulation, airway, and breathing. Effective communication is crucial, and team members should state vital signs every 5 minutes or in response to any change in the patient's condition. Team members should also state when they complete procedures and medication administration.

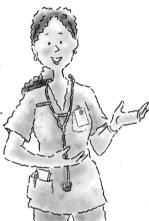

> During resuscitation, the team leader needs to keep the team focused on the basics of circulation, airway, and breathing.

Maintenance

The maintenance component begins when vital signs have stabilized. During this time, team members need to maintain the patient's condition by focusing on the CABs and staying ready for any new or renewed problems.

Family notification

This component directs members of the team to inform the family of the patient's condition. Whether you're bearing good or bad news, this notification must be done promptly, honestly, and with sensitivity. If family members are present, they may wish to watch the resuscitation efforts because these may be the final moments for the patient. If the family does observe, a practitioner should remain with them to answer questions, explain procedures, and direct them where to stand. The practitioner can also watch for signs of major discomfort or distress in the family members and end the observation, if necessary.

Transfer

The transfer component occurs when the resuscitation team transfers the patient to another team. When transferring the patient and all relevant information, you should be concise, complete, and well organized.

Debriefing

Every emergency situation should finish with a debriefing of the event. This debriefing exercise should occur away from the crisis situation. It allows for self-assessment, identification of areas for self-improvement, and reflection on positive and negative outcomes as well as the opportunity to defuse emotions when dealing with volatile situations.

> Using treatment algorithms can help you recall which steps to take in an emergency situation.

Treatment algorithms

The AHA uses treatment algorithms as educational tools for learning ACLS. Algorithms are flowcharts that can serve as memory tools for carrying out the steps involved in different emergency situations.

It's important to remember that real-life patient care rarely corresponds exactly to any particular algorithm. Therefore, algorithms provide a useful guide but can't replace a flexible, thorough understanding of patient care. (For specific algorithms, see Chapter 8, Emergency cardiac care.)

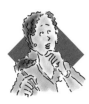

Quick quiz

1. The link in the chain of survival that's most likely to improve the patient's survival rate is:
    A.   immediate recognition and activation.
    B.   early CPR.
    C.   rapid defibrillation.
    D.   effective ACLS.

Answer: C. When performed correctly, rapid defibrillation is the link in the chain of survival that's the most important to patient survival because it's ultimately the only way to reverse cardiac arrest resulting from VF. However, all links in the chain are important for successful resuscitation.

2. When confronted with a possible cardiac arrest, which action is important to perform prior to beginning the initial CABD steps?
    A.   Call for help and activate the EMS.
    B.   Clear the area.
    C.   Notify the family.
    D.   Call the practitioner.

Answer: A. Steps that are important to take prior to the initial CABD steps include assessing unresponsiveness, calling for help

Key points

Summary points
• Immediate recognition and activation of emergency medical services personnel for all cardiac arrest patients
• Early cardiopulmonary resuscitation (CPR) using "CAB" (circulation, airway, breathing)
• Rapid defibrillation
• Minimization of interruptions in CPR to perform advanced coronary life support interventions
• Incorporation of a multidisciplinary approach to care for the patient after return of spontaneous circulation

and activating the emergency response team, positioning the patient, and positioning the rescuer (yourself).

3. ACLS treatment algorithms are:
   A. mathematical equations used in ACLS.
   B. ACLS educational tools.
   C. flowcharts to guide ACLS treatment.
   D. the second link in the chain of survival.

Answer: C. Treatment algorithms are flowcharts that guide ACLS treatment. They're designed to be a memory tool; however, they aren't absolute because every patient needs to be assessed according to their response to treatment and individual circumstances.

4. Determining a differential diagnosis is part of the:
   A. initial CABD steps.
   B. progressive CABD steps.
   C. patient history.
   D. discharge summary.

Answer: B. The progressive CABD steps include C (circulation), A (airway), B (breathing), and D (differential diagnosis).

5. Effective communication among team members is key during which component of the organized team approach?
   A. Entry
   B. Maintenance
   C. Resuscitation
   D. Transfer

Answer: C. Effective communication is key during the resuscitation component. The team members should state vital signs every 5 minutes or in response to any change in the monitored parameters. Team members should also state when procedures and medication administration are complete.

6. After establishing unresponsiveness and assessing ineffective breathing, compressions begin:
   A. at a ratio of 15 compressions to two breaths.
   B. at a ratio of 30 compressions to one breath.
   C. at a rate of at least 100/minute interrupted by pauses for ventilations.
   D. at a rate of at least 100/minute continuously without interruption for ventilation.

Answer: C. After establishing unresponsiveness and ineffective breathing, deliver compressions at a rate of at least 100/minute interrupted by pauses for ventilation.

Scoring

☆☆☆ If you answered all six questions correctly, outstanding! Your chain of survival is strong.

☆☆ If you answered four or five questions correctly, great job! You're "primarily" on the right track.

☆ If you answered fewer than four questions correctly, good effort! With a bit more study, you'll master the ABCs of ACLS in no time.

Recognizing cardiac arrhythmias

Just the facts

In this chapter, you'll learn:

♦ normal cardiac conduction

♦ application of cardiac rhythm monitoring devices

♦ methods to interpret cardiac rhythms

♦ characteristics of cardiac arrhythmias.

The importance of interpretation

An essential component of advanced cardiac life support (ACLS) is the rapid recognition of cardiac arrhythmias. Frequently, identification of an arrhythmia is what triggers an ACLS response, especially in the hospital setting. Accurate interpretation of a cardiac arrhythmia guides appropriate treatment and may help prevent hemodynamic deterioration.

Understanding cardiac conduction

The cardiovascular system contains specialized pacemaker cells that enable the heart to generate a precise rhythm. These cells have four unique characteristics:

• automaticity—the ability to spontaneously initiate an electrical impulse

• conductivity—the ability to transmit the impulse to the next cell

• contractility—the ability to shorten the fibers in the heart when receiving the impulse

• excitability—the ability to respond to an electrical stimulus.

An essential component of ACLS is rapid recognition of cardiac arrhythmias.

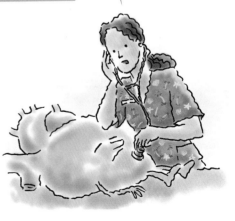

Cardiac conduction system

In normal conduction, each electrical impulse travels from the sinoatrial (SA) node through the atria along the internodal and interatrial tracts. The impulse slows momentarily as it passes through the atrioventricular (AV) junction to the bundle of His. Then it descends the left and right bundle branches and finally down the Purkinje fibers.

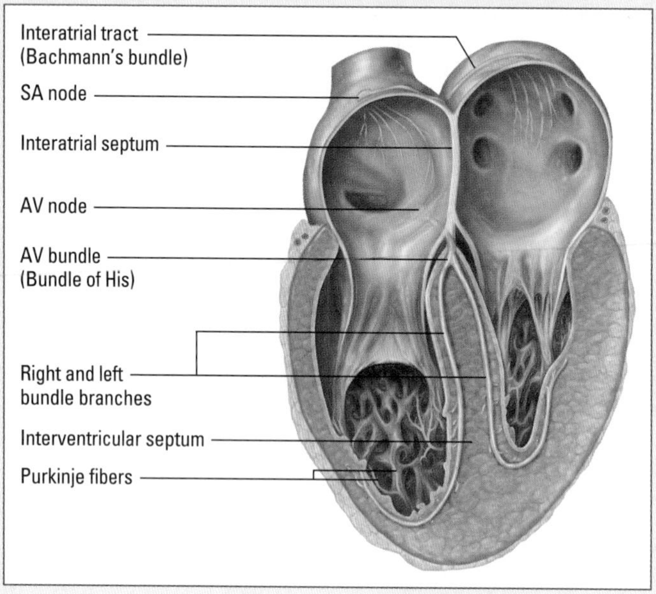

Interatrial tract
(Bachmann's bundle)

SA node

Interatrial septum

AV node

AV bundle
(Bundle of His)

Right and left
bundle branches

Interventricular septum

Purkinje fibers

Cardiac conduction begins in the sinoatrial (SA) node and proceeds through the cardiac conduction system. (See *Cardiac conduction system*)

Sinoatrial node

The SA node is the heart's natural pacemaker. It's located on the endocardial surface of the right atrium near the superior vena cava. When the SA node fires, it sends an impulse throughout the right and left atria that results in an atrial contraction. Normally, the SA node generates an impulse 60 to 100 times/minute.

Atrioventricular node

The atrioventricular (AV) node slows impulse conduction between the atria and the ventricles. Situated low in the septal wall of the right

Key points

Cardiac conduction
- SA node—normal pacemaker
- AV node—impulse conduction.
- AV node will generate impulse if SA node fails.
- Ventricles will generate impulse if SA and AV nodes fail.

atrium, this "resistor" node provides time for the contracting atria to fill the ventricles with blood before the lower chambers contract.

From the AV node to the myocardium

The impulse from the AV node travels to the bundle of His (modified muscle fibers), branching off to the right and left bundle branches. Then it travels to the distal portions of the bundle branches called the *Purkinje fibers*. These fibers fan across the surface of the ventricles from the endocardium to the myocardium. As the impulse spreads, it signals the blood-filled ventricles to contract.

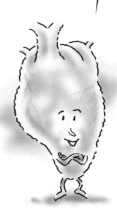

My SA and AV nodes take a lickin'—but my ventricles just keep on tickin'!

Safety mechanisms

The conduction system has two built-in safety mechanisms. If the SA node fails to fire, the AV node will generate an impulse 40 to 60 times/minute. If the SA node and AV node both fail, the ventricles can generate their own impulse 20 to 40 times/minute.

Abnormal impulses

Abnormal impulse conduction results from disturbances in automaticity, conduction, or both.

It's automatic

Automaticity can increase or decrease. For example, increased automaticity of pacemaker cells below the SA node commonly causes tachycardia. Likewise, decreased automaticity of cells in the SA node can cause bradycardia or an escape rhythm.

Conduction junction

Conduction may occur too quickly, as in Wolff-Parkinson-White (WPW) syndrome, or too slowly, as in AV block. Atrial tachycardia with a 4:1 block is an example of a combined automaticity and conduction disturbance.

Monitoring cardiac rhythms

An electrocardiogram (ECG) is used to monitor the precise sequence of electrical events in the cardiac cycle. There are two types of ECG recordings: the 12-lead and the single lead, commonly known as a *rhythm strip*.

You'll want to get this complex

An ECG complex reflects the electrical events occurring in one cardiac cycle. Each complex consists of five waveforms, labeled with the letters P, Q, R, S, and T. The middle three letters—Q, R, and S—are collectively referred to as the *QRS complex*. (See *ECG waveform components*.)

Typically, you identify cardiac arrhythmias by recognizing their effects on the ECG waveform. However, ECG interpretation doesn't replace the need for keen assessment skills. Always remember that ECG findings should correlate with the patient's physical condition.

ECG waveform components

An electrocardiogram (ECG) waveform has three basic components: the P wave, the QRS complex, and the T wave. These elements can be further divided into the PR interval, J point, ST segment, U wave, and QT interval.

P wave and PR interval

The P wave represents atrial depolarization. The PR interval represents the time it takes an impulse to travel from the atria through the atrioventricular nodes and the bundle of His. The PR interval measures from the beginning of the P wave to the beginning of the QRS complex.

QRS complex

The QRS complex represents ventricular depolarization (the time it takes for the impulse to travel through the bundle branches to the Purkinje fibers).

The Q wave appears as the first negative deflection in the QRS complex; the R wave as the first positive deflection. The S wave appears as the second negative deflection or

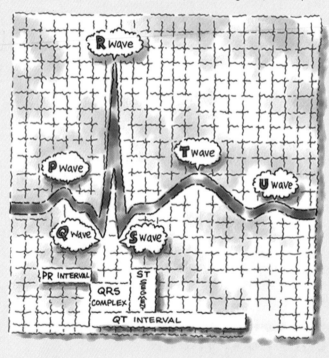

the first negative deflection after the R wave.

J point and ST segment

The J point marks the end of the QRS complex and also indicates the beginning of the ST segment. The ST segment represents part of ventricular repolarization; it's measured from the end of the S wave to the beginning of the T wave.

T wave and U wave

The T wave represents ventricular repolarization and usually follows the same deflection pattern as the P wave. The U wave follows the T wave; however, because the U wave signifies a problem, it isn't seen in most patients.

QT interval

The QT interval represents ventricular depolarization and repolarization. It extends from the beginning of the QRS complex to the end of the T wave.

Applying monitoring devices

An ECG monitor is a tool that provides continuous information about the heart's electrical activity. Electrodes applied to the patient's chest pick up the heart's electrical activity and display it on the monitor.

Commonly monitored leads include the three bipolar leads—I, II, and, III—and MCL_1 and MCL_6, which are modified versions of leads V_1 and V_6. You may use a three-, four-, or five-electrode system for cardiac monitoring. (See *Using a five-leadwire system.*)

Technique matters

To ensure accurate lead monitoring, you must apply the electrodes correctly. Follow these steps for accurate lead placement:
- Clip dense hair at each site.
- Prepare the skin by briskly rubbing each site until the skin reddens using the rough patch on the back of the electrode or a dry gauze pad.

Peak technique

Using a five-leadwire system

This illustration shows the correct placement of leadwires for a five-leadwire system. The chest electrode shown is located in the V_1 position, but you can place it in any of the chest lead positions. Each lead's color is included in the key.

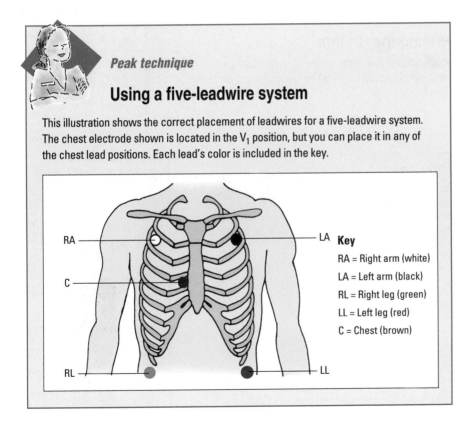

Key

RA = Right arm (white)

LA = Left arm (black)

RL = Right leg (green)

LL = Left leg (red)

C = Chest (brown)

- Remove the backing from the electrodes and apply one to each prepared site by pressing it against the patient's skin (the electrode gel should be moist in order to conduct properly).
- Attach leadwires or cable connections by clipping them to the electrodes. (If you're using a snap-on leadwire, attach it to the electrode before placing the electrode on the patient's chest to prevent patient discomfort.)
- Turn on the monitor.
- Select the lead you wish to view following the monitor's instructions.

Let me get this straight — you attach electrodes and wires to the chest and then we get this?

That's right. The rhythm strip from an ECG monitor tells us all about your electrical activity.

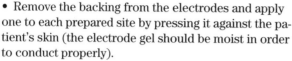

Interpreting rhythm strips: An eight-step method

You can learn to analyze and interpret ECGs systematically and correctly by using this eight-step method. First, scan the entire strip and identify the waveform components. Then follow these steps.

Step 1: Determine the rhythm

To determine the heart's atrial and ventricular rhythms, use either the paper-and-pencil method or the calipers

These 8 steps will lead you to success in analyzing and interpreting rhythm strips.

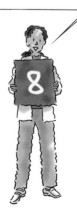

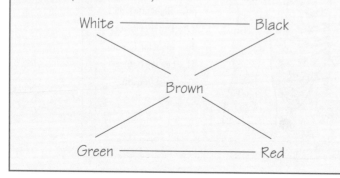

Memory jogger

To help you remember where to place electrodes in a five-electrode configuration, think of the phrase "White, upper right." Then think of snow over trees (white above green), and smoke over fire (black above red). And, of course, chocolate (brown electrode) lies close to the heart!

White ———————— Black

Brown

Green ———————— Red

method. (See *Methods of measuring rhythm.*) Then ask yourself, "Does the rhythm appear to be regular or irregular?"

Step 2: Determine the rate

Next, calculate the heart's atrial and ventricular rates, using the times ten method, the 1,500 method, or the sequence method. (See *Calculating heart rate*, page 26.)

Peak technique

Methods of measuring rhythm

You can use either of the following methods to determine atrial and ventricular rhythm.

Paper-and-pencil method
Place the electrocardiogram (ECG) strip on a flat surface. Then position the straight edge of a piece of paper along the strip's baseline. Move the paper up slightly so the straight edge is near the peak of the R wave. With a pencil, mark the paper at the R waves of two consecutive QRS complexes, as shown. This is the R-R interval.

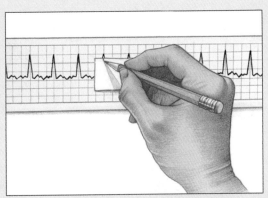

Next, move the paper across the strip and line up those two marks with succeeding R-R intervals. If the distance for each R-R interval is the same, the ventricular rhythm is regular. If the distance varies, the rhythm is irregular.

Use the same method to measure the distance between the P waves (the P-P interval) and determine whether the atrial rhythm is regular or irregular.

Calipers method
With the ECG strip on a flat surface, place one point of the calipers on the peak of the R wave of two consecutive QRS complexes. Then adjust the legs and place the other point on the peak of the next R wave, as shown. This distance is the R-R interval.

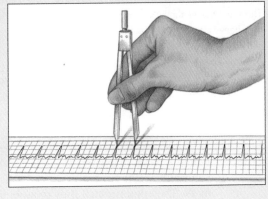

Next, pivot the first point of the calipers toward the third R wave and note whether it falls on the peak of that wave. Check succeeding R-R intervals in the same way. If they're all the same distance, the ventricular rhythm is regular. If the distance varies, the rhythm is irregular.

Using the same method, measure the P-P intervals to determine whether the atrial rhythm is regular or irregular.

Peak technique

Calculating heart rate

You can use one of three methods—the times ten method, the 1,500 method, or the sequence method—to determine atrial and ventricular heart rates from an electrocardiogram waveform.

Times ten method

The simplest, quickest, and most common technique, the times ten method is particularly useful if the patient's heart rhythm is irregular. First, obtain a rhythm strip. Then locate the small markings at the top of the strip. Each marking represents 3 seconds. Count the number of P waves (to determine atrial rate) or R waves (to determine ventricular rate) over a 6-second time period (two 3-second markings). Multiply by 10.

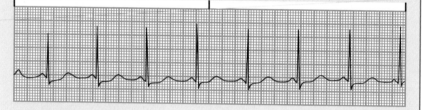

1,500 method

Use the 1,500 method only if the patient's heart rhythm is regular. First, identify two consecutive P waves on the rhythm strip. Next, select identical points in each wave and count the number of small squares between the points. Then divide 1,500 by the number of small squares counted (1,500 small squares equal 1 minute) to get the atrial rate. To calculate the ventricular rate, use the same procedure but with two consecutive R waves instead of P waves.

Sequence method

The sequence method gives you an estimated heart rate. First, find a P wave that peaks on a heavy black line. Assign the following numbers to the next six heavy black lines: 300, 150, 100, 75, 60, and 50, respectively.

Then find the next P wave peak and estimate the atrial rate based on the number assigned to the nearest heavy black line. Estimate the ventricular rate following the same procedure but use the R wave instead of the P wave.

Determine if the rate is within normal limits (60 to 100 beats/minute). Next, determine if the atrial (P-P interval) rate and ventricular (R-R interval) rate are continually the same measurement. Then determine if they're associated with each other.

Step 3: Evaluate the P wave

Look at the rhythm strip and ask these questions:
• Are P waves present?
• Do the P waves have a normal shape (usually upright and rounded)?
• Are the P waves similar in size and shape?
• Do all the P waves point in the same direction? Are they all upright, inverted, or diphasic?
• Do the P waves and QRS complexes have a one-to-one relationship?
• Is the distance between each P wave and its QRS complex the same?

Step 4: Determine the duration of the PR interval

After you've determined the duration of the PR interval (normal duration is 0.12 to 0.20 second), determine if the PR interval is constant.

Step 5: Determine the duration of the QRS complex

Look at the rhythm strip again and ask these questions:
• Are all the QRS complexes the same size and shape?
• What's the duration of the QRS complex? (Normal duration is 0.06 to 0.10 second.)
• Are all the QRS complexes the same distance from the T waves that follow them?
• Do all the QRS complexes point in the same direction?
• Do any QRS complexes appear different from the others on the strip? (If so, measure and describe each one individually.)

Step 6: Evaluate the T wave

Examine the strip once more and ask these questions:
• Are T waves present?
• Do all the T waves have the same size and shape?
• Could a P wave be hidden in a T wave?
• Do the T waves point in the same direction as the QRS complexes?

Step 7: Determine the duration of the QT interval

Note whether the duration of the QT interval falls within normal limits (0.36 to 0.44 second, or 9 to 11 small squares).

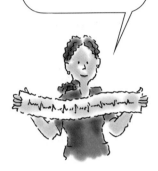

P waves, and T waves, and QRS complexes, oh my! When reading ECG strips, remember to take it one step at a time.

Step 8: Evaluate other components

Finally, observe other components on the ECG strip, including ectopic or aberrantly conducted beats and other abnormalities. Check the ST segment for any abnormalities, such as elevation above or depression below the isoelectric line, and look for a U wave. Note your findings.

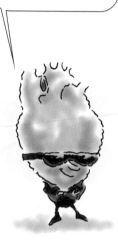

I'm so proud of myself! My normal sinus rhythm is a model of classic cardiac conduction.

Recognizing normal sinus rhythm

Before you can recognize an arrhythmia, you must be able to recognize a normal sinus rhythm (NSR). NSR is a heart rhythm that starts in the SA node and progresses to the ventricles through a normal conduction pathway—from the SA node to the atria and AV node, through the bundle of His to the bundle branches, and on to the Purkinje fibers. NSR is the standard against which all other rhythms are compared.

In NSR:
• atrial and ventricular rhythms are regular
• atrial and ventricular rates are 60 to100 beats/minute
• P wave is normally shaped (upright and rounded in lead II) (All P waves are similar in size and shape; there's a P wave for every QRS complex.)
• PR interval is within normal limits (0.12 to 0.20 second)
• QRS complex is within normal limits (0.06 to 0.10 second)
• T wave is normally shaped (upright and rounded in lead II)
• QT interval is within normal limits (0.36 to 0.44 second).

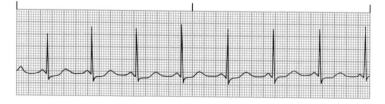

Recognizing narrow complex tachycardias

Narrow complex tachycardias are arrhythmias that involve an accelerated heart rate and a narrow QRS complex. They include sinus tachycardia, atrial fibrillation, atrial flutter, atrial tachycardia, multifocal atrial tachycardia (MAT), WPW syndrome, and junctional tachycardia.

Sinus tachycardia

Sinus tachycardia involves the accelerated firing of the SA node beyond its normal discharge rate, resulting in a heart rate of 100 to 150 beats/minute. The rate rarely exceeds 160 beats/minute, except during strenuous exercise.

Pesty tachy may persist

Persistent sinus tachycardia, especially with acute myocardial infarction (MI), may lead to ischemia and myocardial damage by raising oxygen requirements.

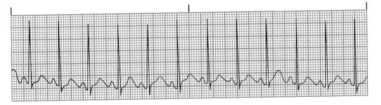

What the ECG tells you

- *Rhythm:* Atrial and ventricular rhythms are regular.
- *Rate:* Atrial and ventricular rates are greater than 100 beats/minute (usually between 100 and 150 beats/minute).
- *P wave:* Normal size and configuration; P wave precedes each QRS complex.
- *PR interval:* Within normal limits and constant.
- *QRS complex:* Normal duration and configuration.
- *T wave:* Normal size and configuration.
- *QT interval:* Within normal limits but commonly shortened.

What causes it

- Caffeine, nicotine, and alcohol ingestion
- Digoxin toxicity
- Hypothyroidism and hyperthyroidism
- Normal cardiac response to demand for increased oxygen during exercise, fever, stress, pain, and dehydration
- Any occurrence that decreases vagal tone and increases sympathetic tone
- Inflammatory response after MI (In acute MI, it may be one of the first signs of heart failure, cardiogenic shock, pulmonary embolism, or infarct extension.)
- Adrenergics
- Anticholinergics
- Antiarrhythmics

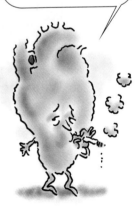

Maybe all this nicotine has pushed my discharge rate over the top...

What to look for

- Usually no symptoms
- Rapid, regular pulse 100 to 150 beats/minute
- Palpitations or angina caused by increased myocardial oxygen consumption and reduced coronary blood flow

How it's treated

- Treatment aims to correct the underlying cause.
- If the patient is symptomatic, a beta-adrenergic blocker such as metoprolol (Lopressor) may be given.

Atrial fibrillation

Atrial fibrillation, usually called *A-fib*, is defined as chaotic, asynchronous, electrical activity in atrial tissue. It stems from the firing of a number of impulses in reentry pathways. Atrial fibrillation results in a loss of atrial kick. The ectopic impulses may fire at a rate of 400 to 600 times/minute, causing the atria to quiver instead of contract.

Help! I think atrial fibrillation is making me lose my atrial kick.

On impulse

The ventricles respond only to those impulses that make it through the AV node. On an ECG, atrial activity is no longer represented by P waves but by erratic baseline waves called *fibrillatory waves*, or *f waves*. This rhythm may be either sustained or paroxysmal (occurring in bursts). It can be preceded by or the result of premature atrial contractions (PACs). The patient may develop an atrial rhythm that frequently varies between a fibrillatory line and flutter waves. This is called *A-fib/flutter*.

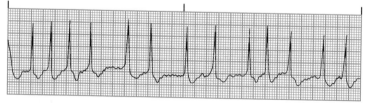

What the ECG tells you

- *Rhythm:* Atrial and ventricular rhythms are grossly irregular.
- *Rate:* The atrial rate (almost indiscernible) usually exceeds 400 beats/minute. The ventricular rate usually varies from 40 to 250 beats/minute.
- *P wave:* Absent. Erratic baseline f waves appear instead. These chaotic f waves represent atrial tetanization from rapid atrial depolarizations.

- *PR interval:* Indiscernible.
- *QRS complex:* Duration and configuration are usually normal.
- *QT interval:* Unmeasurable.

What causes it

- Rheumatic heart disease, valvular disorders (especially mitral stenosis), hypertension, MI, coronary artery disease (CAD), heart failure, cardiomyopathy, and pericarditis
- Thyrotoxicosis
- Chronic obstructive pulmonary disease (COPD)
- Drugs such as digoxin (Lanoxin)
- Cardiac surgery
- Occasional increased sympathetic activity from exercise

What to look for

- Irregular pulse rhythm with a normal or rapid rate ("palpitations"); peripheral pulse commonly slower than apical pulse
- Signs and symptoms of decreased cardiac output (if ventricular rate is rapid)

How it's treated

- If the patient is hemodynamically unstable, perform synchronized cardioversion immediately (initially, 120 to 200 joules or the biphasic equivalent). If using monophasic energy, start at 200 joules and increase in a stepwise fashion as indicated.
- For patients with a rapid rate, consult a practitioner and administer a beta-adrenergic blocker, such as esmolol I.V., or a calcium channel blocker, such as diltiazem (Cardizem), to control ventricular rate.
- For patients with atrial fibrillation of 48 hours or less duration, administer amiodarone (Cordarone), ibutilide (Corvert), propafenone (Rhythmol), flecainide (Tambocor), or digoxin to control the rhythm, as ordered by the practitioner.
- Consider anticoagulants when deciding how quickly to correct atrial fibrillation that has been present longer than 48 hours because rapid conversion may cause blood clots.

Atrial flutter

Atrial flutter is characterized by an atrial rate of 250 to 400 beats/minute, although it's generally about 300 beats/minute. Originating in a single atrial focus, this rhythm results from reentry and, possibly, increased automaticity.

Fast flutter, slow kick

The significance of atrial flutter depends on the acceleration of the ventricular rate. The faster the ventricular rate, the more dangerous the arrhythmia. Like atrial fibrillation, atrial flutter results in a loss of atrial kick. Even a small rise in the ventricular rate can cause angina, syncope, hypotension, heart failure, and pulmonary edema. Atrial fibrillation or flutter may appear.

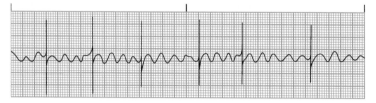

What the ECG tells you

• *Rhythm:* Atrial rhythm is regular. Ventricular rhythm depends on the AV conduction pattern; it's usually regular, although cycles may alternate. An irregular pattern may signal atrial fibrillation or indicate a block.
• *Rate:* Atrial rate is 250 to 400 beats/minute. Ventricular rate depends on the degree of AV block; usually it's 60 to 100 beats/minute but it may accelerate to 125 to 150 beats/minute.
• *P wave:* Saw-toothed or picket fence appearance (called *flutter waves*).
• *PR interval:* Unmeasurable.
• *QRS complex:* Duration is usually within normal limits but the complex may be widened if flutter waves are buried within.
• *T wave:* Not identifiable.
• *QT interval:* Unmeasurable.

What causes it

• Acute or chronic cardiac disorder, mitral or tricuspid valve disorder, cor pulmonale, and cardiac inflammation such as pericarditis
• MI (transient complication)
• Digoxin toxicity
• Hyperthyroidism
• Alcoholism
• Cardiac surgery

What to look for

• Absence of symptoms or palpitations
• Cardiac, cerebral, and peripheral vascular effects (if ventricular filling and coronary artery blood flow are compromised)

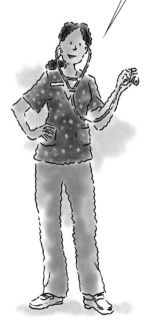

In patients with atrial flutter even a small increase in ventricular rate can cause angina, syncope, hypotension, heart failure, and pulmonary edema.

How it's treated

- If the patient is hemodynamically unstable, perform synchronized cardioversion immediately, beginning with, 50 to 100 joules of biphasic energy. Increase energy in a stepwise fashion if the intial shock fails. If a monophasic device is used, begin with 200 joules and increase the energy in a stepwise fashion if necessary.
- For patients with a rapid rate, consult a practitioner and administer a beta-adrenergic blocker, such as esmolol I.V., or a calcium channel blocker, such as diltiazem, to control ventricular rate.
- Follow the orders of the practitioner for rhythm control.
- Consider anticoagulants when deciding how quickly to correct atrial flutter that has been present longer than 48 hours because rapid conversion may cause blood clots.

Atrial tachycardia

In atrial tachycardia, the atrial rhythm is ectopic and the atrial rate ranges from 150 to 250 beats/minute. Benign in a healthy person, this arrhythmia can be dangerous in a patient with an existing cardiac disorder.

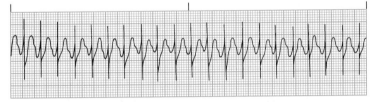

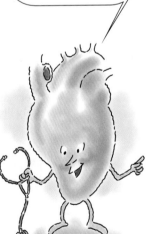

Atrial tachycardia is benign in a healthy person. I sure hope I'm healthy!

What the ECG tells you

- *Rhythm:* Atrial and ventricular rhythms are regular.
- *Rate:* The atrial rate is characterized by three or more successive ectopic atrial beats at a rate of 150 to 250 beats/minute. The rate rarely exceeds 250 beats/minute. The ventricular rate depends on the AV conduction ratio.
- *P wave:* Usually upright, the P wave may be aberrant or hidden in the previous T wave. If visible, it precedes each QRS complex.
- *PR interval:* May be unmeasurable if the P wave can't be distinguished from the preceding T wave.
- *QRS complex:* Duration and configuration are usually normal.
- *T wave:* Usually distinguishable but may be distorted by the P wave.
- *QT interval:* Usually within normal limits but may be shortened because of the rapid rate.

What causes it

• Digoxin toxicity (most common cause)
• Primary cardiac disorders, such as MI, cardiomyopathy, pericarditis, valvular heart disease, and WPW syndrome
• Secondary cardiac problems, such as hyperthyroidism, cor pulmonale, and systemic hypertension
• COPD
• In healthy people, physical or psychological stress, hypoxia, hypokalemia, excessive use of caffeine or other stimulants, and marijuana use

What to look for

• Rapid apical or peripheral pulse rates
• Signs and symptoms of decreased cardiac output, such as hypotension, syncope, and blurred vision

How it's treated

• Attempt vagal stimulation.
• Administer adenosine (Adenocard).
• If the patient is hemodynamically unstable, perform synchronized cardioversion immediately (initially, 50 to 100 joules of biphasic or monophasic energy).

Multifocal atrial tachycardia

MAT results from the extreme rapid firing of multifocal ectopic sites. Very rare in healthy people, this arrhythmia is usually found in acutely ill patients with pulmonary disease or elevated atrial pressures.

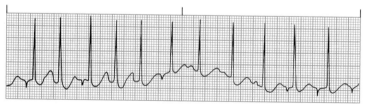

What the ECG tells you

• *Rhythm:* Atrial and ventricular rhythms are irregular.
• *Rate:* Atrial and ventricular rates range from 100 to 250 beats/minute.
• *P wave:* Configuration varies, usually with at least three unique P waves.

- *PR interval:* Varies.
- *QRS complex:* Duration and configuration are usually normal but may become aberrant if the arrhythmia persists.
- *T wave:* Usually distorted.
- *QT interval:* May be indiscernible.

What causes it

- Atrial distention from elevated pulmonary pressure (usually seen in patients with COPD)

What to look for

- Palpitations
- Rapid apical or peripheral pulse rates
- Signs and symptoms of decreased cardiac output, such as blurred vision, syncope, and hypotension

How it's treated

- First, distinguish MAT from atrial fibrillation because both may cause an irregular rhythm.
- For a patient with a rapid rate, consult a practitioner and administer a calcium channel blocker (verapamil [Calan] or diltiazem) or a beta-adrenergic blocker (use cautiously in patients with pulmonary disease).
- MAT is *not* responsive to cardioversion.

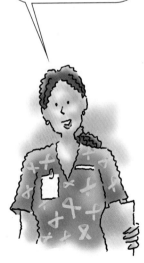

You must distinguish MAT from atrial fibrillation because both can cause an irregular rhythm.

Wolff-Parkinson-White syndrome

Seen mostly in young children and adults ages 20 to 35, WPW syndrome occurs when an anomalous atrial bypass tract (bundle of Kent) develops outside the AV junction, which connects the atria and ventricles. This pathway can conduct impulses either to the ventricles or atria. With retrograde conduction, reentry can arise, resulting in reentrant tachycardia.

The delta wave is the hallmark of WPW syndrome. The syndrome may cause abrupt episodes of premature supraventricular tachycardia (SVT), atrial fibrillation, and atrial flutter with a rate as fast as 300 beats/minute.

No tachy, no problem

WPW syndrome is usually considered insignificant if tachycardia doesn't occur or if the patient has no associated cardiac disease.

When tachycardia does occur in WPW syndrome, decreased cardiac output may develop.

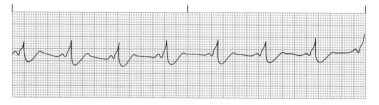

What the ECG tells you

- *Rhythm:* Atrial and ventricular rhythms are regular.
- *Rate:* Atrial and ventricular rates are within normal limits, except when SVT occurs.
- *P wave:* Normal in size and configuration.
- *PR interval:* Short (less than 0.12 second).
- *QRS complex:* Duration greater than 0.10 second; beginning of the QRS complex may be slurred, producing a delta wave.
- *ST segment:* Usually normal but may go in a direction opposite the QRS complex.
- *QT interval:* Usually within normal limits.
- *T wave:* Usually normal but may be deflected in a direction opposite the QRS complex.

What causes it

- Commonly congenital in origin

What to look for

- Usually no symptoms
- If tachyarrhythmias develop with a high ventricular response, palpitations, sudden onset of chest pain, shortness of breath and, possibly, syncope

How it's treated

- If the patient is hemodynamically unstable, perform synchronized cardioversion immediately (initially, 50 to 100 joules of biphasic energy).
- For patients with a rapid rate, consult a practitioner and consider administering amiodarone to control the rate.
- For patients with atrial fibrillation and WPW syndrome, consult a practitioner and prepare for synchronized cardioversion or to administer procainamide.

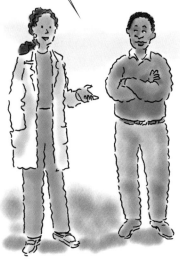

WPW syndrome is usually insignificant if the patient has no signs of tachycardia.

- Consider anticoagulants when deciding how quickly to correct atrial fibrillation with WPW syndrome that has been present longer than 48 hours because rapid conversion may cause blood clots.

Junctional tachycardia

Considered an SVT, junctional tachycardia is characterized by three or more premature junctional contractions in a row. This happens when an irritable focus from the AV junction has enhanced automaticity and overrides the SA node's function as the heart's pacemaker. The atria depolarize by retrograde conduction, and conduction through the ventricles is normal. Usually, the heart rate measures between 100 and 200 beats/minute.

Well, that depends

The significance of junctional tachycardia depends on the rate, the underlying cause, and the severity of the accompanying cardiac disease. At higher ventricular rates, junctional tachycardia may compromise cardiac output by affecting ventricular filling.

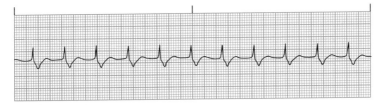

What the ECG tells you

- *Rhythm:* Atrial and ventricular rhythms are usually regular. The atrial rhythm may be difficult to determine if the P wave is absent or hidden in the QRS complex or preceding T wave.
- *Rate:* Atrial and ventricular rates exceed 100 beats/minute (usually between 100 and 200 beats/minute). Atrial rate may be difficult to determine if the P wave is hidden in the QRS complex or if it precedes the T wave.
- *P wave:* Usually inverted; it may occur before or after the QRS complex or be hidden in the QRS complex.
- *PR interval:* If the P wave precedes the QRS complex, the PR interval is shortened (less than 0.12 second); otherwise, the PR interval can't be measured.
- *QRS complex:* Duration within normal limits; usually normal configuration.

- *T wave:* Usually normal configuration but may be abnormal if the P wave is hidden in the T wave. Fast rate may make the T wave indiscernible.
- *QT interval:* Usually within normal limits.

What causes it

- Digoxin toxicity (most common cause)
- Cardiomyopathy
- Enhanced automaticity
- Hypoxia
- Inferior wall MI and ischemia
- Myocarditis
- Vagal stimulation
- Valve replacement surgery

What to look for

- Pulse rate greater than 100 beats/minute
- Usually no symptoms if the patient can compensate
- Possibly signs and symptoms of decreased cardiac output if compensation is poor

How it's treated

- Discontinue digoxin therapy.
- Administer beta-adrenergic blockers or calcium channel blockers to control rate.

What do you mean "junctional tachycardia"? I feel fine.

Recognizing wide complex tachycardias

Wide complex tachycardias are arrhythmias that involve an accelerated heart rate and a wide QRS complex. They include premature ventricular contractions (PVCs), monomorphic ventricular tachycardia, polymorphic ventricular tachycardia, torsades de pointes, and ventricular fibrillation.

Premature ventricular contractions

PVCs are ectopic beats that originate low in the ventricles and occur earlier than expected. PVCs may occur singly, in pairs, in threes, or in fours; in many cases, they're followed by a compensatory pause. PVCs that occur every other beat are

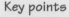

Key points

Surviving cardiac arrest
Early identification and treatment of ventricular tachycardias greatly increase a patient's chances of surviving cardiac arrest. The highest survival rates are reported among patients of all ages who have had:
- a witnessed arrest
- an initial rhythm of pulseless ventricular tachycardia or ventricular fibrillation
- early defibrillation
- early, effective chest compressions.

known as *bigeminy;* those that occur every third beat are known as *trigeminy.* Those that occur every fourth beat are known as *quadrigeminy.* Two PVCs that occur together are called a *couplet.*

PVCs may be uniform, arising from the same ectopic focus, or they may be multiform, arising from different ventricular sites or from one site with changing patterns of conduction. (See *When PVCs spell danger,* page 40.)

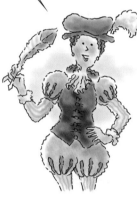

Two PVCs that occur together are called a couplet.

Are you serious?

The significance of PVCs depends on how well the ventricles function and how long the arrhythmia lasts. Cardiac output diminishes because of insufficient ventricular filling time.

Generally, PVCs are more serious if they occur in a patient with heart disease. In an ischemic or damaged heart, PVCs are more likely to develop into ventricular tachycardia, flutter, or fibrillation.

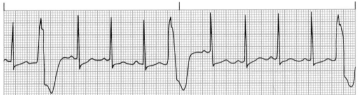

What the ECG tells you

• *Rhythm:* Atrial and ventricular rhythms are irregular during PVCs; the underlying rhythm may be regular.
• *Rate:* Atrial and ventricular rates reflect the underlying rhythm.
• *P wave:* Usually absent in the ectopic beat; however, may appear after the QRS complex with retrograde conduction to the atria. Usually normal if present in the underlying rhythm.
• *PR interval:* Unmeasurable, except in the underlying rhythm.
• *QRS complex:* Occurs earlier than expected; duration exceeds 0.12 second; bizarre configuration.
• *T wave:* Occurs in direction opposite QRS complex. A horizontal baseline, called a *compensatory pause,* may follow the T wave. (A compensatory pause exists if the P-P interval encompassing the PVC has twice the duration of a normal sinus beat's P-P interval.)
• *QT interval:* Not usually measured.

What causes it

• Caffeine, tobacco, and alcohol ingestion
• Digoxin toxicity
• Exercise
• Hypocalcemia

When PVCs spell danger

Here are some examples of dangerous patterns that occur with premature ventricular contractions (PVCs).

Multiple PVCs

Two PVCs in a row are called a *pair,* or couplet (see shaded areas). A pair can produce ventricular tachycardia because the second contraction usually meets refractory tissue. A salvo (three or more PVCs in a row) is considered a run of ventricular tachycardia.

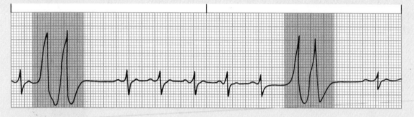

Multiform PVCs

PVCs that look different from one another and arise from different sites or from the same site with abnormal conduction (see shaded areas) are called *multiform PVCs.* Multiform PVCs may indicate severe heart disease or digoxin toxicity.

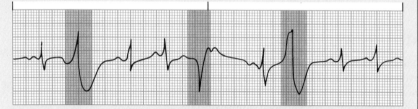

Bigeminy and trigeminy

PVCs that occur every other beat (bigeminy) or every third beat (trigeminy) can cause ventricular tachycardia or ventricular fibrillation (see shaded areas).

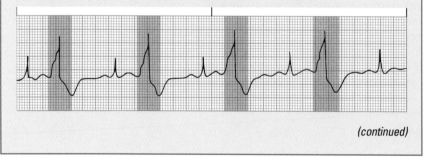

(continued)

When PVCs spell danger *(continued)*

R-on-T phenomenon

In R-on-T phenomenon, the PVC occurs so early that it falls on the T wave of the pre-ceding beat (see shaded areas). Ventricular tachycardia or ventricular fibrillation may occur because the cells haven't fully repolarized.

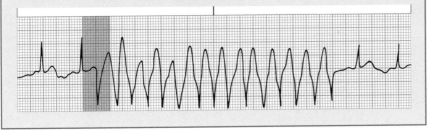

- Hypokalemia
- Myocardial irritation by pacemaker electrodes or pulmonary artery catheter
- Myocardial ischemia and infarction
- Sympathomimetic drugs (such as epinephrine and isoproterenol [Isuprel])
- Antiarrhythmics (proarrhythmic effect)

What to look for

- Possibly no symptoms
- A longer than normal pause immediately after the premature beat
- Signs of decreased cardiac output if PVCs are frequent
- Palpitations

How it's treated

- Treatment is required only when PVCs are frequent or the patient becomes symptomatic.
- Administer oxygen.
- Correct electrolyte imbalances.
- Administer amiodarone, procainamide, or sotalol. Lidocaine may be administered as a second-choice drug.

Monomorphic ventricular tachycardia

Monomorphic ventricular tachycardia is the most common form of ventricular tachycardia. In this life-threatening arrhythmia, all the QRS complexes have the same morphology, indicating that they originate from the same location in the ventricles. Three or more PVCs occur in succession at a rate of more than 100 beats/minute. The arrhythmia may be paroxysmal or sustained.

Taking the plunge

Because atrial and ventricular activities are dissociated and ventricular filling time is short, cardiac output may drop sharply. Monomorphic ventricular tachycardia may lead to ventricular fibrillation.

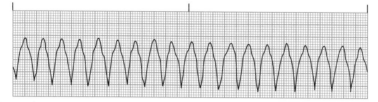

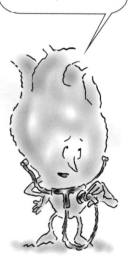

Monomorphic ventricular tachycardia is the most common form of ventricular tachycardia.

What the ECG tells you

• *Rhythm:* Atrial rhythm is unmeasurable. Ventricular rhythm is usually regular but may be slightly irregular.
• *Rate:* Atrial rate is unmeasurable. Ventricular rate is usually rapid (100 to 250 beats/minute).
• *P wave:* Usually absent; may be obscured by and is dissociated from the QRS complex. Retrograde P waves may be present.
• *PR interval:* Unmeasurable.
• *QRS complex:* Duration greater than 0.12 second; bizarre appearance, usually with increased amplitude.
• *T wave:* Occurs in opposite direction of QRS complex.
• *QT interval:* Unmeasurable.

What causes it

• Usually, myocardial irritability and circuit reentry, precipitated by a PVC that occurs in the vulnerable period of ventricular repolarization (R-on-T phenomenon)
• Acute MI
• Cardiomyopathy
• CAD
• Drug toxicity
• Electrolyte imbalance
• Heart failure
• Mitral valve prolapse
• Pulmonary embolism
• Rheumatic heart disease

What to look for

• Palpitations, dizziness, chest pain, and shortness of breath (if the patient is conscious)

- Signs and symptoms of low cardiac output, such as decreased blood pressure or syncope
- Loss of consciousness and hemodynamic collapse

How it's treated

- Identify and treat the underlying cause. If the patient is hemo-dynamically stable, consider administering adenosine (may help distinguish a wide-complex SVT from ventricular tachycardia [VT]). If adenosine is ineffective, give amiodarone, procainamide, or sotalol.
- If the patient is hemodynamically unstable, prepare for imme-diate synchronized cardioversion (initially, 100 joules of mono-phasic or biphasic energy; if no response, increase joules in a stepwise fashion: 200, 300, 360).
- If pulseless VT is present, initiate cardiopulmonary resuscita-tion (CPR), prepare for immediate defibrillation (360 joules mono-phasic energy or 120 to 200 joules of biphasic energy), and then resume CPR for 2 minutes. Defibrillate again at 360 or 200 joules, resume CPR, and then administer epinephrine or vasopressin (Pitressin). Then resume attempts at CPR and defibrillation and consider other antiarrhythmics such as amiodarone.

Polymorphic ventricular tachycardia

Polymorphic ventricular tachycardia is a form of VT in which the QRS complex morphology is unstable, continually varying because the site of origin changes throughout the ventricle. Polymorphic ventricular tachycardia is associated with a poorer prognosis than monomorphic ventricular tachycardia.

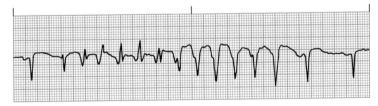

What the ECG tells you

- *Rhythm:* Atrial rhythm is unmeasurable. Ventricular rhythm is irregular.
- *Rate:* Atrial rate is unmeasurable. Ventricular rate is usually rapid (100 to 250 beats/minute).
- *P wave:* Absent.
- *PR interval:* Unmeasurable.
- *QRS complex:* Duration varies but is greater than 0.12 second; bizarre appearance, possibly with increased amplitude.

In polymorphic ventricular tachycardia, the QRS complex is unstable.

- *T wave:* Abnormal morphology.
- *QT interval:* Unmeasurable.

What causes it

- Acute MI
- CAD

What to look for

- Palpitations, dizziness, chest pain, and shortness of breath (if the patient is conscious)
- Signs and symptoms of low cardiac output, such as decreased blood pressure or syncope
- Loss of consciousness and hemodynamic collapse

How it's treated

- Administer amiodarone and then perform synchronized cardioversion (120 to 200 joules biphasic energy or 360 joules monophasic energy).
- If the patient is unstable, prepare for defibrillation because as the rhythm deteriorates and the patient becomes unstable, the rhythm may not respond to synchronized cardioversion. If the rhythm persists, perform CPR for 2 minutes if necessary and administer epinephrine or vasopressin before the next defibrillation attempt.

Torsades de pointes

A life-threatening arrhythmia, torsades de pointes (or simply "torsades") is a polymorphic ventricular tachycardia characterized by prolonged QT intervals and QRS polarity that seems to spiral around the isoelectric line. Any condition that causes a prolonged QT interval can also cause torsades de pointes. Torsades may be paroxysmal, starting and stopping suddenly.

Although sinus rhythm sometimes resumes spontaneously, torsades de pointes usually degenerates into ventricular fibrillation.

> Torsades de pointes may start and stop suddenly.

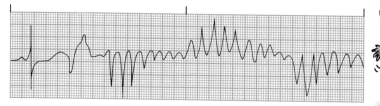

What the ECG tells you

- *Rhythm:* Atrial rhythm can't be determined. Ventricular rhythm is regular or irregular.
- *Rate:* Atrial rate can't be determined. Ventricular rate is 150 to 250 beats/minute.
- *P wave:* Not identifiable because it's buried in the QRS complex.
- *PR interval:* Not applicable because the P wave can't be identified.
- *QRS complex:* Usually wide with a phasic variation in its electrical polarity, shown by complexes that point downward for several beats and then turn upward for several beats and vice versa.
- *T wave:* Not discernible.
- *QT interval:* Prolonged (indicating delayed ventricular repolarization) while the patient is in sinus rhythm.

What causes it

- AV block
- Drug toxicity (particularly sotalol, quinidine [Novoquinidin], procainamide, and related antiarrhythmics such as disopyramide [Norpace])
- Electrolyte imbalance (hypokalemia, hypocalcemia, and hypomagnesemia)
- Hereditary QT prolongation syndrome
- Myocardial ischemia
- Psychotropic drugs (phenothiazines and tricyclic antidepressants)
- SA node disease that results in profound bradycardia

What to look for

- Palpitations, dizziness, chest pain, and shortness of breath (if the patient is conscious)
- Rapidly occurring signs or symptoms of low cardiac output, such as hypotension and altered level of consciousness (LOC)
- If rapid and prolonged torsades, loss of consciousness, pulse, and respirations

Dizziness is one symptom of torsades de pointes.

How it's treated

- If the patient is stable, correct the electrolyte imbalance, if present. Administer one of the following agents: magnesium, isoproterenol, or lidocaine. Overdrive pacing may be necessary.
- If a specific drug is causing torsades, discontinue it.
- If torsades is associated with cardiac arrest, consider giving magnesium sulfate.
- If torsades persists and the patient has no pulse, perform defibrillation at 120 to 200 joules biphasic energy or

360 joules monophasic energy, perform CPR for 2 minutes, and then defibrillate again and resume CPR. Then administer epinephrine or vasopressin. Resume attempts at CPR and defibrillation and consider other antiarrhythmics such as amiodarone.

Ventricular fibrillation

Commonly called *V-fib*, ventricular fibrillation is a chaotic pattern of electrical activity in the ventricles in which electrical impulses arise from many different foci. It produces no effective muscular contraction and no cardiac output.

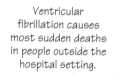

Ventricular fibrillation causes most sudden deaths in people outside the hospital setting.

Of coarse

Coarse fibrillation indicates more electrical activity in the ventricles than fine fibrillation. The fibrillatory waves become finer as acidosis and hypoxemia develop. If fibrillation continues, it eventually leads to ventricular asystole. Ventricular fibrillation causes most sudden cardiac deaths in people who aren't hospitalized.

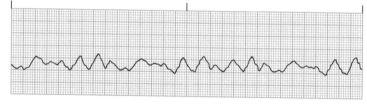

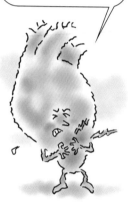

What the ECG tells you
- *Rhythm:* Atrial rhythm is unmeasurable. Ventricular rhythm has no pattern or regularity.
- *Rate:* Atrial and ventricular rates are unmeasurable.
- *P wave:* Absent.
- *PR interval:* Unmeasurable.
- *QRS complex:* Duration unmeasurable.
- *T wave:* Unmeasurable.
- *QT interval:* Unmeasurable.

What causes it
- Myocardial ischemia
- Acute MI
- Untreated VT
- Underlying heart disease
- Acid–base imbalance
- Electric shock

- Severe hypothermia
- Electrolyte imbalances, such as hypokalemia, hyperkalemia, and hypercalcemia

What to look for

- Absent pulse, heart sounds, and blood pressure
- Dilated pupils
- Loss of consciousness
- Rapid development of cyanosis
- Seizures (occasional)

How it's treated

- Perform CPR until a defibrillator or an automated external defibrillator is available. Then perform defibrillation (120 to 200 joules biphasic energy or 360 joules monophasic energy).
- If you're unsuccessful in correcting the rhythm, continue CPR for 2 minutes, defibrillate again, resume CPR, and administer epinephrine or vasopressin. If vasopressin is used first and is ineffective, follow with epinephrine.
- Resume attempts at CPR and defibrillation.
- Consider antiarrhythmics such as amiodarone. If the patient is hypomagnesemic, administer magnesium.
- Continue attempts at defibrillation, if necessary.

Recognizing atrioventricular blocks

AV blocks result from interruption in the conduction of impulses between the atria and the ventricles. They can be partial, total, or involve only a delay of conduction. Blocks can occur at the AV node, bundle of His, or bundle branches.

Three degrees of separation

The clinical effect depends on how many impulses are completely blocked, how slow the ventricular rate is, and how the block affects the heart. Blocks with slow rates can decrease cardiac output. AV blocks are classified as first-, second-, or third-degree.

First-degree AV block

A first-degree AV block occurs when impulses from the atria are consistently delayed during conduction through

You can classify AV blocks as first-, second-, or third-degree.

the AV node. It can be temporary and is the least dangerous of the AV blocks; however, it can progress to a more severe block.

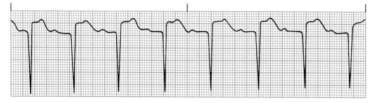

What the ECG tells you

- *Rhythm:* Atrial and ventricular rhythms are regular.
- *Rate:* Atrial and ventricular rates are the same and within normal limits.
- *P wave:* Normal size and configuration.
- *PR interval:* Prolonged (exceeding 0.20 second) but constant. (If you see an exceptionally long PR interval, look for hidden P waves; these may indicate a second-degree AV block.)
- *QRS complex:* Duration usually remains within normal limits if the conduction delay occurs in the AV node. If the QRS duration exceeds 0.12 second, the conduction delay may be in the His-Purkinje fibers.
- *T wave:* Normal size and configuration unless the QRS complex is prolonged.
- *QT interval:* Usually within normal limits.

What causes it

- Toxicity from drugs, such as digoxin, propranolol, verapamil, or procainamide
- Chronic degenerative disease of the conduction system and inferior-wall MI
- Hypokalemia and hyperkalemia
- Hypothermia
- Hypothyroidism

What to look for

- Usually no symptoms (however, the patient's peripheral pulse rate will be normal or slow with a regular rhythm)
- Signs and symptoms of decreased cardiac output, such as hypotension, syncope, and blurred vision, if the patient has a slow rate

How it's treated

- Correct the underlying cause.
- Monitor for worsening heart block, especially if myocardial damage is present.

Second-degree AV block (type I)

In type I (Wenckebach or Mobitz I) second-degree AV block, diseased tissues in the AV node delay conduction of impulses to the ventricles. As a result, each successive impulse arrives increasingly earlier in the refractory period. After several beats, an impulse arrives during the absolute refractory period when the tissue can't conduct it. The next impulse arrives during the relative refractory period and is conducted normally. The cycle then repeats. Usually distinguished by group beating, type I second-degree AV block is referred to as the *footprints of Wenckebach.*

Type I second-degree AV block is usually transient. An asymptomatic patient has a good prognosis; however, the block may progress to a more serious type.

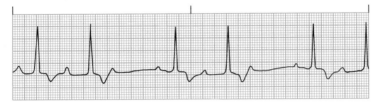

What the ECG tells you

• *Rhythm:* Atrial rhythm is regular, whereas ventricular rhythm is irregular. The R-R interval shortens progressively until a P wave appears without a QRS complex; the cycle then repeats.
• *Rate:* The atrial rate exceeds the ventricular rate, but both usually remain within normal limits.
• *P wave:* Normal size and configuration.
• *PR interval:* Typically progressively longer (only slightly) with each cycle until a P wave appears without a QRS complex; the PR interval after the nonconducted beat is shorter than the interval preceding it.
• *QRS complex:* Duration usually remains within normal limits because the block commonly lies above the bundle of His; the complex is absent periodically.
• *T wave:* Normal size and configuration but its deflection may be opposite that of the QRS complex.
• *QT interval:* Usually within normal limits.

What causes it

• CAD
• Inferior-wall MI
• Rheumatic fever
• Digoxin toxicity and use of beta-adrenergic blockers, calcium channel blockers, quinidine, or procainamide

> Type I second-degree AV block is known as the *footprints of Wenckebach.*

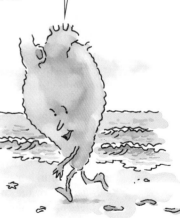

What to look for

- Usually no symptoms
- Possibly a first heart sound that becomes progressively softer with intermittent pauses
- Hypotension or syncope (if ventricular rate is low)

How it's treated

- For most patients, treat the underlying cause.
- If hemodynamically symptomatic bradycardia is present, prepare to administer atropine.
- If atropine fails to increase the heart rate, transcutaneous pacing or infusions of either dopamine or epinephrine are indicated

Second-degree AV block (type II)

Produced by a conduction disturbance in the His-Purkinje fibers, a type II (Mobitz II) second-degree AV block causes an intermittent conduction delay or block. On the ECG, you won't see any warning before a beat is dropped as you would with type I second-degree AV block.

Don't drop the beat

In type II second-degree AV block, the PR and R-R intervals remain constant before the dropped beat. The arrhythmia frequently progresses to third-degree, or complete, heart block.

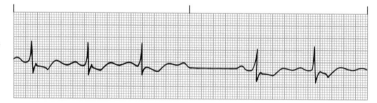

What the ECG tells you

- *Rhythm:* The atrial rhythm is regular. The ventricular rhythm can be regular or irregular. Pauses correspond to the dropped beat. If the block is intermittent, the rhythm is often irregular; if the block stays constant (for example, 2:1 or 3:1), the rhythm is regular.
- *Rate:* The atrial rate is usually within normal limits. The ventricular rate, slower than the atrial rate, may be within normal limits.
- *P wave:* Normal size and configuration but some P waves aren't followed by a QRS complex.

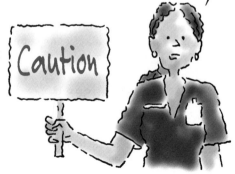

Be careful. With type II second-degree AV block, you won't see a warning on the ECG before a dropped beat.

Caution

- *PR interval:* Within normal limits or prolonged but always constant for the conducted beats.
- *QRS complex:* Duration is within normal limits if the block occurs at the bundle of His; prolonged if it occurs below the bundle of His. The complex is absent periodically.
- *T wave:* Usually normal size and configuration.
- *QT interval:* Usually within normal limits.

What causes it

- Acute anterior-wall MI
- Degenerative changes in the conduction system
- Severe CAD
- Acute myocarditis

What to look for

- Normal or slow peripheral pulse rate
- Signs and symptoms of decreased cardiac output (if pulse rate is slow)

How it's treated

- If the patient is asymptomatic, immediate treatment usually isn't needed.
- If hemodynamically symptomatic bradycardia is present, atropine may be given as a temporary measure.
- If atropine fails to increase the heart rate, prepare to apply a transcutaneous pacemaker or administer a dopamine or epinephrine infusion.
- Prepare for transvenous pacing.

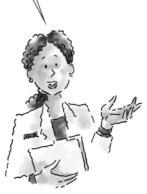

If symptomatic bradycardia is present with second-degree AV block, apply a transcutaneous pacemaker.

Third-degree AV block

When all supraventricular impulses are prevented from reaching the ventricles, the patient has third-degree AV block, also known as *complete heart block.* Just how significant the block is depends on the patient's response to any decline in ventricular rate and the stability of the escape rhythm.

Some rhythms are better than others

Junctional escape rhythms are typically stable and may produce adequate cardiac output. However, ventricular escape rhythms are slower and less stable, posing a risk for intermittent or permanent ventricular standstill.

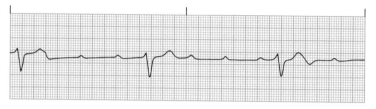

What the ECG tells you

• *Rhythm:* Atrial and ventricular rhythms are regular but aren't related.
• *Rate:* Atrial rate, which is usually within normal limits, exceeds ventricular rate. A ventricular escape rhythm ranges from 20 to 40 beats/minute. A junctional escape rhythm usually ranges from 40 to 60 beats/minute.
• *P wave:* Normal size and configuration.
• *PR interval:* Not applicable or measurable because the atria and ventricles beat independently (AV dissociation).
• *QRS complex:* Configuration depends on where the ventricular beat originates. A high AV junctional pacemaker produces a narrow QRS complex; a ventricular pacemaker produces a wide, bizarre QRS complex.
• *T wave:* Normal size and configuration unless the QRS complex originates in the ventricle.
• *QT interval:* May be within normal limits.

What causes it

• Digoxin toxicity
• Beta-adrenergic blockers
• Calcium channel blockers
• Anterior- or inferior-wall MI
• Cardiac catheterization
• Myocarditis caused by Lyme disease
• Cardiac surgery
• Congenital heart defect
• Degenerative changes in the myocardial system

What to look for

• Slow peripheral pulse rate, usually less than 40 beats/minute, but a regular rhythm
• Signs and symptoms of decreased cardiac output, such as decreased blood pressure or altered LOC, if the patient has a slow peripheral pulse rate

How it's treated

- If hemodynamically symptomatic bradycardia is present, atropine may be given as a temporary measure.
- If atropine is ineffective, prepare to apply a transcutaneous pacemaker or administer a dopamine or epinephrine infusion.
- Prepare the patient for insertion of a transvenous pacemaker, if indicated.

Recognizing other arrhythmias

Other common arrhythmias include sinus bradycardia, premature atrial contractions (PACs), pulseless electrical activity (PEA), and asystole.

Sinus bradycardia

In sinus bradycardia, the sinus rate is below 60 beats/minute and all impulses come from the SA node. This arrhythmia's significance depends on the symptoms and underlying cause.

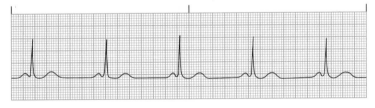

What the ECG tells you

- *Rhythm:* Atrial and ventricular rhythms are regular.
- *Rate:* Atrial and ventricular rates are less than 60 beats/minute.
- *P wave:* Normal size and configuration; P wave precedes each QRS complex.
- *PR interval:* Within normal limits and constant.
- *QRS complex:* Normal duration and configuration.
- *T wave:* Normal size and configuration.
- *QT interval:* Within normal limits but may be prolonged.

What causes it

- A well-conditioned heart (in athletic people)
- Hyperkalemia
- Increased intracranial pressure

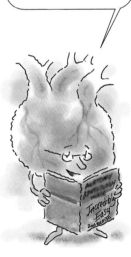

The significance of sinus bradycardia depends on the patient's symptoms and its underlying cause.

• Increased vagal tone that accompanies straining at stool, vomiting, intubation, mechanical ventilation, sick sinus syndrome, hypothyroidism, or hard physical exertion
• Possible result of inferior MI involving the right coronary artery, which supplies blood to the SA node
• Treatment with beta-adrenergic blockers, sympatholytic drugs, digoxin, or morphine

What to look for

• Possibly no symptoms
• Heart rate less than 60 beats/minute
• Fatigue, light-headedness, syncope, and palpitations
• Chest pain and premature beats (if heart disease exists and coronary blood flow is decreased)

How it's treated

• If the patient normally has a low heart rate, treatment may not be needed.
• Administer oxygen.
• Administer atropine if the patient is hemodynamically unstable (use cautiously in patients with acute myocardial ischemia or MI because atropine may cause excessive increases in heart rate, worsening ischemia, or increase of the infarction zone).
• If atropine is ineffective, prepare to apply a transcutaneous pacemaker or administer epinephrine or dopamine.
• Transvenous pacing may be indicated.

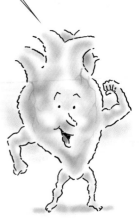

Bradycardia may produce no symptoms in athletes.

Premature atrial contractions

Originating outside the SA node, PACs usually arise from an irritable focus in the atria that supersedes the SA node as the pacemaker for one or more beats. PACs can occur in groups of two or every other beat (bigeminy).

A PAC is usually followed by a pause as the SA node is reset, which may be noncompensatory, compensatory, or longer than compensatory. Commonly, the pause is noncompensatory. PACs may also be blocked, with only an early P wave present. The most common cause of a pause is a blocked PAC.

Precipitous PACs

PACs may precipitate a more serious arrhythmia, such as atrial flutter or atrial fibrillation, in patients with heart disease. If PACs occur with an acute MI, they may signal heart failure or an electrolyte imbalance.

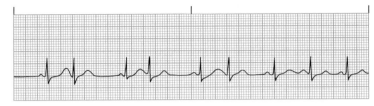

What the ECG tells you

- *Rhythm:* Atrial and ventricular rhythms are irregular as a result of the PACs but the underlying rhythm may be regular.
- *Rate:* Atrial and ventricular rates vary with the underlying rhythm.
- *P wave:* Premature and abnormally shaped; possibly lost in the previous T wave.
- *PR interval:* Usually within normal limits; may be shortened or slightly prolonged for the ectopic beat, depending on where the ectopic focus originates.
- *QRS complex:* Duration and configuration are usually normal. If no QRS complex follows the P wave, a nonconducted PAC has occurred. With nonconducted PACs, the P wave is seen in a distorted T wave.
- *T wave:* Usually has a normal configuration; however, if the P wave is hidden in the T wave, the T wave may be distorted.
- *QT interval:* Usually within normal limits.

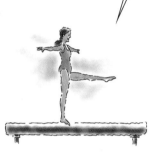

When PACs occur with acute MI, they may signal heart failure or an electrolyte imbalance.

What causes it

- Acute respiratory failure
- Heart failure
- Drugs that prolong the SA node's absolute refractory period, such as digoxin, quinidine, and procainamide
- Excessive use of caffeine, tobacco, and alcohol
- Ischemic heart disease
- Stress, fatigue, and overeating

What to look for

- Possibly no symptoms
- Irregular pulse
- Palpitations

How it's treated

- Typically, no treatment is necessary.
- Eliminate known causes, such as caffeine, tobacco, and alcohol.

Pulseless electrical activity

In PEA, formerly known as *electromechanical dissociation*, isolated electrical activity occurs sporadically without any evidence of effective myocardial contraction. Typically, a flat line tracing occurs within a few minutes, indicating asystole. PEA may be caused by clinical conditions that can be reversed when identified quickly and treated appropriately.

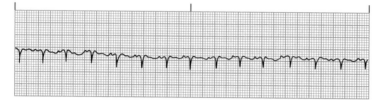

What the ECG tells you

• *Rhythm:* Atrial and ventricular rhythms are the same as the underlying rhythm. They eventually become irregular as the rate slows.
• *Rate:* Atrial rate reflects the underlying rhythm. Ventricular rate also reflects the underlying rhythm but gradually decreases.
• *P wave:* Same as the underlying rhythm but gradually flattens and disappears.
• *PR interval:* Same as the underlying rhythm but eventually disappears as the P wave disappears.
• *QRS complex:* Same as the underlying rhythm but eventually becomes progressively wider.
• *T wave:* Same as the underlying rhythm but eventually becomes indiscernible.
• *QT interval:* Same as the underlying rhythm but eventually becomes indiscernible.

What causes it

• Failure in the calcium transport mechanism
• Extensive myocardial damage, such as rupture of the left ventricular wall or massive MI
• Additional causes (see *The Five H's and T's of PEA*)

What to look for

• Apnea and sudden loss of consciousness
• No blood pressure and pulse
• Cardiac rhythm change

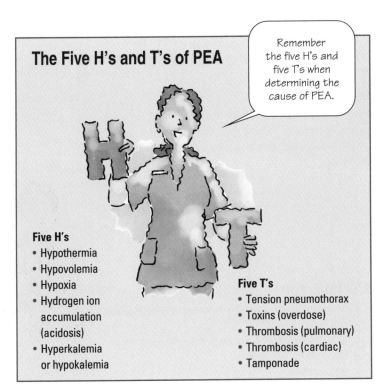

The Five H's and T's of PEA

Remember the five H's and five T's when determining the cause of PEA.

Five H's
- Hypothermia
- Hypovolemia
- Hypoxia
- Hydrogen ion accumulation (acidosis)
- Hyperkalemia or hypokalemia

Five T's
- Tension pneumothorax
- Toxins (overdose)
- Thrombosis (pulmonary)
- Thrombosis (cardiac)
- Tamponade

How it's treated

- Begin CPR immediately and check rhythm every 2 minutes. Establish an airway and IV or intraosseous access with minimal CPR interruption. Monitor airway with continuous waveform capnography.
- Administer epinephrine every 3 to 5 minutes
- Identify the cause of PEA and treat accordingly. The patient may need volume infusion for hypovolemia from hemorrhage; pericardiocentesis for cardiac tamponade; needle decompression or chest tube insertion for tension pneumothorax; surgery or thrombolytic therapy for massive pulmonary embolism; or ventilation for hypoxemia.

Asystole

Asystole refers to the total absence of ventricular activity. Some activity may be evident in the atria, but atrial impulses aren't conducted to the ventricles. Without ventricular electrical activity, ventricular contraction doesn't occur. As a result, no cardiac output or perfusion occurs. The ECG waveform is almost a flat line.

Asystole is associated with a low rate of survival, so the only hope for your patient is to identify and reverse the underlying cause immediately. As an ACLS provider, you'll need to focus on whether you should begin resuscitation and when you should stop if you do initiate it.

Asystole by any other name...

It's important to distinguish asystole from fine ventricular fibrillation, which may mimic it. Make sure that you place all ECG leads properly; otherwise, the resulting waveform may also resemble asystole.

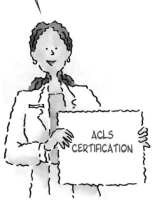

As an ACLS provider, you'll want to make sound, informed decisions during your rescue efforts.

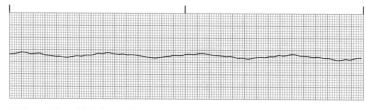

What the ECG tells you

- *Rhythm:* Atrial rhythm is indiscernible. No ventricular rhythm is present.
- *Rate:* Atrial rate is indiscernible. No ventricular rate is present.
- *P wave:* May or may not be present.
- *PR interval:* Unmeasurable.
- *QRS complex:* Absent or occasional escape beats.
- *T wave:* Absent.
- *QT interval:* Unmeasurable.

What causes it

- Severe metabolic deficit
- Acute respiratory failure
- Extensive myocardial damage, possibly from myocardial ischemia, MI, or ruptured ventricular aneurysm

What to look for

- Loss of consciousness
- Absence of peripheral pulses, blood pressure, and respirations
- Absence of cardiac rhythm on the cardiac monitor

How it's treated

- Confirm that the patient is in asystole by checking for a pulse and verifying the rhythm in another lead, along with checking lead and cable connections.
- Begin CPR and establish a patent airway and IV or intraosseous access with minimal CPR interruption.
- Identify and treat reversible causes.
- Administer epinephrine every 3 to 5 minutes.
- If asystole persists, consider stopping resuscitation.

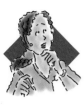

Quick quiz

1. Identify the characteristics and interpret the rhythm strip below.

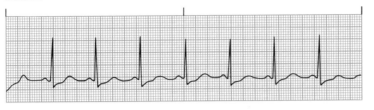

Rhythm: _____

Rate: _____

P wave: _____

PR interval: _____

QRS complex: _____

T wave: _____

QT interval: _____

Interpretation: _____

Answer:
   Rhythm: Atrial and ventricular rhythms are both regular.
   Rate: Atrial and ventricular rates are both 79 beats/minute.
   P wave: Normal size and configurations.
   PR interval: 0.12 second.
   QRS complex: 0.08 second; normal size and configuration.
   QT interval: 0.44 second.
   Interpretation: NSR.

2. A patient with symptomatic sinus bradycardia at a rate of 40 beats/minute typically experiences:
   A. high blood pressure.
   B. chest pain and dyspnea.
   C. facial flushing and ataxia.
   D. no perceptible symptoms.

Answer: B. A patient with symptomatic bradycardia suffers from low cardiac output, which may produce chest pain and dyspnea. The patient may also have crackles, an S_3 heart sound, and a sudden onset of confusion.

3. Immediate treatment of ventricular fibrillation includes:
   A. epinephrine, defibrillation, and procainamide.
   B. defibrillation, CPR, atropine, and lidocaine.
   C. epinephrine, defibrillation, and atropine.
   D. defibrillation, CPR, defibrillation, CPR, epinephrine or vasopressin, and resume CPR and defibrillation.

Answer: D. Perform defibrillation, resume CPR for 2 minutes, defibrillate, and then resume CPR. Then administer epinephrine or vasopressin. Resume attempts at CPR and defibrillation.

4. The preferred treatment for symptomatic third-degree AV block is:

A. atropine.
B. a pacemaker.
C. epinephrine.
D. dopamine.

Answer: B. Use of either a transcutaneous or transvenous pacemaker is recommended for symptomatic third-degree AV block until a permanent pacemaker can be inserted.

5. In the strip that follows, the ventricular rhythm is irregular, the ventricular rate is 130 beats/minute, the P wave is absent, the PR interval and QT interval aren't measurable, the QRS complex is wide and bizarre with varying duration, and the T wave is opposite the QRS complex. You would interpret this rhythm as:

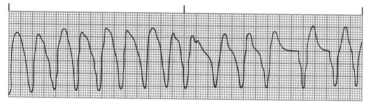

A. ventricular fibrillation.
B. ventricular tachycardia.
C. idioventricular rhythm.
D. sinus bradycardia.

Answer: B. This strip shows ventricular tachycardia: the rhythm is irregular, the rate is from 100 to 200 beats/minute, the P wave is absent, the PR and QT intervals are unmeasurable, the QRS complex is wide and bizarre, and the T wave is opposite the QRS complex.

Scoring

★★★ If you answered all five questions correctly, brilliant! You're really in rhythm with arrhythmias.

★★ If you answered four questions correctly, super job! At this junction, you're doing fine.

★ If you answered fewer than four questions correctly, not to worry! A quick review will help you get the beat.

Airway management

Just the facts

In this chapter, you'll learn:

♦ anatomy of the respiratory system

♦ effective techniques to open the airway

♦ use of airway, ventilation, and barrier devices

♦ use of oxygen administration devices.

Respiratory system basics

The major function of the respiratory system is gas exchange. Air is taken into the body on inhalation and travels through respiratory passages to the lungs. Oxygen in the lungs replaces carbon dioxide in the blood, and the carbon dioxide is expelled from the body on exhalation. (See *A close look at the respiratory system,* page 62.)

No interruptions, please

When respiratory function is interrupted, the whole body becomes compromised. Brain damage occurs within 5 minutes, and brain cell death occurs within 10 minutes. Therefore, maintaining a patent airway and restoring respiratory function are vital to advanced cardiac life support (ACLS) success.

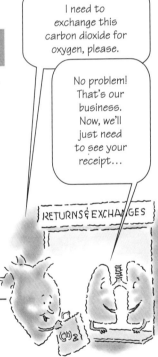

Conducting airways

The conducting airways allow air into and out of the lungs. Conducting airways include the upper and lower airways.

You take the high road...

The upper airway consists of the nose, mouth, pharynx, and larynx. These structures allow air to flow into and out of the lungs.

A close look at the respiratory system

Get to know the basic structures and functions of the respiratory system so you can perform a comprehensive respiratory assessment and identify abnormalities. The major structures of the upper and lower airways are illustrated below. The pulmonary airway is shown in more detail in the inset.

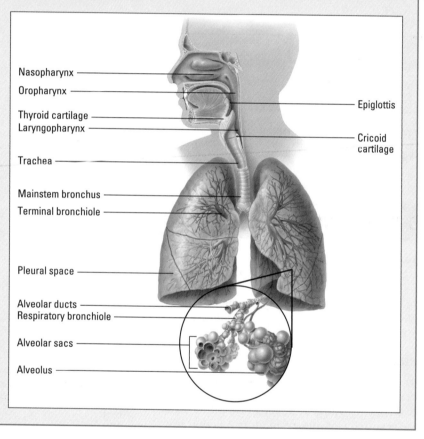

Nasopharynx

Oropharynx

Thyroid cartilage

Laryngopharynx

Trachea

Mainstem bronchus

Terminal bronchiole

Pleural space

Alveolar ducts

Respiratory bronchiole

Alveolar sacs

Alveolus

Epiglottis

Cricoid cartilage

Key points

Basics of conducting airways
• The upper airway consists of the nose, mouth, pharynx, and larynx.
• The upper airway warms, humidifies, and filters inspired air.
• The lower airway consists of the trachea, right and left mainstem bronchi, five secondary bronchi, and bronchioles.
• The lower airways facilitate gas exchange.
• Upper and lower airway obstruction occurs when a structure becomes partially or totally blocked.

They warm, humidify, and filter inspired air and protect the lower airway from foreign matter.

Upper airway obstruction occurs when the nose, mouth, pharynx, or larynx becomes partially or totally blocked. Upper airway obstruction can stem from trauma, tumors, or foreign objects.

...And I'll take the low road

The lower airway consists of the trachea, right and left mainstem bronchi, five secondary bronchi, and bronchioles. These structures facilitate gas exchange. Each bronchiole descends from a lobule and contains terminal bronchioles, alveolar ducts, and alveoli. Terminal bronchioles are anatomic dead spaces because they don't participate in gas exchange. Conversely, the alveoli are the chief units of gas exchange.

The lower airway can become partially or totally blocked as a result of inflammation, tumors, foreign bodies, or trauma.

Airway management steps

Steps in airway management include proper positioning and manual techniques to open the patient's airway. Without an open, or patent, airway, attempts to ventilate and oxygenate the patient won't be successful.

Proper positioning

When you approach a patient in possible cardiopulmonary compromise, the first step in airway management is proper positioning of both yourself and the patient. Without proper positioning, it's difficult to assess the patient's breathing and ensure a patent airway. You should be at the patient's side, at about the level of his upper chest. From this position, you can perform both rescue breathing and chest compressions.

Proper positioning of both yourself and the patient is key to ensuring correct assessment and a patent airway.

Supine is superlative

Initially, place the patient in a supine position on a firm, flat surface. You may find a patient lying face down or on his side. If so, roll the patient so that his head, shoulders, and torso move together. Avoid twisting the patient's body. If you suspect the patient has a neck injury, use manual spine motion restriction to keep his head, neck, and spine in alignment and ensure that they don't move. After the patient is in a supine position with his arms along his body, you can begin to assess him.

Opening the airway

A patient's airway can become obstructed or compromised by vomitus, food, edema, his tongue or teeth, saliva, or a foreign object. The most common cause of airway obstruction is the tongue. Muscle tone decreases when a person is unconscious or unresponsive, which increases the potential for the tongue and epiglottis to obstruct the pharynx.

Assess airway patency. Check to see if the chest rises with inspiration and falls with expiration. Wheezing; suprasternal, supraclavicular, or intracostal retractions; and cyanosis may all point to airway obstruction.

Open for business

If rescue ventilations are indicated, open the airway using the head-tilt, chin-lift maneuver or the jaw-thrust maneuver. Use the head-tilt, chin-lift maneuver to relieve an upper airway obstruction caused by the patient's tongue or epiglottis. (See *Using the head-tilt, chin-lift maneuver*.) If you suspect a neck injury, use the jaw-thrust maneuver. (See *Using the jaw-thrust maneuver*, page 65.) If the jaw-thrust maneuver isn't effective in opening the airway, use the head-tilt, chin-lift maneuver because opening the airway and providing adequate ventilation is a priority in cardiopulmonary resuscitation (CPR).

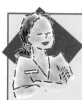

Peak technique

Using the head-tilt, chin-lift maneuver

If the patient doesn't appear to have a neck injury, use the head-tilt, chin-lift maneuver to open his airway.

First, place your hand closest to the patient's head on his forehead. Then apply firm pressure—firm enough to tilt the patient's head back.

Next, place the fingertips of your other hand under the bony portion of the patient's lower jaw, near his chin. Then lift the patient's chin, making sure to keep his mouth partially open (as shown).

Avoid placing your fingertips on the soft tissue under the patient's chin because this may inadvertently obstruct the airway you're trying to open.

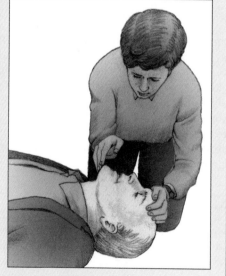

Peak technique

Using the jaw-thrust maneuver

If you suspect a neck injury, or if the head-tilt, chin-lift maneuver is unsuccessful, use the jaw-thrust maneuver.

Kneel at the patient's head with your elbows on the ground. Rest your thumbs on the patient's lower jaw near the corners of his mouth, pointing your thumbs toward his feet.

Then place your fingertips around the lower jaw. To open the airway, lift the lower jaw with your fingertips (as shown).

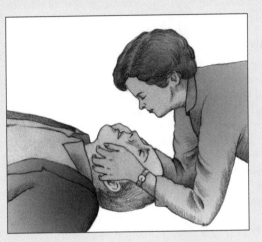

Obstinate obstructions

Address foreign body airway obstruction if the patient's chest doesn't rise with ventilations. Check the patient's mouth to see if the foreign body is visible. If so, remove it. If it isn't, remove the foreign object by using subdiaphragmatic abdominal thrusts or chest thrusts (on a pregnant or obese patient). Recheck the patient's mouth to see if the foreign body is visible. If so, remove it.

Free and clear

After you clear the airway, the patient may begin breathing spontaneously. If so, deliver supplemental oxygen in the most effective but least invasive manner possible. If spontaneous breathing doesn't occur, initiate rescue breathing using a barrier device until an advanced airway can be inserted.

Once you've opened the airway, if the patient's chest doesn't rise with ventilations, you'll need to check for foreign body obstruction.

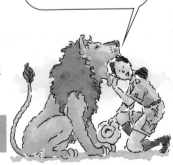

Airway devices

If manual steps such as the head-tilt, chin-lift maneuver aren't enough to maintain the patient's airway, you may need to use an advanced airway device. Always follow standard precautions and wear personal protective equipment, as needed, when using airway devices. Typically, these devices are used in an unconscious patient who has no gag reflex because insertion in a conscious patient would stimulate the gag reflex and increase the risk of aspiration. When it becomes necessary to use an advanced airway device in a conscious patient, administer sedation before insertion.

This invasion saves lives

Advanced airway devices include the endotracheal (ET) tube, supraglottal airways (esophageal-tracheal tube airway, laryngeal tube airway, and laryngeal mask [LMA] airway), nasopharyngeal airway, and oropharyngeal airway. If the use of these advanced airway devices is unsuccessful or inappropriate, a transtracheal catheter or a surgical cricothyroidotomy may be necessary. These techniques may be explained during ACLS instruction; however, they are considered beyond the scope of practice of most ACLS providers.

During a cardiac arrest, the best device to use to manage the airway depends upon the patient's condition, the provider's experience, the health care facility, and the emergency response system available.

Staff training and the continual monitoring of skills, complications, and success are essential components of airway management.

Endotracheal tube

ET intubation involves inserting a tube through the patient's mouth or nose into the trachea to obtain or maintain a patent airway. In the past, ET intubation was considered the gold standard of advanced airway control. Studies have shown, however, that the rate of complications due to staff inexperience may be unacceptably high. Frequent staff training, experience, and monitoring are required.

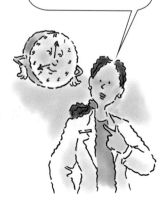

ET tube insertion should occur in less than 10 seconds.

10 seconds on the clock

Only health care practitioners trained and experienced in ET tube insertion should perform the procedure. First, you'll ventilate the patient with 100% oxygen via a bag-mask device. During CPR, chest compressions should be interrupted only for the time required for the intubating provider to visualize the vocal cords and insert the ET tube, ideally in less than 10 seconds.

Intubation indications

ET intubation should be performed when a patient who's unable to maintain adequate spontaneous ventilation has ineffective airway protective reflexes. It's used in patients receiving general anesthesia and in those with:

- cardiopulmonary arrest
- respiratory distress or failure
- persistent apnea
- obstructive angioedema (edema involving the deeper layers of the skin, subcutaneous tissue, and mucosa)
- upper airway hemorrhage
- risk of increased intracranial pressure
- laryngeal or upper airway edema
- absent swallowing or gag reflexes.

What you need

- Sedative, if appropriate
- Laryngoscope, comprised of a handle (where the batteries for the light source are housed) and a blade (curved or straight) with a light bulb
- ET tube of proper size and type (for average adult men, use size 8 mm; for average adult women, use size 7.5 mm); also have available ET tubes that are 0.5 mm and 1 mm smaller than the selected size for cases in which the initial size you choose is inappropriate for the patient; tubes with low-pressure cuffs are used in patients older than age 8
- Stylet of appropriate size for tube to facilitate proper tube insertion; plastic-coated for ease of insertion into the tube (may be lubricated with water-soluble lubricant); must end $1/2$" (1.3 cm) before it reaches the distal end of the tube
- 10-cc syringe to inflate tube cuff
- Magill forceps to assist with tube placement or to remove foreign matter from the airway
- Water-soluble lubricant
- Suction device (both rigid and soft devices should be available)
- Bag-mask device and oxygen source
- Oral airway or bite block
- Tape or tube holder
- Extra laryngoscope batteries and bulbs
- Equipment to assist with detecting proper placement (pulse oximeter, end-tidal carbon dioxide [ETco$_2$] detector, waveform capnography, if available, and stethoscope)
- Personal protective equipment (gown, gloves, and goggles)

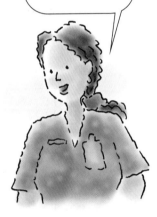

Don't forget, you'll need equipment to detect proper tube placement.

How it's done

Begin by assembling the equipment and checking it for proper functioning. Select the proper size and type of blade, either the straight (Miller) blade or the curved (Macintosh) blade, according to the patient's size. Attach the blade to the laryngoscope and snap it to a right angle to test the light.

Inflate the tube cuff to detect air leaks and check the tube lumen for patency, keeping it in the sterile wrapper until you use it. Check that the adapter fits snugly into the ET tube's proximal end.

Next, prepare the patient:

• Assess respiratory status and color.
• Place the patient's head in the sniffing position to align the airway and visualize the larynx. Remove the patient's dentures, if present. (See *Essential anatomic landmarks*.)
• Preoxygenate using a bag-mask device and 100% oxygen.
• Administer a pharmacologic agent, if appropriate (such as a sedative to induce sleep and relax the patient and a paralyzing agent to prevent movement, if necessary).
• Perform hand hygiene and put on personal protective equipment.

Now begin the procedure to insert the tube:

• Hold the laryngoscope in your left hand.

Essential anatomic landmarks

Locate the landmarks shown here when inserting an endotracheal tube through the oral cavity. These landmarks will help you ensure proper tube placement.

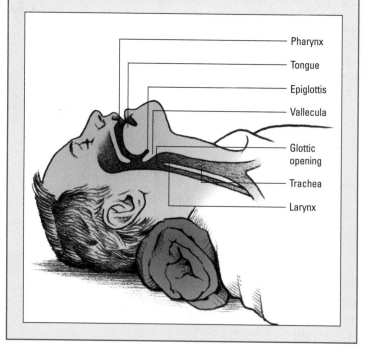

• Hold the ET tube in your right hand.
• Insert the lubricated blade into the right side of the patient's mouth, and advance it midline to the base of his tongue.
• After visualizing the arytenoid cartilage, lift the epiglottis directly with the straight blade or indirectly by inserting the curved blade into the vallecula. (See *Varying technique with blade type* and *Structures seen during direct laryngoscopy,* page 70.)
• Expose the larynx by pulling the handle of the laryngoscope in the direction toward which it points (90 degrees to the blade); don't cock the handle (especially with the straight blade) because doing so may fracture teeth.
• Lift forward and upward to expose the glottis.
• Insert the ET tube to the right of the laryngoscope and into the trachea, passing through the vocal cords.
• If you can visualize the arytenoid cartilage but not the glottis, have another person apply cricoid pressure or use a curved stylet to direct the tube anteriorly. (See *Applying cricoid pressure,* page 71.) During a cardiac arrest, cricoid pressure shouldn't be used routinely because it can impede ventilation.
• Remove the laryngoscope while holding the tube in place.

Peak technique

Varying technique with blade type

You need to vary your laryngoscope technique during intubation depending on the type of blade used.

Curved blade
If you use a curved blade, apply upward traction with the tip of the blade in the vallecula. This displaces the epiglottis anteriorly (as shown).

Straight blade
If you use a straight blade, lift the epiglottis anteriorly, exposing the opening of the glottis.

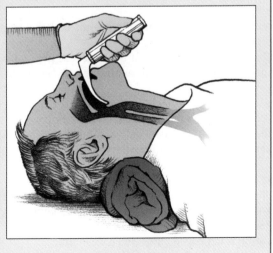

Structures seen during direct laryngoscopy

Locating anatomic structures with a laryngoscope is the key to successful intubation. This illustration shows the anatomic structures of the larynx.

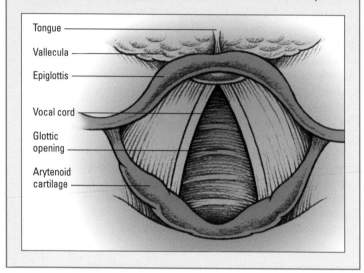

- Tongue
- Vallecula
- Epiglottis
- Vocal cord
- Glottic opening
- Arytenoid cartilage

- Remove the stylet.
- Look for tube depth marks between the 19- and 23-cm marks at the front teeth.
- Inflate the cuff using a cuff manometer to verify the correct amount of pressure.
- Attempt to ventilate the patient using the bag-mask device with an adapter attached to the ET tube.
- Insert an oral airway or a bite block, if necessary, to prevent occlusion of the airway caused by the patient biting and occluding the tube.

Now assess for placement. Check that:
- the patient's chest rises and falls with each ventilation
- breath sounds are auscultated using a five-point check (left and right anterior chest, left and right midaxillary points, and over the epigastrium)
- $ETCO_2$ measurement indicates the presence of carbon dioxide (CO_2), confirming that the tube is in the trachea
- continuous waveform capnography confirms ET placement by CO_2 detection (see *Waveform capnography*, page 72)
- oxygen saturation is improved using pulse oximetry.
- Obtain a chest x-ray to confirm proper ET placement above the carina.

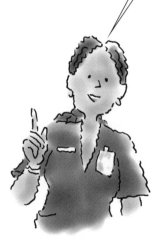

After intubating the patient, you must assess the tube's placement and check for proper cuff inflation.

Inflation in moderation

Overinflation of the balloon can affect its integrity, resulting in an air leak. To check for proper cuff inflation, make sure that no audible leaks are present. If you detect a leak, remove air from the balloon and reinflate. If the leak persists, you must replace the ET tube.

Overinflation can also result in tracheal damage. Too much pressure can injure the tracheal mucosa, which can lead to tracheal necrosis if not corrected. Use a cuff manometer to verify the correct amount of pressure.

Strive for stability

Next, stabilize the ET tube. You may use a commercially produced ET tube holder or tape or ties to secure the tube so that it's immobile. If you use a commercial product, follow the manufacturer's directions. If you use tape:
• Tear about 2' (60 cm) of tape, split both ends in half about 4" (10 cm), and place it adhesive-side up on a flat surface.

Peak technique

Applying cricoid pressure

Also called the Sellick maneuver, the cricoid pressure technique involves applying pressure to the patient's cricoid cartilage, which displaces the trachea posteriorly, compressing the esophagus.

Cricoid pressure may help prevent gastric inflation, reducing the risk of vomiting and aspiration. It's contraindicated in a conscious patient and isn't recommended for routine use during cardiac arrest because it may impede ventilation or interfere with the placement of a supraglottic airway or intubation.

Health care professionals should apply cricoid pressure only when a third rescuer is present.

To apply cricoid pressure:
• Locate the patient's thyroid cartilage with your index finger; then slide your index finger to the base of the thyroid cartilage.
• Palpate the prominent horizontal ring, which is the cricoid cartilage.
• Apply firm but moderate pressure to the cricoid cartilage using the tips of your thumb and index finger (as shown).

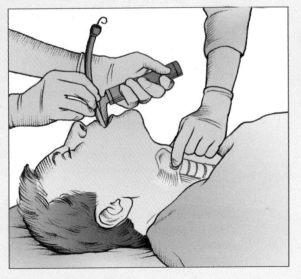

Waveform capnography

Studies of waveform capnography to verify endotracheal (ET) position in victims of cardiac arrest have shown 100% sensitivity and 100% specificity in identifying correct ET tube placement. ET tubes can be easily displaced during such activities as transfer or transport. Continuous waveform capnography is recommended, in addition to clinical assessment, as the most reliable method of confirming and monitoring correct placement of the ET tube.

> Use continuous waveform capnography to confirm and monitor that an ET tube is correctly placed in the patient's trachea.

If waveform capnography isn't immediately available, exhaled carbon dioxide (CO_2) detectors, in addition to clinical assessment, can be used as the initial method for confirming correct tube placement. However, studies of exhaled CO_2 detectors indicate that the accuracy of these devices doesn't exceed that of auscultation and direct visualization of the vocal cords for confirming the tracheal position of an ET tube.

• Tear another piece of tape about 10" (25 cm) long and place it adhesive-side down in the center of the 2" piece.
• Slide the tape under the patient's neck and center it.
• Bring the right side of the tape up and wrap the top split end counterclockwise around the tube; secure the bottom split end beneath the lower lip.
• Bring the left side of the tape up and wrap the bottom split piece clockwise around the tube; secure the top split above the patient's upper lip.

If you're using ties:
• Cut about 2' (60 cm) and place it under the patient's neck.
• Bring both ends up to the tube and cross them at the bottom of the tube near his lips.
• Bring the ends to the top of the tube and tie an overhand knot.
• Bring the ends back to the bottom of the tube, tie another overhand knot, and then secure it with a square knot (right over left, left over right).

> Once you've secured the ET tube, reverify its placement every 5 to 10 minutes.

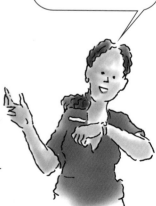

Reconfirm tube placement after you've finished securing the tube. Following ET intubation, monitor continuous waveform capnography to verify ET tube placement. Assess bilateral breath sounds and equal chest movement every 5 to 10 minutes.

Sock it to secretions

Suction the patient, as necessary, through the ET tube to remove secretions. (See *Open tracheal suctioning*, pages 74 and 75.) After the patient is connected to the ventilator, in-line suctioning is the preferred method of ET suctioning. (See *Closed tracheal suctioning*, page 76.)

What to consider

- Practitioners who perform ET intubation need adequate training and frequent experience to reduce the risk of complications, such as oropharyngeal trauma and hypoxemia.
- ET intubation isn't an ideal intubation method for patients with suspected cervical spine injury.
- Awake or uncooperative patients may need a short-acting muscle relaxant before ET intubation while you maintain the airway with a bag-mask device.

Esophageal-tracheal tube airway

The esophageal-tracheal tube airway consists of a plastic tube with two lumens and a ventilation bag attachment port for each lumen. Proximal and distal balloons help secure the tube and prevent ventilation gases from escaping around the tube. Rings on the proximal tube indicate the depth of the tube's insertion and should be at the level of the patient's teeth. The pharyngeal lumen of the tube has the longer primary port (port #1) at the proximal end, holes along the lumen between the balloons for supraglottic ventilation, and a blind distal end. The tracheoesophageal lumen has the shorter secondary proximal port (port #2), is patent between the balloons, and has an open distal end.

Ease and versatility

The tube may be inserted blindly, usually in prehospital cardiac arrest situations, and may be used by those not trained in ET intubation or in place of ET intubation. If used properly, insertion in either the esophagus or trachea provides satisfactory oxygenation. When the tube is inserted blindly, it most commonly enters the esophagus. With esophageal intubation, port #1 of the pharyngeal lumen (blind end) is used to perform supraglottic ventilations, and port #2 of the tracheoesophageal lumen (open

(Text continues on page 75.)

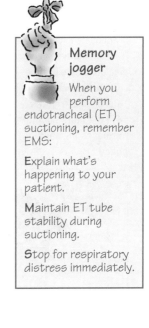

Memory jogger

When you perform endotracheal (ET) suctioning, remember EMS:

Explain what's happening to your patient.

Maintain ET tube stability during suctioning.

Stop for respiratory distress immediately.

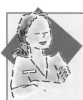

Peak technique

Open tracheal suctioning

Open tracheal suctioning involves the removal of secretions from the trachea. It's performed by inserting a catheter through the mouth, nose, tracheal stoma, and tracheostomy or endotracheal (ET) tube. This procedure helps maintain a patent airway to promote optimal exchange of oxygen and carbon dioxide and can be performed as frequently as the patient's condition warrants. Tracheal suctioning calls for strict aseptic technique and is best performed by two people.

What you need

- Oxygen source
- Portable or wall-mounted suction system
- Connecting tube
- Suction catheter kit or a sterile suction catheter, sterile gloves, and a disposable, sterile solution container
- Sterile water or normal saline solution
- Handheld resuscitation bag

How it's done

When preparing to perform tracheal suctioning:
- Check all equipment for proper functioning.
- Attach the suction canister and tubing to the wall or portable system.
- Set the suction between 80 and 100 mm Hg (this amount is adequate to clear the airway without causing tissue trauma); the suction catheter should be one-half the diameter of the ET tube.
- Open the suction kit or catheter.
- Put on sterile gloves.
- Fill the sterile container with sterile water or normal saline solution, according to your facility's policy.

- Deliver three to six breaths with the handheld resuscitation bag to preoxygenate the patient (as shown), or set the ventilator on 100% oxygen for suctioning (if available).

    To perform tracheal suctioning:
- Remove the catheter from the kit.
- Manipulate the connecting tubing and attach the catheter to the tubing (as shown).

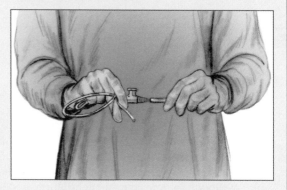

- Hold the catheter with your dominant hand while placing the thumb of your other hand over the control valve (as shown).

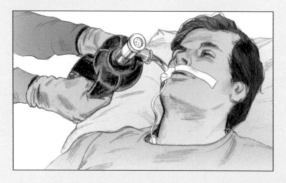

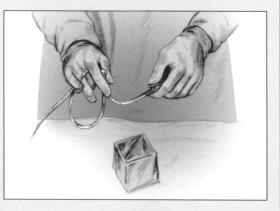

Open tracheal suctioning *(continued)*

• Dip the catheter tip in the sterile solution and suction a small amount of solution through the catheter (as shown).

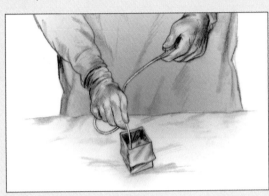

• Disconnect the resuscitation bag from the ET tube.
• Place the catheter into the tube without engaging suction, with the ET tube firmly positioned, and gently advance it until you feel resistance.
• Suction the patient for no longer than 10 seconds: Pull the catheter back about 1 cm, slowly rotate and withdraw it, and use your thumb to intermittently occlude the vent (as shown).

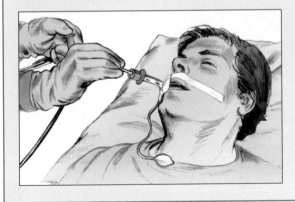

• Deliver breaths with the handheld resuscitation bag between attempts.
    After you've finished suctioning:
• Reconnect the patient to the oxygen source.
• Clean the catheter and tubing by aspirating sterile saline solution.
• Ensure a patent airway and properly dispose of the catheter and gloves.

What to consider
• Remember to explain to the patient what's occurring and observe him for signs of anxiety.
• Maintain ET tube stability during suctioning.
• Report respiratory distress immediately.
• Interrupting ventilation causes decreased lung volume, which may cause hypoxemia and lead to cardiac arrest.
• Suctioning of the oral mucosa may stimulate the gag reflex and cause vomiting, so maintain ET tube cuff inflation to prevent aspiration.
• Prolonged suctioning (more than 15 seconds) may cause hypoxia and can lead to cardiac arrest.
• ET suctioning may stimulate the cough reflex, which can cause an increase in intracranial pressure (ICP), constricting blood flow to the brain. It may also cause displacement of the ET tube if it isn't secured properly.
• Suctioning may increase ICP and blood pressure, produce cardiac arrhythmias, or stimulate a vagal response. Monitor the patient closely.
• Suctioning may cause feelings of suffocation in the patient (be sure to reassure him).
• Suctioning may introduce bacterial infection into the airway if performed incorrectly. Maintain aseptic technique.
• Overzealous suctioning or improper technique may cause tracheal trauma.
• Suctioning should be limited in patients taking anticoagulants (observe for blood in the secretions).

distal end) can then be used to suction gastric contents. If the tube is inserted into the trachea, port #2 of the tracheoesophageal lumen (open distal end) is used to ventilate the patient, similar to using an ET tube.

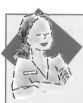

Peak technique

Closed tracheal suctioning

The closed tracheal suction system can ease removal of secretions and reduce patient complications. The system consists of a sterile suction catheter in a clear plastic sleeve (as shown). It allows the patient to remain connected to the ventilator during suctioning.

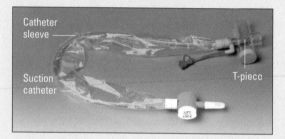

Catheter
sleeve

Suction
catheter

T-piece

LIFT
LOCK

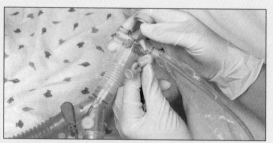

As a result, the patient can maintain the tidal volume, oxygen concentration, and positive end-expiratory pressure delivered by the ventilator while being suctioned. In turn, this reduces the occurrence of suction-induced hypoxemia.

Another advantage of this system is a reduced risk of infection, even when the same catheter is used many times. The caregiver doesn't need to touch the catheter and the ventilator circuit remains closed.

What you need
- Closed suction control valve
- T-piece
- Catheter sleeve (with connections at each end)
- Gloves

How it's done
To perform closed tracheal suctioning, follow these steps:
- Remove the closed suction system from its wrapping; attach the control valve to the connecting tubing.
- Depress the thumb suction control valve and keep it depressed while setting the suction pressure to the desired level.
- Connect the T-piece to the ventilator breathing circuit, making sure that the irrigation port is closed; then connect the T-piece to the patient's endotracheal or tracheostomy tube (as shown above right).

- While one hand keeps the T-piece parallel to the patient's chin, use the thumb and index finger of your other hand to advance the catheter through the tube and into the patient's tracheobronchial tree (as shown).

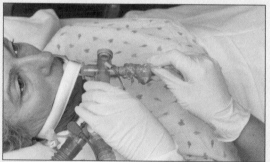

- If necessary, gently retract the catheter sleeve as you advance the catheter.
- While continuing to hold the T-piece and control valve, apply intermittent suction and withdraw the catheter until it reaches its fully extended length in the sleeve. Repeat the procedure as necessary.
- After you finish suctioning, flush the catheter by maintaining suction while slowly introducing normal saline solution or sterile water into the irrigation port.
- Place the thumb control valve in the off position.
- Dispose of and replace the suction equipment and supplies and change the closed suctioning system, according to your facility's policy.

What you need

- Esophageal-tracheal tube (37 French or 41 French; follow manufacturer's instructions for appropriate size tube based on the patient's height)
- 50-cc syringe to inflate proximal balloon
- 15-cc syringe to inflate distal balloon
- Stethoscope to auscultate for proper position
- Suction device
- Bag-mask device
- Oropharyngeal or nasopharyngeal airway
- Oxygen source
- Water-soluble lubricant
- Placement confirmation devices ($ETCO_2$ detector, pulse oximeter, continuous waveform capnography if available)
- Personal protective equipment (gown, gloves, and goggles)

How it's done

To prepare, you should first:
- Determine cuff integrity according to the manufacturer's directions.
- Lubricate the tube, as necessary, with water-soluble lubricant.
- Gather all necessary components and accessories.
- Perform hand hygiene and put on personal protective equipment.
- Inspect the patient's upper airway and remove any visible obstruction.

   To insert the esophageal-tracheal tube
- Position the patient's head in a neutral position.
- Insert the esophageal-tracheal tube in the same direction as the natural curvature of the pharynx.
- Grasp the tongue and lower jaw between your index finger and thumb, and lift upward.
- Insert the esophageal-tracheal tube gently but firmly until the black rings on the tube are positioned between the patient's teeth.
- Place the proximal cuff between the base of the patient's tongue and his hard palate.
- If the tube doesn't insert easily, withdraw it and retry.
- Inflate the large proximal balloon to stop ventilatory gases from exiting through the pharynx to the mouth or nose; inflate the distal cuffs according to the manufacturer's instructions.
- Ventilate through the primary tube.

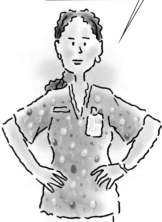

Placement of a supraglottic airway is an alternative to ET intubation and can be done successfully without interrupting chest compressions.

Placement test

Proper tube placement is essential. After attaching the ventilation bag to the primary port (port #1 located on the pharyngeal lumen), check to see if the tube is in the esophagus by attempting to ventilate the patient. Listen for breath sounds and epigastric insufflation sounds, and look for the chest to rise. If breath sounds are present, the chest rises, and no epigastric insufflation sounds are heard, the tube is probably in the esophagus. Confirm tube placement with capnography if it's available. Secure the tube.

Absence doesn't make the heart grow fonder

If breath sounds are negative and the chest doesn't rise but gastric sounds are heard, the tube may be in the trachea. Immediately switch the ventilation bag to the shorter port #2, which is located on the tracheoesophageal lumen (open distal end), attempt to ventilate, and reassess the patient. If the tube is in the trachea, breath sounds should be heard, the chest should rise, and epigastric insufflation sounds should be absent. Tube placement should be confirmed with capnography if it's available. Secure the tube.

If both breath and epigastric sounds are absent using either port:
• Immediately deflate both cuffs.
• Withdraw the tube ¾" to 1¼" (2 to 3 cm), and then reinflate the cuffs.
• Ventilate and reassess for placement by using the $ETco_2$ detector and waveform capnography.

If breath and epigastric sounds are still absent:
• Immediately deflate the cuffs and extubate.
• Suction as necessary.
• Insert an oropharyngeal or nasopharyngeal airway.
• Hyperventilate.
• Continue ongoing respiratory assessment and treatment.

What to consider

• When used by properly trained health care professionals, the esophageal-tracheal tube delivers ventilation and oxygenation comparable to an ET tube.
• This method is only used as a temporary measure.
• The esophageal-tracheal tube is contraindicated in any person with an active gag reflex, esophageal disease, or caustic substance ingestion.
• Esophageal tears and subcutaneous emphysema are possible because of tube insertion or increased pressure distal to the placed tube during CPR.
• You must remove the esophageal-tracheal tube if the patient regains consciousness or his gag reflex.

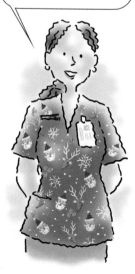

Use an esophageal-tracheal tube as a temporary measure only.

Esophageal-tracheal tube airway

The esophageal-tracheal tube is a supraglottal airway that can be used to manage the airway and reduce the risk of aspiration during cardiac arrest. Ventilation and oxygenation compare favorably to endotracheal tube intubation, and training is easier.

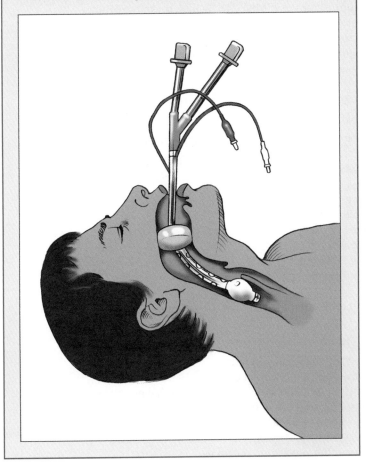

Laryngeal tube airway

The laryngeal tube airway consists of a curved tube with ventilation holes located between two inflatable cuffs. Both cuffs are inflated using a single valve/pilot balloon. The distal cuff is designed to seal the esophagus, while the proximal tube is intended to seal the oropharynx. There is a connector at the proximal tube to connect it to a standard resuscitation bag.

Not so complicated

Like the esophageal-tracheal tube, the laryngeal tube helps prevent aspiration while protecting the patient's airway, and it's more compact and less complicated to insert. During CPR, chest compressions don't have to be interrupted for its insertion. In cardiac arrest situations, the American Heart Association (AHA) has determined that properly trained health care professionals may consider using the laryngeal tube as an alternative to bag-mask ventilation or ET intubation for airway management.

What you need

- Laryngeal tube of appropriate size according to the patient's height
- 10-mL syringe
- Stethoscope
- Suction device
- Bag-mask device
- Oropharyngeal or nasopharyngeal airway
- Oxygen source
- Water-soluble lubricant
- Placement confirmation device (ETco$_2$ detector or waveform capnography)
- Personal protective equipment (gown, gloves, and goggles)

How it's done

To prepare the equipment and patient:
- Be aware of the contraindications for use.
- Assess the cuff for defects. Inject the recommended amount of air into the inflation port, then deflate.
- Apply a water-based lubricant to the beveled distal tip and posterior aspect of the tube, taking care to avoid introducing lubricant in or near the ventilation openings.
- Perform hand hygiene.
- Inspect the patient's upper airway and remove visible obstructions.

To insert the airway:
- Preoxygenate the patient.
- Place the patient in the "sniffing" position.
- Hold the laryngeal tube at the connector with the dominant hand. With the nondominant hand, hold the mouth open and apply the chin-lift maneuver, unless contraindicated.

Laryngeal tube airway

The laryngeal tube airway is a type of supraglottal airway that may be used to manage a patient's airway during cardiac arrest situations. It's less complicated to insert than the esophageal-tracheal tube airway and less likely to enter the trachea.

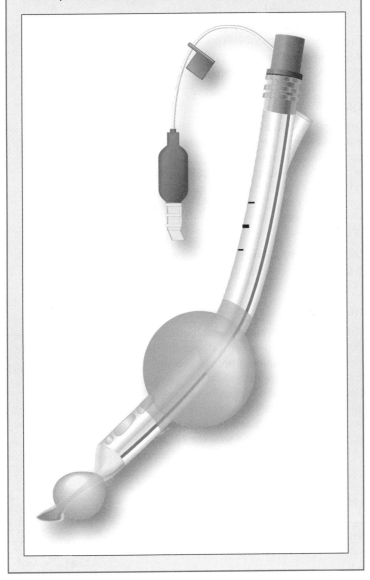

- With the laryngeal tube rotated laterally 45 to 90 degrees (so that the orientation line is touching the corner of the mouth), introduce the tip into the mouth and advance it behind the base of the tongue. Never force the tube into position.
- As the tube passes under the tongue, rotate the tube back to midline (the orientation line should face the chin).
- Without exerting excessive force, advance the tube until the base of the connector aligns with the teeth or gums.
- Use the 10-mL syringe to inject the correct amount of air into the cuff according to the manufacturer's specifications.
- Confirm tube placement by auscultation and by $ETCO_2$ detector or waveform capnography and then secure the tube.

What to consider

- Don't use a laryngeal tube airway for responsive patients with an intact gag reflex, patients with known esophageal disease, or patients who have ingested caustic substances.
- The laryngeal tube hasn't been proven to fully protect the airway from aspiration due to regurgitation of gastric contents.

Laryngeal mask airway

The LMA is a silicone device that combines tracheal intubation and the use of a face mask to maintain a patent airway in an unconscious patient.

When immediacy is needed

The LMA is useful for situations in which intubation attempts have failed, bag-mask ventilation is unsuccessful, and the patient needs immediate airway management. It's simple to use and insert, and may be inserted by nurses, respiratory therapists, and emergency services personnel after receiving adequate training.

For airway management during cardiac arrest, the LMA is an acceptable alternative to bag-mask or ET ventilation. Occasionally, patients can't be adequately ventilated with the LMA after successful insertion. Make sure an alternative ventilation method is available.

What you need

- LMA of appropriate size with syringe to inflate the cuff
- Stethoscope to auscultate for proper position
- Suction device
- Bag-mask device
- Oxygen source
- Water-soluble lubricant

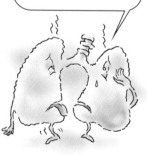

Use an LMA when intubation attempts have failed and your patient needs immediate airway management.

- Placement confirmation devices ($ETco_2$ detector, pulse oximeter, continuous waveform capnography if available).
- Personal protective equipment (gown, gloves, and goggles)

How it's done

Before you begin the procedure:
- Perform hand hygiene and put on personal protective equipment.
- Assess the cuff for defects and the patient for gag reflex.
- Ventilate and oxygenate the patient with a bag-mask or mouth-to-mask device.
- Place the patient in the sniffing position.
    To insert the airway:
- Press the distal tip of the lubricated, deflated LMA cuff against the hard palate using your index finger to guide the tube over the back of the tongue. (Avoid lubricating the anterior surface of the mask because the lubricant may be aspirated.)
- Gently advance the tube until you feel resistance as the upper esophageal sphincter is engaged.
- Without holding the tube, inflate the cuff with the appropriate amount of air.

Laryngeal mask airway

The laryngeal mask airway doesn't require direct visualization of the vocal cords for insertion so it's easier to insert than an endotracheal tube and provides a more secure and reliable means of ventilation than the face mask.

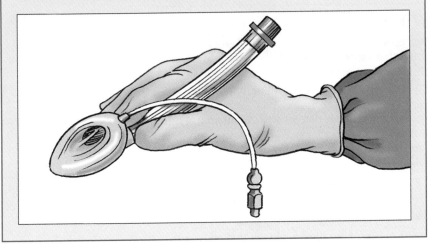

The tube will move outward about $^5/_8$" (1.5 cm) and the cuff will position itself around the laryngeal inlet, resulting in a slight movement of the thyroid and cricoid cartilage. The longitudinal black line on the shaft of the tube should lie in the midline against the upper lip.

In the right place at the right time

Confirm placement using auscultation and an $ETco_2$ detector or waveform capnography. When correctly positioned, the tip of the LMA cuff lies at the base of the hypopharynx against the upper esophageal sphincter; the sides lie in the pyriform fossa; and the upper border of the mask lies at the base of the tongue, pushing it forward.

Once the LMA is correctly placed, ventilate the patient and assess its effect. Pulse oximetry should show an increase in oxygenation. If vomiting occurs, leave the LMA in place, immediately tilt the patient's head down, and suction through the LMA.

What to consider

• Consider using the LMA for patients with suspected cervical injury or when you have limited access to the patient.
• The LMA is contraindicated for patients at risk for aspiration and in patients who are morbidly obese or more than 14 weeks pregnant.
• Don't use the LMA if the patient's mouth can't be opened more than $^5/_8$".

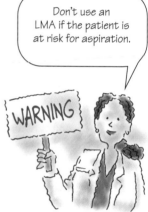

Don't use an LMA if the patient is at risk for aspiration.

WARNING

Nasopharyngeal airway

The nasopharyngeal airway is a soft rubber uncuffed tube with a smooth curvature that's inserted through the nose into the oropharynx. When properly positioned, it creates a wide air channel and permits positive pressure ventilation through the trachea.

A semiconscious or conscious patient with an intact gag reflex can tolerate the nasopharyngeal airway. It's easier to insert than an oral airway and is useful for maintaining an airway in an adult with seizures, trismus (tonic contraction of the muscles involved in chewing), or cervical spine injuries.

What you need

• Personal protective equipment (gown, gloves, and goggles)
• Appropriate size airway
• Water-soluble lubricant

How it's done

Use a nasal tube of the largest diameter size that will fit the patient's nares. Determine the size by measuring from the tip of the nose to the tip of the earlobe. The typical sizes are:
- small adult—6 to 7 mm internal diameter (24 to 28 French)
- medium adult—7 to 8 mm internal diameter (28 to 32 French)
- large adult—8 to 9 mm internal diameter (32 to 36 French).

   Perform hand hygiene, don personal protective equipment, and assess the nares for patency. Place the patient in a supine position and properly position the airway using the head-tilt, chin-lift maneuver.

   Apply a water-soluble lubricant to the distal half of the tube. Then gently insert the tube bevel-side toward the patient's septum. Rotate the tube slightly if resistance occurs but don't force entry.

Peak technique

Inserting a nasopharyngeal airway

First, hold the airway beside the patient's face to make sure it's the proper size (as shown). It should be slightly smaller than the patient's nostril diameter and slightly longer than the distance from the tip of his nose to his earlobe.

   To insert the airway, hyper-extend the patient's neck (unless contraindicated). Then push up the tip of his nose and pass the lubricated airway into his nostril (as shown). Avoid pushing against any resistance to prevent tissue trauma and airway kinking.

   To check for correct airway placement, first close the patient's mouth. Then place your finger over the tube's opening to detect air exchange. Also, depress the patient's tongue with a tongue blade and look for the airway tip behind the uvula.

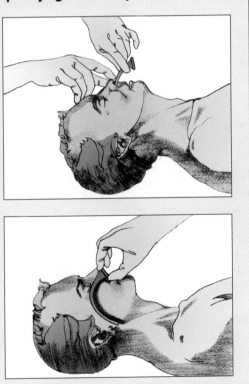

Auscultate the lungs for clear and equal breath sounds after you've inserted the tube. Also be sure to have suction equipment available. (See *Inserting a nasopharyngeal airway, page 85.*)

What to consider

• The nasopharyngeal airway may stimulate laryngospasm, gag reflex, and vomiting.
• Aspiration or improper placement may cause hypoxemia. (If this occurs, check respiration and provide ventilatory assistance as needed.)
• The nasopharyngeal airway may injure nasal mucosa.
• The nasopharyngeal airway is contraindicated when basilar skull fracture is suspected.

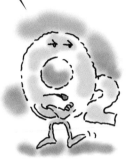

Improper placement of a nasopharyngeal airway may cause hypoxemia.

Oropharyngeal airway

The oropharyngeal (or oral) airway is a C-shaped tubular or channeled device made of firm plastic or flexible vinyl (to prevent occlusion by the teeth). It's inserted between the tongue and the posterior wall of the pharynx to lift the base of the tongue off the hypopharynx and establish an open airway.

The oral airway is generally used:
• during bag-mask ventilation to facilitate lung oxygenation and minimize gastric distention
• as a bite block with ET intubation to prevent accidental occlusion of the tube by biting
• to prevent airway occlusion by the tongue in an unconscious patient with spontaneous breathing.

What you need

• Suction and tonsillar (oral suction) catheter
• Appropriate size oropharyngeal airway:
  – small adult—size 3 (80 mm)
  – medium adult—size 4 (90 mm)
  – large adult—size 5 (100 mm)
• Tongue blade to move the tongue out of the way
• Personal protective equipment (gown, gloves, and goggles)

How it's done

Perform hand hygiene and don personal protective equipment. Before you begin, place the patient in a supine position and, if needed, suction the oropharynx area. Measure the patient for appropriate airway size (from the corner of the mouth to the tip of the earlobe or the bottom angle of the jaw).

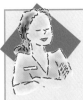

Peak technique

Inserting an oral airway

Hyperextend the patient's head, unless this position is contraindicated, before using either the cross-finger or tongue blade insertion method.

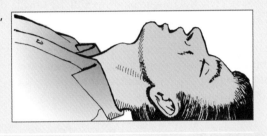

To insert an oral airway using the cross-finger method, place your thumb on the patient's lower teeth and your index finger on his upper teeth. Gently open his mouth by pushing his teeth apart.

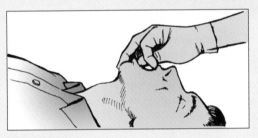

Insert the airway upside down to avoid pushing the tongue toward the pharynx, and slide it over the tongue toward the back of the mouth. As it approaches the posterior wall of the pharynx, rotate the airway so that it points downward.

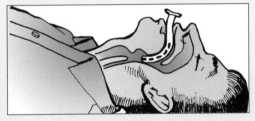

To use the tongue blade technique, open the patient's mouth and depress his tongue with the blade. Guide the airway over the back of the tongue as you did for the cross-finger technique.

To insert the airway, turn the airway upside down and insert it into the patient's mouth. Then turn it 180 degrees into proper position as the end of the airway reaches about the middle of the tongue (one-half of the curved part is in the mouth). The flange should rest on the patient's lips, and the end of the airway should be in place between the base of the tongue and the back of the throat. Auscultate for breath sounds during ventilation. Clear and equal breath sounds indicate proper ventilation. (See *Inserting an oral airway*.)

What to consider

- Trauma is possible to the oral mucosa, lips, tongue, or teeth as well as displacement of the tongue back into the pharynx and airway occlusion from incorrect insertion.
- Elderly patients are at risk for palate injury when an airway is inserted upside down. (Use the tongue blade to pull the tongue to the front and insert the airway right side up into the pharynx, if necessary.)
- Use the oral airway only in unconscious patients because insertion of an oral airway can cause gagging and vomiting or stimulate laryngospasm in patients regaining consciousness, necessitating removal and maintenance of the patent airway.

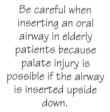

Be careful when inserting an oral airway in elderly patients because palate injury is possible if the airway is inserted upside down.

Ventilation devices

Numerous devices are used to ventilate patients and help deliver oxygen. They include the bag-mask device and automatic transport ventilator (ATV). When in place, these devices are used either to deliver room air or supplemental oxygen. Remember to always follow standard precautions when using ventilation devices.

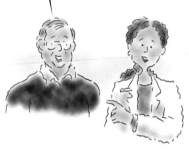

Bag-mask device

The bag-mask device (also called a *bag-valve mask*) is an inflatable handheld resuscitation bag with a reservoir and an adapter that can be directly attached to a face mask, ET tube, or tracheostomy tube. It's used to manually deliver ventilation with room air or supplemental oxygen (if an oxygen source is available) by positive pressure to patients with apnea or inadequate respirations.

A bag-mask device provides manually delivered ventilation with room air or supplemental oxygen.

Seal of approval

When used with a face mask, the bag-mask device should fit tightly, providing a good seal. If you use a device with an inflatable rim, it can be molded to facial contours. A tidal volume of 6 to 7 mL/kg with the bag-mask device should adequately inflate the average adult's lungs while minimizing gastric inflation.

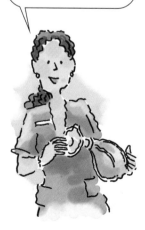

What you need

- Oral or nasal airway, unless the patient is intubated
- Pharyngeal suctioning equipment
- Bag-mask device with oxygen reservoir
- Tubing to connect to oxygen source
- Personal protective equipment (gown, gloves, goggles)

Peak technique

How to apply a bag-mask device

Here's a step-by-step guide for applying a bag-mask device.

Cover the bridge
Place the mask over the patient's face so that the apex of the triangle covers the bridge of his nose and the base lies between his lower lip and chin. Notice the hand in the photo— the practitioner is using the E-C (hand placement) technique to hold the mask to the patient's face (creating a "C" with the thumb and index finger, and creating the "E" with the last three fingers of the hand while lifting the patient's jaw).

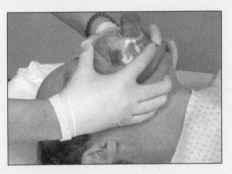

Keep the mouth open
Make sure that the patient's mouth remains open underneath the mask. Attach the bag to the mask and to the tubing leading to the oxygen source.

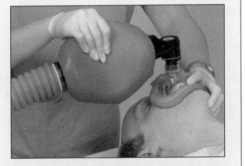

If the patient has a tube
If the patient has a tracheostomy tube or endotracheal tube in place, detach the mask from the bag and attach the handheld resuscitation bag directly to the tube.

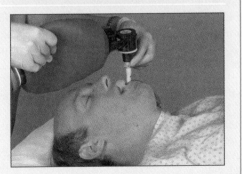

How it's done

To prepare the patient and the device:
- Suction the airway to ensure patency.
- Insert an oral or nasal airway in an unconscious patient.
- Connect the tubing to the oxygen source and set the flow rate between 10 and 15 L/minute (this flow rate should yield from 90% to 100% oxygen).
- Attach the tubing to the oxygen inlet of the device.
- Assess oxygen flow by placing the mask against your hand.
  To attach the device to the patient:
- Place the narrow end of the appropriate size mask over the patient's nose while lifting the patient's lower jaw with the fingers of both your hands (the patient's mouth should be open under the mask, and the tip of the patient's chin should be at the rounded end of the mask). Use the E-C (hand placement) technique if two people aren't available for bag-mask ventilation. (See *How to apply a bag-mask device*, page 89.)
- If the patient is intubated, attach the adapter to the ET tube, esophageal-tracheal tube, laryngeal tube, or LMA.
- Squeeze the bag and observe for the rise and fall of the chest.
- During cardiac arrest, deliver ventilation over 1 second at a rate of 8 to 10 breaths/minute without reference to chest compressions (with a protected airway).

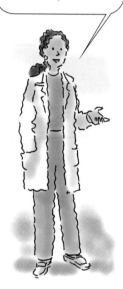

You may need to insert an oral or nasal airway before using a bag-mask device on an unconscious patient.

What to consider

- Watch for inadequate ventilation because of an improper mask seal or improper bag squeezes.
- Gastric distention, which can trigger vomiting and aspiration or pneumothorax, may occur with too hard or too rapid bag squeezing.
- Eye injury caused by direct pressure on the eyes with too large a mask is possible.

Automatic transport ventilator

The ATV provides supplemental oxygen at a constant inspiratory flow rate for an extended time and gives you the freedom to perform other treatment procedures. Here are the basic forms:
- Time-cycled ATVs stop delivery when a preset time for inspiration expires. The timing mechanism can run on oxygen or electricity, and you set the length of inspiration.
- Volume-cycled ATVs deliver a preset amount of oxygen and then stop.
- Pressure-cycled ATVs stop when a preset airway pressure is met during the inspiratory phase.
- Flow-cycled ATVs stop when the inspiratory flow rate drops to a preset critical level.

What you need

- ATV
- Oxygen source
- Suction equipment
- Gloves and goggles

How it's done

To prepare the ATV:
- Check that the device is functioning properly.
- Use a bag-mask device to assist ventilation until the equipment is ready. (Keep the bag-mask device handy in the event that the oxygen supply is diminished.)
- Have suction equipment ready.
    To attach the ATV:
- Turn on the unit and, if necessary, set the tidal volume (12 to 15 mL/kg is the guideline) and rate (8 to 12 breaths/minute).
- Set the peak inspiratory pressure at 60 cm H_2O pressure. (It should have the ability to increase to 80 cm.)
- Attach the device to the proper airway adjunct.
- Observe the patient's respirations for adequate chest expansion. (The tidal volume knob can be adjusted for more or less expansion.)
- Assess for effectiveness using waveform capnography.

What to consider

- Reliable oxygen and electrical sources and backup bag-mask device are necessary.
- Ventilation may stop if the patient fights the equipment, causing increased airway resistance.
- Increased intrathoracic pressure and hypotension caused by decreased blood flow to the heart are possible.
- Increased airway pressure is possible, causing barotrauma to the airway.
- Watch for gastric distention if the patient isn't intubated with an ET tube.

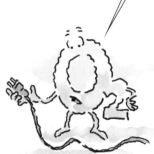

When using an ATV, you must have reliable oxygen and electrical sources available.

Barrier devices

Barrier devices serve as a physical barrier between you and the patient. They're typically used with CPR in such areas as the workplace. Remember to always follow standard precautions when using barrier devices. Two categories of barrier devices are available: the face shield and pocket face mask.

Face shield

The face shield contains a clear plastic or silicone section to prevent direct contact between you and the patient during mouth-to-mouth ventilation.

What you need

- Face shield
- Gloves

How it's done

To use the face shield:
- Establish a patent airway.
- Place the shield over the patient's mouth and nose with the center opening over his mouth.
- Slowly blow a sufficient volume of air into the center opening to make the patient's chest rise.

What to consider

- Obtaining adequate ventilation with a face shield can be difficult.
- A supplemental oxygen source is necessary as soon as possible to prevent hypoxemia.

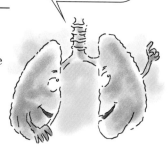

Be careful— adequate ventilation is difficult with a face shield.

Pocket face mask

The pocket face mask (also called *mouth-to-mask*) is used to deliver enriched oxygen to patients with spontaneous, ineffective respirations or to those requiring artificial ventilation. It's made of transparent, moldable plastic that allows visualization so that vomiting can be detected. Its components include an inflatable cushion, an oxygen port, a low-resistance one-way valve, and a disposable filter that prevents contact between you and the patient's secretions. (See *The pocket face mask*.)

Concentrate on oxygen

The pocket face mask delivers 16% oxygen concentration from exhaled air. By connecting the mask to an oxygen source, you can provide a higher concentration.

What you need

- Pocket face mask
- Supplemental oxygen (optional)
- Gloves

The pocket face mask

Portable and easy to use, a pocket face mask is a barrier device that allows you to deliver a breath through a one-way valve while directing the patient's exhaled air away from you. Some devices contain an oxygen administration port that allows you to administer supplemental oxygen.

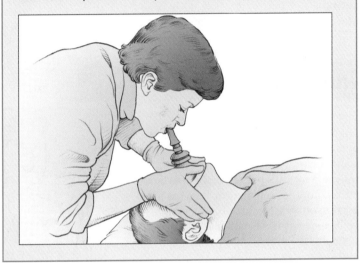

How it's done

To prepare the mask and the patient:
- Establish a patent airway.
- Snap the mask's filter firmly in place; the dome should be popped out.
- Attach the one-way valve to the mask port, directing the exhalation port away from the narrow end.
    To attach the mask:
- Position the mask on the patient's face forming a tight seal, with the narrow end at the bridge of the patient's nose and the rounded end between his lower lip and chin.
- Encircle the mask with your thumbs and index fingers and apply pressure to both sides of the mask with the thumb sides of your hands.
- Use the last three fingers to lift the mandible while maintaining head tilt.
- Blow a sufficient volume slowly into the opening of the mask to make the patient's chest rise.

- Remove your mouth, allowing exhalation to occur.
- Apply the oxygen source at a flow rate of 10 to 15 L/minute for 50% to 80% oxygen concentration as soon as possible.

What to consider

- If the mask isn't sealed tightly to the patient's face it can cause inadequate ventilation.
- A supplemental oxygen source is necessary as soon as possible to prevent hypoxemia.

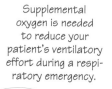

Supplemental oxygen is needed to reduce your patient's ventilatory effort during a respiratory emergency.

Oxygen administration devices

In a respiratory emergency, supplemental oxygen administration reduces the patient's ventilatory effort. In a cardiac emergency, oxygen therapy helps meet the increased myocardial workload as the heart tries to compensate for hypoxemia. It's particularly important for a patient with a compromised myocardium (as in myocardial infarction or arrhythmia). Oxygen administration devices include the nasal cannula, nonrebreather mask, simple face mask, and Venturi mask.

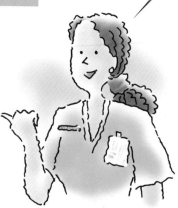

Nasal cannula

The nasal cannula is the most frequently used low-flow oxygen delivery system for a spontaneously breathing patient who doesn't need precise concentrations. It's comfortable, easy to use, and composed of flexible plastic tubing with two nasal prongs (about $5/8$" [1.5 cm] long) and an adjustable strap.

It isn't the heat, it's the humidity

The nasal cannula provides 24% to 44% humidified oxygen concentration with 1 to 6 L/minute flow rates for patients with minimal or no respiratory distress. Every 1 L/minute increase equals a 4% oxygen concentration increase.

What you need

- Nasal cannula
- Oxygen source

How it's done

Assess the patient for nasal airway patency. Then:
- Attach the cannula tubing to the humidified oxygen source.

- Set the flow rate to the desired flow.
- Check the flow by holding the cannula against your hand.
- Place the cannula tubing behind the patient's ears and under his chin.
- Slide the adjuster to secure the tubing in position.

What to consider

- The nasal cannula is contraindicated for patients with nasal obstructions.
- Variable oxygen concentration can occur because of the breathing pattern.
- Flow rates greater than 6 L/minute dry mucous membranes and require a humidity source; they may also cause headaches.
- The nasal cannula is easily dislodged.

Nonrebreather mask

The nonrebreather mask is a face mask with an oxygen reservoir. It provides oxygen concentrations (60% to 90%) to a spontaneously breathing patient with intact gag reflexes.

One-way street

On inhalation, the one-way inspiratory valve opens, directing oxygen from a reservoir bag into the mask. On exhalation, gas exits the mask through the one-way expiratory valves and enters the atmosphere. The patient breathes air only from the bag. (See *Components of a nonrebreather mask*, page 96.)

What you need

- Nonrebreather mask
- Oxygen source

How it's done

To prepare the mask:
- Attach the tubing to the oxygen source and adjust to the desired 12 to 15 L/minute oxygen flow rate.
- Choose a face mask size that fits from the bridge of the patient's nose to the tip of his chin.
- Inflate the reservoir bag by occluding the outlet to the mask.
    To attach the mask:
- Mold the metal nosepiece to conform to the bridge of the patient's nose.

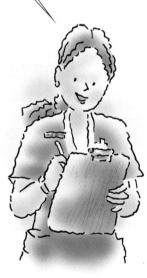

Use a nonrebreather mask for a spontaneously breathing patient with intact gag reflexes.

Components of a nonrebreather mask

This illustration shows the components of a nonrebreather mask.

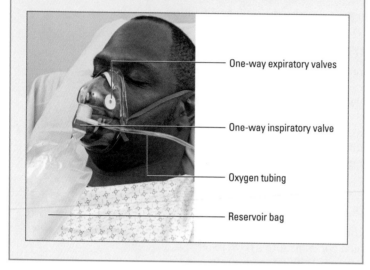

- One-way expiratory valves
- One-way inspiratory valve
- Oxygen tubing
- Reservoir bag

- Place the elastic strap over the patient's head and adjust the strap so that the mask fits comfortably and securely over his chin, cheeks, and nose to prevent the intake of room air, which will dilute oxygen concentration.
- Adjust the oxygen flow so the reservoir bag remains two-thirds inflated during inspiration and expiration, never completely collapsing.
- Don't allow the reservoir bag to kink.

What to consider

- Oxygen concentration varies depending on the manufacturer's design, patient's respiratory pattern, oxygen flow rate, proper fit of the mask, and removal of the one-way valve from side exhalation ports.
- An inhalation valve malfunction or kink in the bag may cause rebreathing of accumulated carbon dioxide.
- The nonrebreather mask can be uncomfortable and hot.
- The mask must be momentarily removed for the patient to eat, drink, or expectorate.
- Patients on nonrebreather masks are at increased risk for aspiration.

Simple face mask

The simple face mask, also called a *basic face mask*, is a low-flow system that allows oxygen to enter through a bottom port and exit through side holes. The face mask is capable of delivering 44% to 60% humidified oxygen concentrations to a patient with adequate spontaneous respiration for short periods. Air is exhaled through holes in the side of the mask.

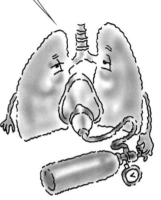

The simple, or basic, face mask allows oxygen to enter through a bottom port and exit through side holes.

Simply adjustable

The simple face mask comes in various standard sizes for adults and children with an adjustable strap to assist with proper fit.

What you need

- Simple face mask
- Oxygen source

How it's done

To prepare the mask:
- Attach the tubing to the oxygen source and adjust to the desired flow rate. (The ideal flow rate is 8 to 10 L/minute with a minimum of 5 L/minute.)
- Choose a face mask size that fits from the bridge of the patient's nose to the tip of his chin.
    To attach the mask:
- Mold the metal nosepiece to conform to the bridge of the patient's nose.
- Place the elastic strap over the patient's head and adjust the strap so that the mask fits comfortably and securely over his chin, cheeks, and nose to prevent the intake of room air, which dilutes oxygen concentration.
- Pad the mask with gauze to promote an airtight seal if the seal can't be secured because of facial contour.

What to consider

- A less desirable fit is possible because of generic, standard sizes, which can cause dilution of the oxygen concentration delivered.
- Air may enter and dilute the oxygen concentration delivered if the mask is improperly placed.
- Depending on the flow rate and the patient's respirations, delivered oxygen concentration may vary.
- The mask must be momentarily removed for the patient to eat, drink, or expectorate.
- Patients on simple face masks are at increased risk for aspiration.

Venturi mask

The Venturi mask is a face mask designed to mix room air with oxygen. It allows you to administer varying percentages of oxygen at a constant concentration of 24% to 50%, regardless of the patient's respiratory rate.

Magnificent mix

The Venturi mask increases the spontaneous breathing efficiency of patients with chronic lung disease without drying mucous membranes. A wide-bore flexible tube attaches between the adapters and the mask, allowing inhaled oxygen and room air to mix. The mask has a perforated cuff that allows exhaled air to flow into the atmosphere. Adapters can change the size of the orifice and oxygen flow. (See *Components of the Venturi mask.*)

What you need

- Venturi mask
- Color-coded adapter
- Oxygen source

> The Venturi mask delivers a mixture of room air and oxygen at varying percentages.

> Take a deep breath and join the oxygen movement

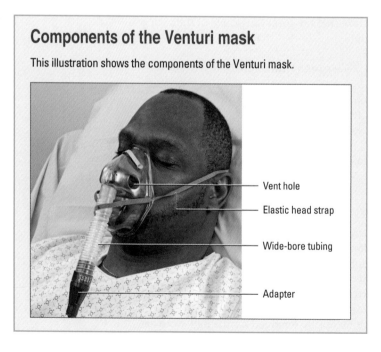

Components of the Venturi mask

This illustration shows the components of the Venturi mask.

- Vent hole
- Elastic head strap
- Wide-bore tubing
- Adapter

How it's done

To prepare the mask:
• Attach the appropriate color-coded adapter to the flexible tube, and then attach the oxygen source.
• Turn the oxygen flowmeter to the prescribed rate (indicated on adapter).
• Check that flow is occurring.
    To attach the mask, position the mask on the patient's face, adjusting the elastic strap as necessary.

What to consider

• Maintain a good seal for proper oxygen concentration delivery.
• If intake ports are obstructed, altered oxygen delivery concentration may occur.
• The mask must be momentarily removed for the patient to eat, drink, or expectorate.

Quick quiz

1.   Which is the preferred method for opening the airway of an unconscious patient who may have suffered a neck injury?
    A.   Head-tilt, chin-lift maneuver
    B.   Chin-lift maneuver
    C.   Jaw-thrust, chin-lift maneuver
    D.   Jaw-thrust maneuver

Answer: D. The jaw-thrust maneuver is the preferred method for opening an airway in an unconscious patient if a neck injury is suspected. However, if you're unable to open the airway using this method, use the head-tilt, chin-lift maneuver.

2.   After performing ET intubation, you auscultate the patient's chest. You find that breath sounds aren't audible. Based on this finding, you've most likely:
    A.   intubated the esophagus.
    B.   intubated the left mainstem bronchus.
    C.   intubated the right mainstem bronchus.
    D.   wedged the tube against the carina.

Answer: A. If breath sounds aren't audible after ET intubation, you've most likely intubated the patient's esophagus. Remove the tube and oxygenate the patient with 100% oxygen for 1 minute and then reattempt ET intubation.

3.   The preferred tidal volume when delivering ventilation with a bag-mask device is:
   A.   6 to 7 mL/kg.
   B.   7 to 10 mL/kg.
   C.   10 to 15 mL/kg.
   D.   15 to 20 mL/kg.

Answer: A. A tidal volume of 6 to 7 mL/kg with the bag-mask device adequately inflates the average person's lungs while minimizing gastric inflation.

4.   The most common cause of airway obstruction is:
   A.   food.
   B.   the patient's tongue.
   C.   small toys.
   D.   false teeth.

Answer: B. The tongue is the most common cause of airway obstruction. The tongue may slide into the airway as a person's neck muscles relax, causing an obstruction. When a person is unconscious, the tongue loses muscle tone and the muscles of the lower jaw relax, allowing the tongue to remain in an obstructed position.

5.   What is the most reliable method of both confirming and monitoring correct placement of an ET tube?
   A. CO_2 detector
   B.   Pulse oximeter
   C.   Continuous waveform capnography
   D.   Breath sounds

Answer: C. According to the AHA's guidelines, continuous waveform capnography is the most reliable method of confirming and monitoring the correct placement of an ET tube.

Scoring

☆☆☆   If you answered all five questions correctly, excellent! You managed to ace the test.

☆☆   If you answered four questions correctly, good work! You're managing quite well.

☆   If you answered fewer than four questions correctly, don't despair! Take a deep breath and review the chapter to manage a perfect score next time.

Electrical therapy

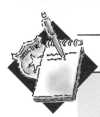

Just the facts

In this chapter, you'll learn:

♦ the procedure for defibrillation

♦ the procedure for cardioversion

♦ techniques for inserting pacemakers

♦ techniques for evaluating pacemaker function.

Defibrillation

Defibrillation is used to deliver a large amount of electric current to a patient over a brief period of time. It's the standard treatment for ventricular fibrillation (VF) and pulseless ventricular tachycardia (VT).

A defibrillation shock aims to temporarily depolarize the heart when the rhythm is chaotic. It does so by completely depolarizing the myocardium, producing a momentary asystole. This provides an opportunity for the heart's natural pacemaker centers to restore a normal rhythm.

CPR before and after is better

According to the 2010 American Heart Association (AHA) *Guidelines for Cardiopulmonary Resuscitation and Emergency Cardiovascular Care*, the foundation of successful advanced cardiac life support (ACLS) is high-quality cardiopulmonary resuscitation (CPR) and, for VF or pulseless VT, attempted defibrillation within moments of arrest. For monitored hospital patients, the time from VF to defibrillation should be less than 3 minutes and CPR should be performed while the defibrillator is readied. This is because effective chest compressions help deliver blood to the coronary arteries and brain.

Key points

Defibrillation
• Delivery of electric shocks to depolarize irregular heartbeat and allow coordinated conteractile activity to resume
• Treatment for ventricular fibrillation and unstable tachycardia
• Early defibrillation most effective

It's also important to perform CPR immediately after defibrillation because the patient may experience a period of asystole or pulseless electrical activity, which CPR may help convert to a perfusing rhythm. However, basic CPR can't convert VF to a normal rhythm. The only way to end VF and restore normal rhythm is electrical defibrillation.

A real need for speed

Defibrillation is significantly more effective when VF is recognized and treated quickly. When defibrillation is performed within the first 5 minutes of cardiac arrest, the survival rate is 50%. This survival rate decreases by 7% to 10% for each minute that the patient is in VF.

When performing defibrillation, you can use either an automated external defibrillator (AED) or a conventional defibrillator.

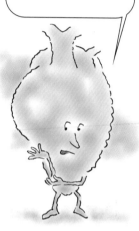

There's a 50% survival rate for patients when defibrillation is performed within the first 5 minutes of cardiac arrest.

Automated external defibrillators

The AED is a portable defibrillator with a microcomputer that senses and analyzes a patient's heart rhythm and then gives you step-by-step directions on how to proceed if defibrillation is indicated.

Form and function

All AED models have the same basic functions but offer different operating options. For example, all AEDs communicate directions by displaying messages on a screen, giving voice commands, or both. Some AEDs simultaneously display a patient's heart rhythm. All devices record your interactions with the patient during defibrillation and some may have an integral printer for immediate event documentation.

Two types of AEDs currently exist:
• the fully automated AED, which delivers a shock if VF is present
• the semiautomatic AED, which requires you to press an ANALYZE control to start the rhythm analysis; it then audibly or visually prompts you to press a SHOCK control to deliver a shock if warranted. (See *Understanding AEDs*.)

With either device, the electrical shock is delivered through two adhesive electrode pads applied to the patient (upper-right sternal border, lower-left ribs over the cardiac apex). The adhesive pads have two functions: to transmit the patient's rhythm and to deliver the shock.

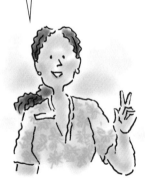

AED adhesive pads have two functions: to transmit the patient's rhythm and to deliver the shock.

Understanding AEDs

Automated external defibrillators (AEDs) vary with the manufacturer but the basic components for each device are similar. This illustration shows a typical AED and proper electrode placement.

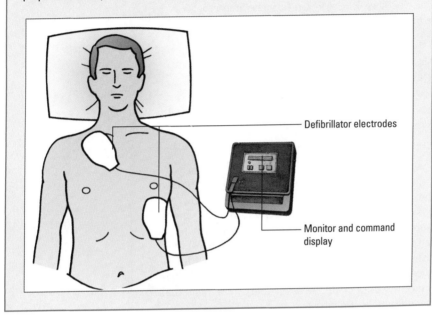

Defibrillator electrodes

Monitor and command display

How it's done

For a person who has collapsed and is unconscious, initiate CPR immediately and use an AED as soon as it's available. Perform five cycles (2 minutes) of CPR before checking the electrocardiogram (ECG) rhythm and attempting defibrillation.

To perform defibrillation with an AED:
- Open the packets containing the two electrode pads.
- Expose the patient's chest.
- Remove the plastic backing film from the electrode pads. Follow the manufacturer's instructions for pad placement and connection to the cable. (The correct pad placement is usually illustrated on the pads.)
- Press the ON button and wait while the machine performs a self-test. (Most AEDs signal their readiness by a computerized voice that says, "Stand clear" or by emitting a series of loud beeps. When that occurs, the machine is ready to analyze the patient's heart rhythm.)

Key points

Automated external defibrillators
- Contain cardiac rhythm analysis systems
- May be fully or semi-automated
- For patients with no pulse and no respirations
- Less training needed to operate
- Faster speed of operation and delivery
- Hands-free-technique
- Energy level = 200 to 360 joules

How AEDs sense rhythm

The accuracy of the automated external defibrillator (AED) in rhythm analysis is considered very high. A microprocessor analyzes features of the patient's electrocardiogram signal for frequency, amplitude, and integration of frequency and amplitude. A safety filter checks for false signals, such as those deriving from radio transmissions, poor electrode contact, 60-cycle interference, or loose electrodes.

Multiple analyses

In addition, the AED takes multiple looks—each lasting a few seconds—at the rhythm being analyzed. Several analyses must confirm the presence of a shockable rhythm, and other checks must be consistent with a nonperfusing cardiac status. The fully automated AED will then charge and deliver a shock; the semiautomatic AED will signal the operator that a shock is advised.

• Ask all personnel to stand clear, then press the ANALYZE button when the machine prompts; don't touch or move the patient while the AED is in analysis mode. Analysis takes 5 to 15 seconds, depending on the machine. (See *How AEDs sense rhythm.*)
• If a shock isn't needed, the AED will display or say "No shock indicated" and then prompt you to immediately resume CPR starting with chest compressions. If the patient needs a shock, the AED will announce a "stand clear" message and emit a beep that changes to a steady tone as it charges.
• When the AED is fully charged and ready to deliver a shock, it will prompt you to press the SHOCK button.
• Make sure no one is touching the patient or bed and call out "Stand clear." Then press the SHOCK button on the AED.
• After you deliver the first shock, immediately resume CPR, performing five cycles (about 2 minutes).

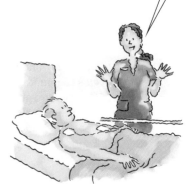

Don't touch the patient or the bed while the AED is analyzing the rhythm, charging its capacitors, or delivering a shock.

Data entry

• The AED should then analyze the rhythm and prompt you to deliver another shock if needed. When the patient is stable, remove the computer memory module or tape from the AED and transcribe it, or prompt the AED to print a rhythm strip with code data.

What to consider

• The patient can't be touched while the AED analyzes the rhythm, charges its capacitors, and delivers the shock.
• You must stop chest compressions and ventilations while the device is operating.

Safety tips for defibrillation

You must take precautions when defibrillating a patient with an implantable cardio-verter-defibrillator (ICD) or pacemaker or for a patient who's wearing a transdermal medication patch. You must also be careful when defibrillating a patient who's in contact with water.

Defibrillating a patient with an ICD or pacemaker
Avoid placing the defibrillator paddles or pads directly over the implanted device. Place them at least 1"(2.5 cm) away from the device.

Defibrillating a patient with a transdermal medication patch
Avoid placing electrodes directly on top of a transdermal medication patch, such as nitroglycerin, nicotine, analgesics, or hormone replacements. The patch can block delivery of energy and cause a small burn to the skin. Remove the medication patch and quickly wipe the area clean before defibrillation.

Defibrillating a patient near water
Water is a conductor of electricity and may provide a pathway for energy from the defibrillator to the rescuers treating the patient. Remove the patient from free-standing water and quickly dry his chest before defibrillation.

- You'll need to modify your actions for patients with implanted pacemakers, implantable cardioverter-defibrillators, transdermal medication patches, and for those being resuscitated around water. (See *Safety tips for defibrillation.*)

Conventional defibrillators

The conventional defibrillator is commonly used in most health care facilities. Unlike an AED, it requires you to analyze the rhythm, select the energy level to be administered, apply the paddles or "hands off" pads to the patient's chest, and discharge the current by pressing both paddle buttons simultaneously or by pressing the SHOCK button on the defibrillator.

Two types of conventional defibrillators exist: mono-phasic and biphasic. (See *Monophasic and biphasic defibrillators*, page 106.)

How it's done

For a quick look at the patient's cardiac rhythm, place the paddles on the patient's chest while you have someone place the defibrillator's monitoring leads and defibrillator pads on

> When using a conventional defibrillator, you'll need to analyze the patient's cardiac rhythm.

Monophasic and biphasic defibrillators

Two types of defibrillators are available: monophasic and biphasic.

Monophasic defibrillators

Monophasic defibrillators deliver a single current of electricity that travels in one direction between the two pads or paddles on the patient's chest. To be effective, a large amount of electrical current is required for monophasic defibrillation.

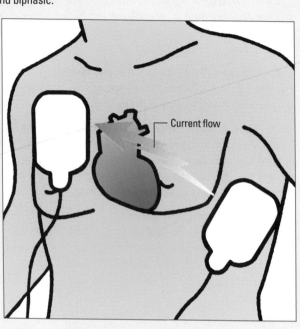

Biphasic defibrillators

For biphasic defibrillators, pad or paddle placement is the same; however, the discharged electrical current travels in a positive direction for a specified duration and then reverses and flows in a negative direction for the remaining time of the electrical discharge, thereby delivering two currents of electricity. Using two currents lowers the defibrillation threshold of the heart muscle, increasing the likelihood for successful defibrillation of ventricular fibrillation with smaller amounts of energy. Biphasic defibrillators also adjust for differences in impedance or resistance, which reduces the number of shocks needed. Most newer defibrillators are biphasic.

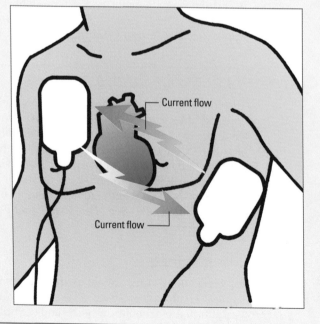

the patient. Assess the patient and the rhythm on the defibrillator monitor. If the patient is in VF or pulseless VT, defibrillation is appropriate.

Conventional wisdom

To perform defibrillation with a conventional defibrillator:
• Expose the patient's chest.
• Apply conductive material—gel to the paddles or conduction pads to the chest wall. You can also use remote defibrillation "hands-off" pads, which connect directly to the defibrillator.
– For anterolateral pad placement: Place one pad to the right of the upper sternum, just below the right clavicle, and the other over the fifth or sixth intercostal space at the left anterior axillary line.
– For anteroposterior pad placement: Place the anterior pad directly over the heart at the precordium to the left of the lower sternal border; place the posterior pad under the patient's body beneath the heart and immediately below the scapula.
• Turn on the defibrillator.
• Set the monophasic defibrillator energy level to 360 joules, or set the biphasic energy level, following manufacturer and facility recommendations, to 120 to 200 joules for an adult patient. If you don't know which type of defibrillator you're using, set the energy level to 200 joules.
• Place the paddles over the conductive pads and press firmly against the patient's chest using 25 lb of pressure. If you're using gel, place the paddles in the appropriate positions; if you're using the "hands off" pads, don't touch the paddles.
• Charge the defibrillator by pressing the CHARGE buttons, located either on the machine or on the paddles themselves. If you're using remote defibrillator pads, press the CHARGE button on the machine.
• When the machine is fully charged, instruct everyone to stand clear of the patient and the bed. Also, instruct someone to turn off any oxygen flow.
• Discharge the current by simultaneously pressing the CHARGE buttons on both paddles. If you're using remote defibrillator pads, press the DISCHARGE or SHOCK button on the machine.

After the first shock is delivered, immediately resume CPR, beginning with chest compressions, performing five cycles (about 2 minutes). Reassess the patient's cardiac rhythm on the monitor and, if necessary, prepare to defibrillate a second time if appropriate.

After successful defibrillation, you'll need to assess and monitor the patient's blood pressure, heart rhythm, and respiratory rate.

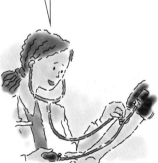

Restoration station

If defibrillation restores cardiac rhythm and return of spontaneous circulation:

• Check the patient's central and peripheral pulses.
• Obtain a blood pressure reading, treat hypotension, and monitor the patient's heart rhythm and respiratory rate.
• Assess the patient's level of consciousness (LOC), breath sounds, skin color, and urine output.
• Obtain baseline arterial blood gas levels and a 12-lead ECG.
• Treat hypoxemia and provide supplemental oxygen, ventilation, and medications, as needed.
• Be prepared to provide therapeutic hypothermia for comatose patients, if appropriate.
• Check the patient's chest for electrical burns and treat them, as ordered.
• Use a shift checklist to prepare the defibrillator for immediate reuse.

What to consider

• Be sure to familiarize yourself with your facility's equipment and policies for a quicker response in cardiac arrest situations.
• A defibrillator can be a dangerous piece of equipment because it delivers electricity to whatever it's in contact with. To avoid injury to others, be diligent in checking that no one is in contact with the patient or bed before discharging a shock.
• Check defibrillator equipment regularly to make sure that it's in working condition. Keep the defibrillator's battery charged by connecting it to alternating current.
• When delivering a shock using paddles, be sure to maintain full contact with the patient's skin, using firm pressure. If the paddles are lifted off the patient's chest while delivering a shock, a dangerous "arc" of electricity may occur, causing electrical injury. Also, make sure that everyone is clear before delivering the shock.

Cardioversion

Cardioversion (synchronized countershock) is used to treat tachyarrhythmias (such as atrial tachycardia, atrial flutter, atrial fibrillation, and symptomatic VT). It's performed as either an elective or emergency procedure and may be performed when the arrhythmia doesn't respond to drug therapy or vagal maneuvers such as carotid sinus massage. (See *Carotid sinus massage.*)

It's electric

Cardioversion delivers an electrical charge to the myocardium at the peak of the R wave, which causes immediate

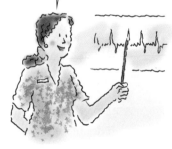

When performing cardioversion, it's important to synchronize the electrical charge with the R wave. Shocking the vulnerable T wave may disrupt repolarization.

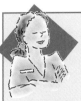

Peak technique

Carotid sinus massage

Carotid sinus massage is used to interrupt paroxysmal atrial tachycardia. Only expert practitioners trained and experienced in this procedure should perform carotid sinus massage. Massaging the carotid sinus stimulates the vagus nerve, which inhibits firing of the sinoatrial (SA) node and slows atrioventricular (AV) node conduction. As a result, the SA node can resume its function as primary pacemaker.

Place the patient in a supine position and turn his head to the left to massage the right carotid sinus (as shown). Firmly massage the patient's carotid sinus for no longer than 5 to 10 seconds. Don't perform carotid massage on both sides simultaneously because you may cause cardiac arrest.

Carotid sinus massage is contraindicated in patients with severe carotid stenosis. Risks of the procedure include decreased heart rate, syncope, sinus arrest, increased degree of AV block, cerebral emboli, stroke, and asystole.

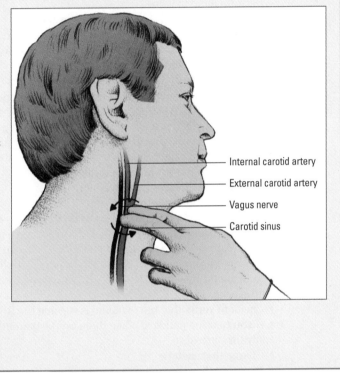

Internal carotid artery

External carotid artery

Vagus nerve

Carotid sinus

depolarization, interrupting reentry circuits and allowing the sino-atrial node to resume control. Synchronizing the electrical charge with the R wave ensures that the current won't be delivered on the vulnerable T wave and disrupt repolarization. This reduces the risk that the current will strike during the relative refractory period of the cardiac cycle and induce VF.

Elective cardioversion

Elective cardioversion is a scheduled procedure that delivers an electric shock to restore normal cardiac rhythm. It's the treatment of choice for arrhythmias that don't respond to drug therapy or vagal maneuvers.

How it's done

Before beginning elective cardioversion:
- Explain the procedure to the patient.
- Verify that the patient has a signed informed consent.
- Withhold food and fluids for 6 to 12 hours before the procedure.
- Perform hand hygiene.
- Obtain a 12-lead ECG to serve as a baseline.
- Connect the patient to a pulse oximeter and blood pressure cuff.
- Obtain I.V. access or check existing I.V. access for patency.
- Administer a sedative, as ordered.
- Place the leads on the patient's chest and assess cardiac rhythm to determine if cardioversion is still appropriate.
- Apply conductive material (gel to the paddles or conduction pads to the chest wall) or apply remote pads; position the pads so that one pad is to the right of the sternum, just below the clavicle, and the other is at the fifth or sixth intercostal space in the left anterior axillary line.

    To perform elective cardioversion:
- Turn on the defibrillator.
- Select the appropriate monophasic energy level—usually between 100 and 200 joules. Biphasic currents generally achieve cardioversion at a lower energy setting, usually 100 joules. (See *Correct amperage for monophasic cardioversion machines.*)
- Activate the synchronize mode by depressing the SYNCHRONIZE button.
- Check to verify that the machine is sensing the R wave correctly.
- If you're using paddles, place them on the patient's chest and apply firm pressure.
- Charge the machine.
- Instruct other personnel to stand clear of the patient and the bed to avoid the risk of an electric shock.
- Discharge the current by pushing the DISCHARGE buttons of both paddles simultaneously or pressing the SHOCK button on

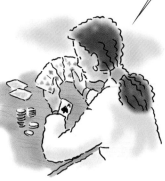

You've got to know when to hold 'em... When performing cardioversion, don't remove the paddles from the patient's chest until the device discharges.

Correct amperage for monophasic cardioversion machines

Use these amperage sequences for cardioversion with a monophasic machine:
- stable, monomorphic VT with a pulse—100, 200, 300, 360 joules
- unstable paroxysmal supraventricular tachycardia—50 to100 joules
- atrial fibrillation with a rapid ventricular response in an unstable patient—100 to 200 joules
- atrial flutter with a rapid ventricular response in an unstable patient—50 to 100 joules.

the machine; don't remove the paddles from the patient's chest until the device discharges. Unlike in defibrillation, the discharge won't occur immediately; you'll notice a slight delay while the defibrillator synchronizes with the R wave.

If at first you don't succeed...

If initial cardioversion is unsuccessful, repeat the procedure up to three more times, as ordered, gradually increasing the energy level with each additional countershock. If normal rhythm is restored, continue to monitor the patient. Obtain an ECG to document successful cardioversion. If the patient's cardiac rhythm changes to VF, switch from the synchronize mode to the defibrillate mode and defibrillate him immediately after charging the machine to the appropriate joules for VF.

What to consider

• Perform cardioversion with a practitioner present.
• Be sure to warn the patient when the shock will be delivered. Explain to him that you may need to deliver additional shocks to achieve cardioversion.
• If the patient's cardiac rhythm converts to polymorphic, unstable VT or VF, defibrillate him with an unsynchronized shock. Make sure that the SYNCHRONIZE button is off or a shock won't be delivered.

Emergency cardioversion

Emergency cardioversion is used to rapidly convert an abnormal cardiac rhythm combined with a deteriorating hemodynamic state to a normal rhythm. If a patient is symptomatic (chest pain, shortness of breath, decreased blood pressure, altered LOC), emergency cardioversion is necessary.

How it's done

Before beginning emergency cardioversion:
• Place cardiac monitor leads on the patient, if they aren't already in place.
• Explain the procedure to the patient, if possible.
• Connect the patient to a pulse oximeter and blood pressure cuff.
• Obtain I.V. access or check existing I.V. access for patency.
• Administer a sedative, if ordered.
• Apply conductive material (gel to the paddles or conduction pads to the chest wall) or apply remote pads; position the pads so that one pad is to the right of the sternum, just below the clavicle, and the other is at the fifth or sixth intercostal space in the left anterior axillary line.

To perform emergency cardioversion:
• Turn on the defibrillator.
• Select the appropriate monophasic energy level—usually between 100 and 200 joules. Biphasic currents generally achieve cardioversion at a lower energy setting, usually 50 to 100 joules.
• Activate the synchronize mode by depressing the SYNCHRONIZE button.
• Check to verify that the machine is sensing the R wave correctly.
• If you're using paddles, place them on the patient's chest and apply firm pressure.
• Charge the machine.
• Instruct other personnel to stand clear of the patient and the bed to avoid the risk of an electric shock.
• Discharge the current by pushing the DISCHARGE buttons of both paddles simultaneously or pressing the SHOCK button on the machine; don't remove the paddles from the patient's chest until the device discharges. Unlike in defibrillation, the discharge won't occur immediately; you'll notice a slight delay while the defibrillator synchronizes with the R wave.

What to consider

• Perform cardioversion with a practitioner present.
• Be sure to warn the patient when the shock will be delivered. Explain to him that you may need to deliver additional shocks to achieve cardioversion.
• If the patient's cardiac rhythm converts to pulseless VT or VF, defibrillate him using an unsynchronized shock. Make sure that the SYNCHRONIZE button is off or a shock won't be delivered.

Temporary pacemakers

The temporary pacemaker, which isn't implanted, is used in an emergency situation if the patient shows signs of decreased cardiac output, such as hypotension or syncope. It's often required for patients with symptomatic bradycardia that's unresponsive to drug therapy. A temporary pacemaker can also serve as a bridge until a permanent pacemaker is inserted.

Initially, a temporary pacemaker is used. Then, if the patient's condition doesn't improve, a permanent pacemaker may be inserted. Pacemakers should be used without delay for an unstable patient with type II second-degree atrioventricular (AV) block or third-degree AV block. They're also typically used for the following conditions:
• hemodynamically symptomatic bradycardia, especially if the patient doesn't respond to drug therapy

- significant bradycardia associated with poisoning or drug overdose
- paroxysmal supraventricular tachycardia.
   Pacemakers are contraindicated in patients with:
- severe hypothermia with a bradycardic rhythm. (Ventricles are more prone to fibrillation and more resistant to defibrillation as core temperature drops.)
- asystolic cardiac arrest because of a poor resuscitation rate.
Types of temporary pacemakers include transcutaneous and transvenous pacemakers.

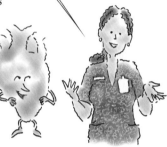

You really have to respect these transcutaneous temp workers. When it's crunch time, they're always available to come in and set the pace.

Transcutaneous pacemakers

The transcutaneous pacemaker, also known as *external pacing*, is the best choice for life-threatening situations when time is critical. It's a temporary noninvasive pacing method that uses the defibrillator to send electrical impulses to the patient's heart by way of electrodes placed on the front and back of the patient's thorax.

Setting the pace

A transcutaneous pacemaker is used until the patient's heart rhythm stabilizes or until a practitioner can institute transvenous pacing or insert a permanent pacemaker.

How it's done

Before transcutaneous pacing:
- If necessary, clip the patient's hair over the areas of electrode placement.
- Attach monitoring electrodes from the defibrillator to the patient in the lead I, II, or III position.
- Set the selector switch to the "Monitor On" position.
- An ECG waveform should be visible on the monitor.
- Adjust the R-wave beeper volume to a suitable level.
- Activate the ALARM ON button; set the alarm for 10 to 20 beats lower and 20 to 30 beats higher than the patient's target pacing rate.
- Press the START/STOP button for a printout of the waveform.
- Make sure the patient's skin is clean and dry to ensure good skin contact.
   To perform transcutaneous pacing:
- Pull the protective strip from the posterior pacing electrode pad marked "Back" and apply it to the left side of the patient's back, just below the scapula and to the left of the spine. (See *Proper pacing electrode pad placement*, page 114.)
- The anterior pacemaker pad marked "Front" has two protective strips. Remove the strip covering the jellied area and apply the pad to the patient's skin in the anterior position, to the left of the

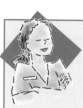

Peak technique

Proper pacing electrode pad placement

For transcutaneous pacing, place the two pacing electrode pads at heart level on the patient's chest and back, as shown. This placement ensures that the electrical stimulus need only travel a short distance to the heart.

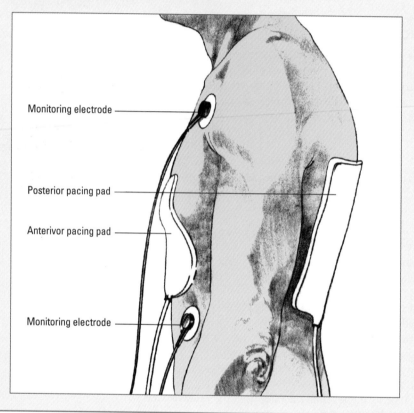

Monitoring electrode

Posterior pacing pad

Anterivor pacing pad

Monitoring electrode

After you've placed the pacing pack, the device is ready to pace the patient's heart.

precordium in the V_2 to V_5 position. Expose the pad's outer rim and firmly press it to the skin. The defibrillator can then begin to pace the heart.

• Make sure the OUTPUT dial is on 0 mA, and connect the pacing cable to the monitor output cable.

• Check the waveform, looking for a tall QRS complex in lead II.

• Turn the selector switch to "Pacer." If the patient is awake, tell him he may feel a twitching sensation and that you can give him medication if he can't tolerate the discomfort.

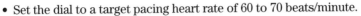

- Set the dial to a target pacing heart rate of 60 to 70 beats/minute.
- Look for pacer artifact or spikes, which will appear as you increase the rate.
- Slowly increase the amount of energy (mA) delivered to the heart by adjusting the OUTPUT dial. Do this until capture is achieved—you'll see a pacer spike followed by a widened QRS complex that resembles a premature ventricular contraction. This is the pacing threshold (the usual pacing threshold is between 40 and 80 mA). To ensure capture, increase output by 10%.
- When full capture is achieved, the patient's heart rate should be about the same as the pacemaker rate set on the machine.

What to consider

- Pacing can cause discanfort. Ensure adequate sedation and analgesia.
- The practitioner may order a transcutaneous pacemaker to be on "stand-by" when the patient has a bradycardic rhythm but doesn't have symptoms of hemodynamic instability.
- Attempt to correct underlying causes for the bradycardia.

Transvenous pacemakers

The transvenous pacemaker is more comfortable for the patient than a transcutaneous pacemaker; however, inserting it is an invasive procedure. It's the most commonly used type of temporary pacemaker.

Pulse power

With a transvenous pacemaker, an electrode catheter is threaded through a large vein into the patient's right atrium or right ventricle. The electrode is then attached to a pulse generator, which can provide an electrical stimulus directly to the endocardium. (See *Pulse generator features*, page 116.)

How it's done

- Attach a cardiac monitor to the patient and obtain a baseline assessment, including the patient's vital signs, oxygen saturation, skin color, LOC, and heart rate and rhythm.
- Ensure that the patient has a patent peripheral I.V. line.
- Put a new battery into the external pacemaker generator and test it to make sure it has a strong charge.
- Connect the bridging cable to the generator and align the positive and negative poles.
- Place the patient in a supine position and perform hand hygiene.

Pulse generator features

This illustration describes the features of a temporary pulse generator.

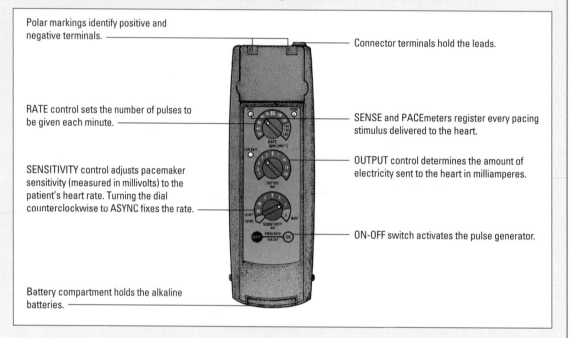

Polar markings identify positive and negative terminals.

Connector terminals hold the leads.

RATE control sets the number of pulses to be given each minute.

SENSE and PACEmeters register every pacing stimulus delivered to the heart.

SENSITIVITY control adjusts pacemaker sensitivity (measured in millivolts) to the patient's heart rate. Turning the dial counterclockwise to ASYNC fixes the rate.

OUTPUT control determines the amount of electricity sent to the heart in milliamperes.

ON-OFF switch activates the pulse generator.

Battery compartment holds the alkaline batteries.

• Put on a sterile gown and gloves and then open the supply tray (maintain a sterile field).
• Using an antibacterial solution, clean the insertion site and cover it with a sterile drape.
• The practitioner will puncture the brachial, femoral, subclavian, or jugular vein and insert the guide wire or introducer, advancing the electrode catheter.
• Watch the cardiac monitor as the catheter is advanced into the heart and treat arrhythmias appropriately.
• When the electrode catheter is in place, attach the catheter leads to the bridging cable, lining up the positive and negative poles.
• Check the battery's charge by pressing the BATTERY TEST button.
• Set the pacemaker, as ordered, adjusting the output and sensitivity until it fires at the preset rate and 100% capture

Your rhythm problems have been widely reported, yet you seem to be pacing yourself nicely now. What's the secret of your success?

Timing! My new pacemaker does the work, and I get the good reviews.

occurs. Each pacemaker spike should be followed by a wide QRS complex.

What to consider

• Monitor the patient's movement and positioning carefully so you don't dislodge the pacemaker wires.
• Monitor cardiac rhythm for pacemaker function.
• Prepare the patient for permanent pacemaker insertion, if appropriate.

Evaluating pacemaker function

As part of performing ACLS, you may need to evaluate a patient's temporary pacemaker. Follow these steps:
• Determine the pacemaker's settings.
• Review the patient's 12-lead ECG.
• Select a monitoring lead that clearly shows the pacemaker spikes.
• When you evaluate the ECG tracing, consider the pacemaker settings and whether symptoms of decreased cardiac output are present. Ask:
  – Is there capture?
  – Is there a P wave or QRS complex after each pacer spike?

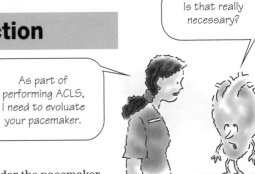

As part of performing ACLS, I need to evaluate your pacemaker.

Is that really necessary?

Pacemaker spikes

Pacemaker impulses (stimuli that travel from the pacemaker to the heart) are visible on the patient's electrocardiogram tracing as spikes. Whether large or small, the spikes appear above or below the isoelectric line. This example shows an atrial and a ventricular pacemaker spike.

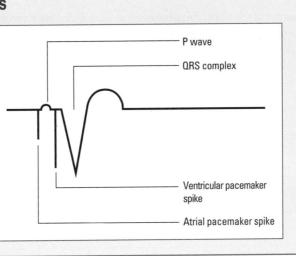

P wave

QRS complex

Ventricular pacemaker spike

Atrial pacemaker spike

– Do P waves and QRS complexes stem from intrinsic activity?

– If intrinsic activity is present, what's the pacemaker's response?

• Determine the rate by quickly counting the number of complexes in a 6-second ECG strip or, more accurately, by counting the number of small boxes between complexes and dividing by 1,500.

After you've evaluated the pacemaker, you can then determine if it's suffering from one of the four common pacemaker problems that can occur with a temporary pacemaker: failure to capture, failure to pace, failure to sense, or oversensing.

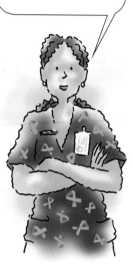

A pacemaker spike without a complex tells you that the pacemaker is failing to stimulate the chamber.

Failure to capture

Failure to capture appears on an ECG as a pacemaker spike without the appropriate atrial or ventricular response (a spike without a complex). Failure to capture indicates the pacemaker's inability to stimulate the chamber. (See *Failure to capture.*)

Causes of failure to capture include:
• acidosis
• electrolyte imbalance
• fibrosis
• incorrect lead position
• low mA setting

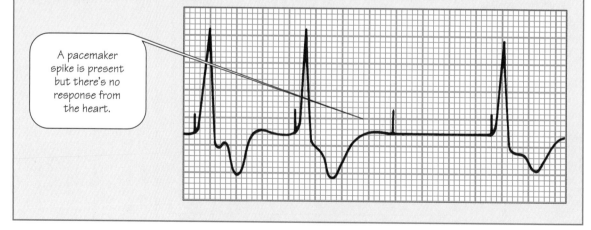

Failure to capture

This illustration shows failure to capture, in which the pacemaker spike is seen but there's no response from the heart.

A pacemaker spike is present but there's no response from the heart.

- battery depletion
- broken or cracked leadwire
- perforation of the leadwire through the myocardium.
    To treat failure to capture:
- Treat metabolic or electrolyte disturbances.
- Change the battery.
- Check all connections and gradually increase mA setting on a temporary pacemaker to see if capture occurs, according to your facility's protocol.
- Obtain a chest X-ray to determine lead placement.

Failure to pace

Failure to pace is seen as no pacemaker activity on an ECG. It can lead to asystole. (See *Failure to pace.*)
    Causes of failure to pace include:
- battery or circuit failure
- cracked or broken leads
    Failure to pace can lead to asystole. To treat failure to pace:
- If the pacing or indicator light of the pluse generator flashes, check the connections to the cable; obtain a chest X-ray to check the position of the pacing electrode for a transvenous pacer.

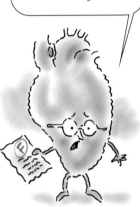

Uh oh! If a temporary pacemaker fails to pace, it could result in asystole.

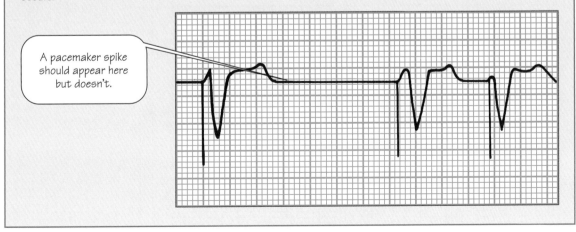

Failure to pace

This illustration shows failure to pace, in which the pacemaker spike isn't seen and no electrocardiogram complex occurs.

A pacemaker spike should appear here but doesn't.

• If the pulse generator is turned on but the indicators aren't flashing, change the battery.
• For a transcutaneous pacer, make sure the pacing pads are adhering adequately to the skin and are in the correct position.

Failure to sense intrinsic beats

Failure to sense, or *undersensing*, is indicated by a pacemaker spike that occurs abnormally when intrinsic cardiac activity is already present. When spikes fall on the T wave, it can result in VT or VF. (See *Failure to sense intrinsic beats*.)

Causes of failure to sense include:
• electrolyte imbalances
• disconnection of a lead
• improper lead placement
• increased sensing threshold from edema or fibrosis at the electrode tip
• drug interactions
• ineffective pacemaker battery.

To treat failure to sense:
• If the pacemaker is undersensing (it fires but at the wrong times or for the wrong reasons), adjust the SENSITIVITY setting, according to your facility's protocol.

Failure to sense intrinsic beats

This illustration shows failure to sense intrinsic beats, in which the pacemaker spike is seen firing at the wrong time or for the wrong reason.

Pacemaker fires anywhere in the cycle.

• Change the battery or pulse generator.
• Remove items in the room that may be causing electromechanical interference.
• Check to ensure that the equipment is grounded.
• If the pacemaker is firing on the T wave and all corrective actions have failed, turn it off. Be prepared to initiate ACLS protocol, depending on the resulting rhythm.

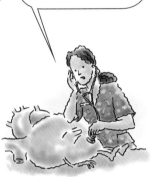

Don't be so sensitive. You might give your pacemaker the wrong idea.

Oversensing

If the pacemaker is too sensitive, it can misinterpret muscle movement or other events in the cardiac cycle as depolarization. It won't pace the patient when needed and his heart rate and AV synchrony won't be maintained.

Causes of oversensing include:
• pacemaker not programmed accurately
• improper lead placement
• disconnection of a lead.

To treat oversensing, adjust the sensitivity setting, according to your facility's protocol.

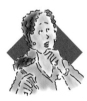

Quick quiz

1. The AED should be used in which situation?
    A. By paramedics, only in situations outside of the hospital
    B. For a patient who has collapsed, isn't breathing, and is unresponsive
    C. For a patient needing cardioversion
    D. After a precordial thump

Answer: B. The AHA recommends that an AED be attached to patients who have collapsed, aren't breathing, and are unresponsive.

2. Cardioversion is used to:
    A. deliver a shock on the T wave.
    B. treat atrial arrhythmias only.
    C. deliver an electrical charge to the myocardium at the peak of the R wave.
    D. generate higher initial energy levels than defibrillation.

Answer: C. Cardioversion delivers an electrical shock to the myocardium during the peak of the R wave.

3. A 68-year-old man is found by emergency rescuers in his home. He has no pulse and is apneic. The rhythm on the cardiac monitor is VF. What are the appropriate monophasic energy levels for the initial defibrillation shock to this patient?
   A.   100 joules
   B.   200 joules
   C.   300 joules
   D.   360 joules
Answer: D. The initial monophasic energy level for the initial defibrillation shock is 360 joules.

4. With a malfunctioning pacemaker, how does failure to capture appear on the ECG?
   A.   Spikes occur where they shouldn't
   B.   A spike without a complex after it
   C.   No pacemaker activity
   D.   Spikes on T waves
Answer: B. A spike occurring without a complex following it indicates that the pacemaker isn't capturing or stimulating the heart chamber.

5. With a malfunctioning pacemaker, how does failure to sense appear on the ECG?
   A.   Lack of a pacemaker spike
   B.   A pacemaker spike in the presence of intrinsic activity
   C.   A pacemaker spike with no cardiac stimulation
   D.   No pacemaker activity
Answer: B. Failure to sense is indicated by a pacemaker spike that occurs abnormally in the presence of intrinsic cardiac activity.

Scoring

★★★ If you answered all five questions correctly, super! Your knowledge is electrifying.

★★ If you answered four questions correctly, good for you! You're pacing yourself very well.

★ If you answered fewer than four questions correctly, don't worry! With just a little stimulus, you'll generate a perfect score next time.

Cardiovascular pharmacology

Just the facts

In this chapter, you'll learn:

♦ guidelines for administering emergency medications

♦ drugs commonly used in advanced cardiac life support (ACLS)

♦ drug indications and dosages

♦ the most common drug interactions encountered in ACLS practice

♦ antidotes for the most common drug overdoses.

Emergency medication administration

Emergency medications used during ACLS are given most frequently by I.V. push or I.V. infusion. If you can't obtain peripheral or central I.V. access, then you may give medications via the intraosseous (I.O.) route (bone marrow cavity is accessed) and some drugs via an endotracheal (ET) tube during cardiac arrest. Depending on the specific situation, you may also give medications subcutaneously, orally, or sublingually.

Here are some general pointers to remember when administering medication:

• Keep in mind that elderly patients usually require smaller dosages than do other adult patients.

• You may need to reduce the dosage for an adult patient with organ impairment (especially kidney or liver) because drug metabolism and excretion may be altered significantly.

• Remember that a patient may be taking over-the-counter (OTC) medications, illegal drugs, or herbal remedies or may be consuming food or beverages that interact with the medication.

- Be aware that a patient may have known or unknown drug allergies; any medication has the potential to cause an anaphylactic or hypersensitivity reaction.
- After you administer a medication, continually monitor the patient for the drug's effects, including adverse reactions. This includes continuous cardiac monitoring; assessing his vital signs before, during, and after giving the medication; and additional assessment indicated by the drug's use.

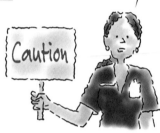

Remember to monitor patients for drug effects, including adverse reactions.

ACE inhibitors

Angiotensin-converting enzyme (ACE) inhibitors are used to reduce mortality and improve left ventricular function in patients with postacute myocardial infarction (MI). They prevent adverse left ventricular remodeling, delay the progression of heart failure, and decrease sudden death and recurrent MI.

Usually given within the first 24 hours after the onset of acute MI symptoms and after blood pressure has stabilized, ACE inhibitors are indicated for suspected MI and ST-segment elevation in two or more precordial leads, hypertension, and heart failure (without hypotension) in patients not responding to digoxin or diuretics. ACE inhibitors should also be used when clinical signs of acute MI with left ventricular dysfunction are present and left ventricular ejection fraction is less than 40%. (See *General precautions for ACE inhibitors.*)

ACE-ing hypertension

ACE inhibitors reduce blood pressure by interrupting the renin-angiotensin-aldosterone cycle. They specifically prevent the conversion of angiotensin I to angiotensin II, a potent vasoconstrictor. Reduced formation of angiotensin II decreases peripheral arterial resistance, thus decreasing aldosterone secretion, sodium and water retention, and blood pressure. ACE inhibitors also decrease systemic vascular resistance (afterload) and pulmonary artery wedge pressure (PAWP; preload), thus increasing cardiac output in patients with heart failure. (See *How ACE inhibitors work*, page 126.)

The ACE inhibitors given during ACLS include captopril, enalapril, lisinopril, and ramipril.

Captopril

Captopril (Capoten) is used to treat hypertension, heart failure, and acute MI. It prevents the conversion of angiotension I to angiotension II, decreasing systemic vascular resistance and

General precautions for ACE inhibitors

Observe these general precautions when you administer angiotensin-converting enzyme (ACE) inhibitors:
• Don't give to pregnant women because fetal injury or death may occur.
• Don't give to patients taking lithium because ACE inhibitors may increase lithium levels and cause toxicity.
• Use with caution in patients with renal impairment.
• Excessive hypotension may occur when used with diuretics or other antihypertensives.
• The risk of hypoglycemia is increased in patients with diabetes.
• The risk of hyperkalemia is increased in patients taking potassium-sparing diuretics.
• Potassium-containing salt substitutes may cause hyperkalemia in patients taking ACE inhibitors.

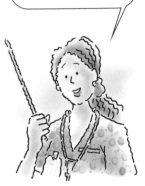

Before you administer a drug, it's important to know the precautions and contraindications.

increasing cardiac output. By reducing aldosterone secretion, captopril promotes sodium and water excretion, which reduces the amount of blood that the heart needs to pump, thus lowering blood pressure.

How to give it

For acute MI, the initial dosage of captopril is 6.25 mg orally in a single dose. Increase to 25 mg three times per day and then to 50 mg three times per day, as tolerated. Several weeks of therapy may be required before beneficial effects are seen.

What can happen

Adverse reactions to captopril include hypotension; tachycardia; angina; angioedema; persistent, dry nonproductive cough; hyperkalemia; leukopenia; and agranulocytosis.

What to consider

• Closely monitor blood pressure response to the drug.
• Monitor the patient's potassium intake and potassium level. Patients with diabetes, those with impaired renal function, and those receiving drugs that may increase the potassium level may develop hyperkalemia.
• Assess renal function before and periodically throughout therapy.
• Aspirin and other nonsteroidal anti-inflammatory drugs (NSAIDs) may decrease the antihypertensive effect of captopril.
• Captopril may increase serum digoxin and lithium levels, leading to toxicity.
• Captopril is contraindicated during pregnancy.

Now I get it!

How ACE inhibitors work

Angiotensin-converting enzyme (ACE) inhibitors reduce blood pressure by interrupting the renin-angiotensin-aldosterone system, which prevents the conversion of angiotensin I to angiotensin II.

The renin-angiotensin-aldosterone system pathway

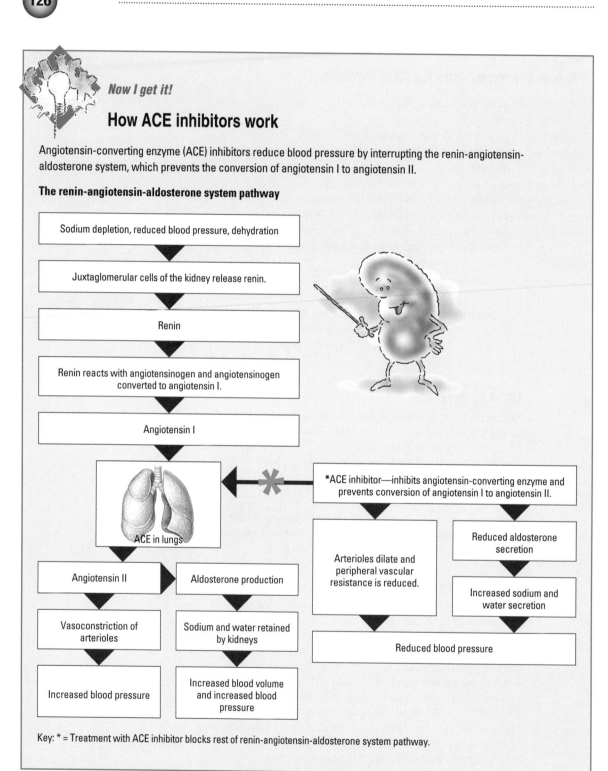

Sodium depletion, reduced blood pressure, dehydration

Juxtaglomerular cells of the kidney release renin.

Renin

Renin reacts with angiotensinogen and angiotensinogen converted to angiotensin I.

Angiotensin I

ACE in lungs

*ACE inhibitor—inhibits angiotensin-converting enzyme and prevents conversion of angiotensin I to angiotensin II.

Angiotensin II

Aldosterone production

Reduced aldosterone secretion

Arterioles dilate and peripheral vascular resistance is reduced.

Increased sodium and water secretion

Vasoconstriction of arterioles

Sodium and water retained by kidneys

Reduced blood pressure

Increased blood pressure

Increased blood volume and increased blood pressure

Key: * = Treatment with ACE inhibitor blocks rest of renin-angiotensin-aldosterone system pathway.

Enalapril

Enalapril (Vasotec) is used to treat hypertension and heart failure. Like captopril, it prevents the conversion of angiotension I to angiotension II, thus reducing blood pressure. You may also give the I.V. form of enalapril—enalaprilat (Vasotec I.V.).

How to give it

Here's how to administer enalapril:
- Orally—Give 2.5 mg as a single dose initially and then increase to 20 mg two times per day.
- I.V.—Give an initial 1.25 mg I.V. dose slowly over 5 minutes, and then 1.25 to 5 mg I.V. every 6 hours. Alternatively, you can dilute the drug in 50 mL of a compatible solution (such as dextrose 5% in water [D_5W], normal saline solution for injection, dextrose 5% in lactated Ringer's solution, dextrose 5% in normal saline solution for injection, or Isolyte E) and infuse it over 15 minutes.

What can happen

Adverse reactions to enalapril include hypotension; tachycardia; angina; angioedema; persistent, dry nonproductive cough; hyperkalemia; leukopenia; and agranulocytosis.

What to consider

- Closely monitor blood pressure response to the drug.
- Monitor the patient's potassium intake and potassium level. Patients with diabetes, those with impaired renal function, and those receiving drugs that may increase the potassium level may develop hyperkalemia.
- Assess renal function before and throughout therapy; monitor the patient for increased blood urea nitrogen (BUN) and creatinine levels.
- Aspirin and other NSAIDs may decrease the antihypertensive effect of enalapril.
- Enalapril is contraindicated during pregnancy and in patients with angioedema or bilateral renal artery stenosis.

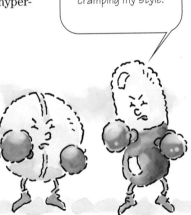

Hey, aspirin! You're really cramping my style.

Lisinopril

Lisinopril (Prinivil, Zestril) is used to treat hypertension and heart failure as well as to improve patient survival after acute MI. Like the other ACE inhibitors, it lowers blood pressure by preventing the conversion of angiotension I to angiotension II.

How to give it

Here's how to administer lisinopril:
- For heart failure—Give 5 mg orally once per day.
- For acute MI—Give 5 mg orally within the first 24 hours of symptom onset, 5 mg after 24 hours, and 10 mg once per day after 48 hours for 6 weeks.

What can happen

Adverse reactions to lisinopril include hypotension; tachycardia; angina; angioedema; persistent, dry nonproductive cough; hyperkalemia; and leukopenia.

What to consider

- Closely monitor blood pressure response to the drug.
- Monitor the patient's potassium intake and potassium level. Patients with diabetes, those with impaired renal function, and those receiving drugs that may increase the potassium level may develop hyperkalemia.
- Use lisinopril cautiously in patients with impaired renal function because hyperkalemia may occur. BUN and creatinine levels may increase.
- Aspirin and other NSAIDs may decrease the antihypertensive effect of lisinopril.
- Lisinopril is contraindicated during pregnancy and for patients with a history of angioedema.

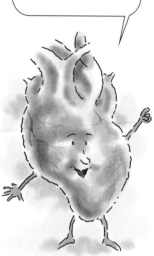

When administering lisinopril, carefully monitor your patient's blood pressure response.

Ramipril

Ramipril (Altace) is used to treat hypertension and heart failure. It prevents the conversion of angiotension I to angiotension II, thus reducing blood pressure.

How to give it

The initial dosage of ramipril is 2.5 mg orally in a single dose. Maintenance dosage is 2.5 to 20 mg daily depending on the indication.

What can happen

Adverse reactions to ramipril include hypotension; tachycardia; angina; angioedema; persistent, dry nonproductive cough; hyperkalemia; and leukopenia.

What to consider

- Closely monitor blood pressure response to the drug.

- Monitor the patient's potassium intake and potassium level. Patients with diabetes, those with impaired renal function, and those receiving drugs that may increase the potassium level may develop hyperkalemia.
- Assess renal function closely during the first few weeks of therapy, especially in patients with severe heart failure or hypertension. BUN and creatinine levels may rise.
- NSAIDs may decrease the antihypertensive effect of ramipril.
- Ramipril is contraindicated during pregnancy.

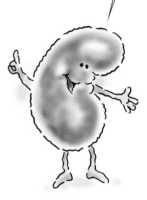

If you're administering ramipril, remember to keep an eye on me. C'mon, how could you miss me? I'm so cute!

Adrenergics

Adrenergic drugs are also called *sympathomimetic drugs* because they produce effects similar to those produced by the sympathetic nervous system (SNS). These drugs are typically used in ACLS as cardiac stimulants to restore heart rate, rhythm, and blood pressure while resuscitating the patient. Adrenergic drugs include dobutamine hydrochloride, dopamine hydrochloride, epinephrine, isoproterenol, and norepinephrine. Vasopressin, or antidiuretic hormone, is a posterior pituitary hormone that has adrenergic properties and is used as an alternative drug to epinephrine to treat adult shock-refractory ventricular fibrillation (VF).

Dobutamine hydrochloride

Dobutamine is used to increase cardiac output in patients experiencing cardiac decompensation with a systolic blood pressure of 70 to 100 mm Hg and no accompanying signs of shock.

Selective stimulator

Dobutamine selectively stimulates beta-1 adrenergic receptors to increase myocardial contractility and stroke volume. This results in increased cardiac output (a positive inotropic effect). Systolic blood pressure and pulse pressure may remain unchanged or may increase as a result of increased cardiac output.

At therapeutic doses, dobutamine decreases peripheral resistance (afterload), reduces ventricular filling pressure (preload), and may facilitate atrioventricular (AV) node conduction.

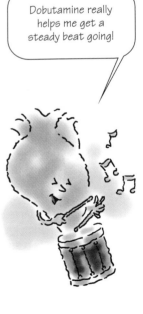

Dobutamine really helps me get a steady beat going!

How to give it

Give an I.V. infusion of 2 to 20 mcg/kg/minute; titrate so that the patient's heart rate isn't greater than 10% of baseline. Remember, you must use an infusion pump or other device to control the flow rate.

What can happen

Adverse reactions to dobutamine include tachycardia, fluctuations in blood pressure (hypertension, hypotension), bronchospasm, headache, and nausea.

What to consider

• Before giving dobutamine, use the appropriate plasma volume expanders to correct hypovolemia.
• Monitor the patient's heart rate and rhythm and blood pressure response to the drug; hemodynamic monitoring is recommended to monitor the drug's effect.
• Avoid administering dobutamine when systolic blood pressure is less than 100 mm Hg and signs of shock exist.
• Don't give dobutamine if poisoning or drug-induced shock is suspected.
• Don't give beta-adrenergic blockers with dobutamine because these drugs may cause increased peripheral resistance.
• Don't give tricyclic antidepressants with dobutamine because these drugs may potentiate pressor response and cause arrhythmias.
• Don't give in the same I.V. line with other drugs.
• Tissue necrosis and sloughing may occur if the I.V. medication leaks into surrounding tissue.

> **Key points**
>
> **Dobutamine hydrochloride**
> • Increases cardiac output
> • Indications: cardiac decompensation situation with systolic blood pressure of 70 to 100 mm Hg and no signs of shock
> • Continuous I.V. infusion: 2 to 20 mcg/kg/minute, titrated so that cardiac rate isn't greater than 10% of baseline

Dopamine hydrochloride

Although it's an adrenergic, dopamine is also classified as a vasopressor. Dopamine is used as a secondary drug (after atropine) for symptomatic bradycardia. It's also used to treat hypotension accompanied by signs and symptoms of shock.

Dopamine stimulates the dopaminergic, beta-adrenergic, and alpha-adrenergic receptors of the SNS. It has a direct stimulating effect on beta-1 receptors and little or no effect on beta-2 receptors.

Dose dependence

The effects of dopamine are dose-dependent. In I.V. doses of 0.5 to 5 mcg/kg/minute, it acts on dopaminergic receptors (dopaminergic response), causing vasodilation in the renal, mesenteric, coronary, and intracerebral vascular beds. Low to moderate doses (5 to 10 mcg/kg/minute) produce a beta effect, which results in cardiac stimulation. In I.V. doses greater than 10 mcg/kg/minute, it

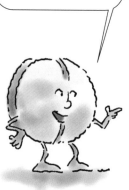

Dopamine stimulates beta-1 receptors and has little or no effect on beta-2 receptors.

stimulates alpha receptors, which results in increased peripheral resistance and renal vasoconstriction.

How to give it

Give an I.V. infusion of 2 to 20 mcg/kg/minute and titrate to the patient's response; taper the infusion slowly.

Livin' large

Remember to administer dopamine on an infusion pump into a large vein (central venous access is recommended) to prevent the possibility of extravasation. (Phentolamine 5 to 10 mg in 10 to 15 mL of normal saline solution is used to infiltrate the area to minimize tissue necrosis if extravasation occurs in a peripheral site. Infiltration must be done within 12 hours of extravasation.) Adjust the dosage to meet individual patient needs and to achieve the desired response. Reduce the dosage as soon as the patient's hemodynamic condition is stabilized.

> Administer dopamine into a large vein to help prevent extravasation.

What can happen

Adverse reactions to dopamine include bradycardia, tachycardia, ventricular arrhythmias, conduction disturbances, hypertension, anxiety, and dyspnea. Severe hypotension may result with abrupt withdrawal of dopamine; remember to taper the dosage gradually.

What to consider

- Before giving dopamine, use the appropriate plasma volume expanders to correct hypovolemia.
- Monitor the patient's heart rate and rhythm and blood pressure response to drug.
- Don't give dopamine to patients with uncorrected tachyarrhythmias, pheochromocytoma, or VF.
- Use caution when giving beta-adrenergic blockers with dopamine because these drugs may antagonize cardiac effects.
- Use caution when giving phenytoin (Dilantin) with dopamine because it may cause hypotension and bradycardia.
- Dopamine is incompatible with alkaline solutions (sodium bicarbonate).
- Tissue necrosis medication may occur if the I.V. medication leaks into surrounding tissue.

Key points

Dopamine hydrochloride
- Vasopressor and adrenergic
- Indications: symptomatic bradycardia, hypotension with signs and symptoms of shock
- Continuous I.V. infusion: low dose, 0.5 to 5 mcg/kg/minute; cardiac dose, 5 to 10 mcg/kg/minute; vasopressor dose, 10 to 20 mcg/kg/minute

Epinephrine

Epinephrine is a naturally occurring catecholamine used for its bronchodilator, vasopressor, and cardiac stimulant effects. It's used to treat cardiac arrest (VF, pulseless ventricular tachycardia [VT], asystole, and pulseless electrical activity [PEA]), symptomatic bradycardia (after atropine), severe hypotension, and severe allergic reactions (when combined with large fluid volumes, corticosteroids, or antihistamines).

Epinephrine acts directly by stimulating alpha- and beta-adrenergic receptors in the SNS. Its main therapeutic effects include relaxation of bronchial smooth muscle, cardiac stimulation, and the dilation of skeletal muscle vasculature.

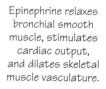

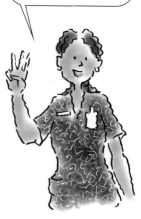

Epinephrine relaxes bronchial smooth muscle, stimulates cardiac output, and dilates skeletal muscle vasculature.

Relax...

Epinephrine relaxes bronchial smooth muscle by stimulating beta$_2$-adrenergic receptors and constricts bronchial arterioles by stimulating alpha-adrenergic receptors, resulting in relief of bronchospasm, reduced congestion and edema, and increased tidal volume and vital capacity. By inhibiting histamine release, it may reverse bronchiolar constriction, vasodilation, and edema.

...Stimulate

As a cardiac stimulant, epinephrine produces positive chronotropic and inotropic effects by acting on beta$_1$ receptors in the heart and increasing cardiac output, myocardial oxygen consumption, and the force of contraction.

How to give it

- Here's how to administer epinephrine:
- During resuscitation—Give 1 mg (10 mL of 1:10,000 solution) I.V. push or I.O. every 3 to 5 minutes; follow each dose with a 20-mL I.V. flush and elevate the arm for 10 to 20 seconds if administering via a peripheral I.V. line in the arm. Dosages of up to 0.2 mg/kg may be considered and used with caution.
- For continuous infusion—Add a 1-mg dose (1 mL of 1:1,000 solution) to 500 mL of normal saline solution or D$_5$W; use an initial I.V. infusion rate of 1 mcg/minute; increase to 2 to 10 mcg/minute.
- For profound bradycardia or hypotension—Add 1 mg of 1:1,000 solution to 500 mL of normal saline solution and infuse at a titrated dosage of 2 to 10 mcg/minute.

You can also give epinephrine via an ET tube with confirmed placement by administering 2 to 2.5 mg diluted in 10 mL of normal saline solution followed by several positive pressure ventilations.

You may give epinephrine via an ET tube if the tube's placement is confirmed.

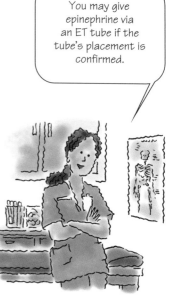

What can happen

Adverse reactions to epinephrine include anxiety, excitability, angina, cardiac arrhythmias, palpitations, hyperglycemia, hypertension, hypertensive crisis, and cerebral hemorrhage.

When epinephrine is given with antihistamines or tricyclic antidepressants, adverse cardiac effects may be potentiated; avoid concomitant use. When used with beta-adrenergic blockers, the cardiac and bronchodilating effects of epinephrine may be antagonized. Additionally, cardiac glycosides may sensitize the myocardium to the effects of epinephrine, causing arrhythmias.

What to consider

- Monitor the patient's heart rate and rhythm and blood pressure response to the drug. Increased heart rate and blood pressure may cause myocardial ischemia.
- Use with caution in patients with myocardial ischemia and hypoxia because epinephrine increases myocardial oxygen demand.
- Don't administer epinephrine with alpha-adrenergic blockers because its vasoconstriction and hypertensive effects may be counteracted.
- Dosage adjustments may be necessary if the patient is taking antidiabetics because the effect of epinephrine may be decreased.
- Monitor the patient's serum glucose levels because epinephrine may cause hyperglycemia.
- Higher doses of epinephrine (up to 0.2 mg/kg) may result in postresuscitation myocardial dysfunction.
- Epinephrine is incompatible with alkaline solutions (sodium bicarbonate).
- Tissue necrosis and sloughing may occur if the I.V. medication leaks into surrounding tissue.

Key points

Epinephrine
- Produces positive chronotropic and inotropic effects by action on $beta_1$-receptors in the heart
- Indications: cardiac arrest, symptomatic bradycardia, severe hypotension, severe allergic reaction
- Administer 1 mg (10 mL of 1:10,000 solution) I.V. every 3 to 5 minutes during resuscitation
- May be given via endotracheal tube: 2 to 2.5 mg in 10 mL normal saline solution

Isoproterenol

Isoproterenol (Isuprel) is used cautiously as a temporary measure for treating symptomatic bradycardia if atropine is ineffective and an external pacemaker isn't available. It's also used to treat torsades de pointes that doesn't respond to magnesium sulfate, for temporary control of bradycardia in heart transplant patients, and for counteracting beta-adrenergic blocker poisoning. Isoproterenol is contraindicated in cardiac arrest.

Quite an actor

Isoproterenol acts on $beta_1$ adrenergic receptors in the heart, producing a positive chronotropic and inotropic effect. It usually increases cardiac output. In patients with AV block, isoproterenol

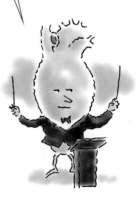

I hear isoproterenol shortens the heart's conduction time. Good thing! I could really use an intermission about now.

shortens conduction time and the refractory period of the AV node and increases the rate and strength of ventricular contraction.

How to give it

For continuous infusion, add a 1-mg dose to 250 mL of D_5W and give an I.V. infusion rate of 2 to 10 mcg/minute; titrate to an adequate heart rate. For torsades de pointes, titrate until the rhythm is suppressed. Always use an infusion pump.

    Because of the danger of arrhythmias, the infusion rate is usually decreased or temporarily stopped if the patient's heart rate exceeds 110 beats/minute. The order for the I.V. infusion rate should include specific guidelines for regulating the flow or terminating the infusion in relation to heart rate, premature beats, electrocardiogram (ECG) changes, myocardial ischemia, blood pressure, and urine output.

What can happen

Adverse reactions to isoproterenol include anxiety, excitability, angina, cardiac arrhythmias, palpitations, and hypertension.

What to consider

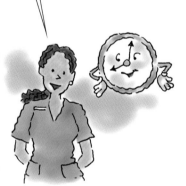

If you're using epinephrine or another adrenergic with isoproterenol, allow 4 hours between administration of the two drugs.

- Remember that isoproterenol doesn't replace the administration of blood, plasma, fluids, or electrolytes in patients with blood volume depletion.
- Monitor the patient's heart rate and rhythm and blood pressure response to the drug. Increased heart rate and blood pressure may cause myocardial ischemia.
- Don't give isoproterenol to patients with tachycardia caused by digoxin toxicity, preexisting arrhythmias (other than those that may respond to treatment with isoproterenol), and angina pectoris.
- Giving isoproterenol with epinephrine or another adrenergic may cause additive reactions and result in VT and VF; allow for at least 4 hours to elapse between administrating the two drugs.
- The patient is at increased risk for arrhythmias when isoproterenol is used with cardiac glycosides, potassium-depleting drugs, and other drugs that affect cardiac rhythm. Additionally, beta-adrenergic blockers antagonize the effects of isoproterenol.

Norepinephrine

Norepinephrine (Levophed) is used to treat severe cardiogenic shock and significant hypotension with low total peripheral resistance. It's the medication of last resort for the management of ischemic heart disease and shock but hasn't been proven to increase neurologically intact survival when compared to epinephrine in cardiac arrest.

Norepinephrine stimulates alpha- and beta-1 receptors within the SNS. It primarily produces vasoconstriction and cardiac stimulation.

How to give it

For continuous infusion, add a 4-mg dose to 250 mL of D_5W or dextrose 5% in normal saline solution titrated to the desired effect; 0.5 to 1 mcg/minute I.V. infusion rate is usually titrated to improve blood pressure. Maintenance dosage is 2 to 4 mcg/minute. You may need to give a higher dosage to achieve adequate perfusion in patients with poison-induced hypotension.

Centrally speaking

Remember to administer norepinephrine via a central venous catheter using an infusion pump to minimize the risk of extravasation. (Phentolamine 5 to 10 mg in 10 to 15 mL of normal saline solution is used to infiltrate the area to minimize tissue necrosis if extravasation occurs in a peripheral site; must be done within 12 hours of extravasation.)

What can happen

Adverse reactions to norepinephrine include anxiety, excitability, angina, cardiac arrhythmias, palpitations, hypertension, hypertensive crisis, and cerebral hemorrhage.

What to consider

- Administering norepinephrine isn't a substitute for blood or fluid replacement therapy. If the patient has a volume deficit, replace fluid before administering vasopressors.
- Monitor the patient's heart rate and rhythm and blood pressure response to the drug.
- Monitor the patient's extremities for color and temperature.
- Don't give alpha-adrenergic blockers with norepinephrine because these drugs may antagonize its effects.
- Severe hypotension may occur when norepinephrine is used with monoamine oxidase inhibitors, methyldopa, or tricyclic antidepressants.
- Norepinephrine is incompatible with alkaline solutions (sodium bicarbonate).
- Tissue necrosis and sloughing may occur if the I.V. medication leaks into surrounding tissue.

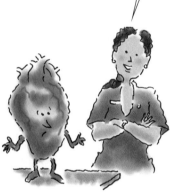

Don't worry, there's still hope. Norepinephrine is the drug of last resort for managing ischemic heart disease and shock.

> **Key points**
>
> **Norepinephrine**
> - Primarily produces vasoconstriction and cardiac stimulation
> - Indications: severe cardiogenic shock, significant hypotension, ischemic heart disease, and shock
> - Continuous infusion: 0.5 to 1 mcg/minute titrated to desired blood pressure (to maximum rate of 30 mcg/minute)

Vasopressin

Vasopressin (antidiuretic hormone) is a nonadrenergic peripheral vasoconstrictor that also causes coronary and renal vasoconstriction. It's used to treat adult shock-refractory VF as an alternative to epinephrine. It may be useful as an alternative to epinephrine for asystole or PEA. Vasopressin may also provide hemodynamic support in vasodilatory shock by maintaining coronary perfusion pressure. When given at high doses, vasopressin is a powerful vasoconstrictor of capillaries and small arterioles.

Totally tubular

Vasopressin acts at the renal tubular level to increase cyclic adenosine monophosphate (cAMP), which, in turn, increases water permeability at the renal tubule and collecting duct. This results in increased urine osmolality and a decreased urine flow rate.

How to give it

Give 40 units by I.V. push or I.O. to replace the first or second dose of epinephrine during cardiac arrest. Although vasopressin can be given endotracheally, the I.V. or I.O. route is preferred because the pharmacologic effects are more predictable. Because of the risk of necrosis and gangrene, remember to use extreme caution to avoid extravasation.

What can happen

Adverse reactions to vasopressin include cardiac ischemia, angina, bronchoconstriction, and water intoxication.

What to consider

• Monitor the patient's heart rate and rhythm and blood pressure response to the drug. Potent vasoconstrictor drug effects may cause myocardial ischemia.
• Assess for hypersensitivity reactions, including urticaria, angioedema, bronchoconstriction, and anaphylaxis.

> **Key points**
>
> **Vasopressin**
> • In the large dose used for advanced cardiac life support, vasopressin is a powerful vasoconstrictor
> • Indications: adult shock-refractory ventricular fibrillation, vasodilatory shock
> • Cardiac arrest: 40 units I.V. push or I.O. only once

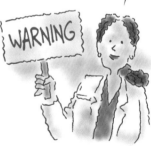

Vasopressin is a potent vasoconstrictor and may cause myocardial ischemia.

Analgesics

Morphine sulfate is the analgesic used in patients with ST-elevation myocardial infarction (STEMI) to help alleviate chest pain unrelieved by nitrates. It should be used with caution in patients with unstable angina and non-STEMI. It's also used to promote relaxation.

Morphine sulfate

The most commonly used analgesic in ACLS, morphine is an opi-oid agonist. It's a schedule II controlled substance indicated for chest pain that doesn't respond to nitrates. Morphine is also given to patients with acute pulmonary edema (if blood pressure is ade-quate) because it dilates peripheral blood vessels and decreases preload, thus reducing pulmonary congestion and relieving short-ness of breath.

The doors of perception

As an opium alkaloid, morphine is thought to work through opiate receptors, altering the patient's perception of pain. It also has a central depressant effect on respiration and the cough reflex center.

How to give it

Give 2 to 4 mg I.V. over 1 to 5 minutes; repeat every 5 to 30 min-utes and titrate to the desired effect. Rapid I.V. administration of morphine may result in overdose because of the delay in maxi-mum central nervous system (CNS) effect (30 minutes).

What can happen

Adverse reactions to morphine include respiratory depression, hypotension, bradycardia, shock, cardiac arrest, tachycar-dia, and hypertension. Apnea and respiratory arrest may also occur. Additionally, morphine may cause hypotension in volume-depleted patients. Correct hypovolemia before giving morphine.

What to consider

• Use morphine with caution in patients with a compromised respiratory state because it may compromise respirations.
• Don't give CNS depressants with morphine because these drugs may potentiate its respiratory, sedative, and hypotensive effects.
• If needed, reverse the effects of morphine with naloxone.

> **Key points**
>
> **Morphine sulfate**
> • Opioid agonist that alters the perception of pain
> • Indications: pain, acute pulmonary edema
> • 2 to 4 mg I.V. over 1 to 5 minutes; repeat every 5 to 30 minutes and titrate to effect

Administering morphine rapidly through an I.V. line may result in overdose.

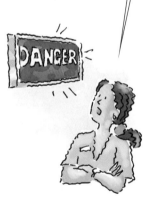

Antiarrhythmics

In general, antiarrhythmics are used to treat, suppress, or prevent three major mechanisms of arrhythmias: increased automaticity, decreased conductivity, and reentry. (See *Antiarrhythmic drugs and the action potential*, page 138.)

Now I get it!

Antiarrhythmic drugs and the action potential

Each class of antiarrhythmic drugs acts on a different phase of the action potential and alters the heart's electrophysiology. Here's a summary of the four classes of antiarrhythmics and how each class affects the action potential.

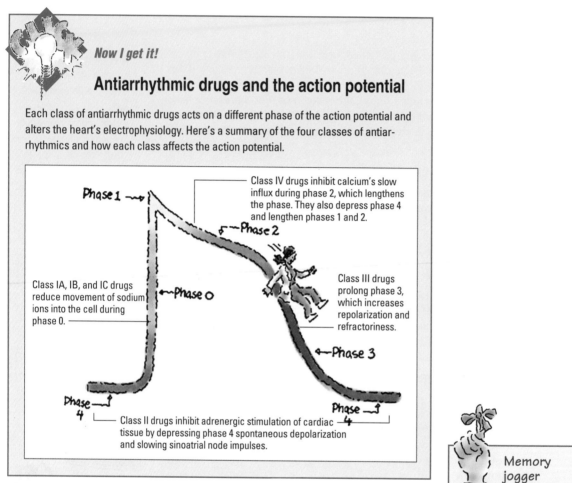

Class IV drugs inhibit calcium's slow influx during phase 2, which lengthens the phase. They also depress phase 4 and lengthen phases 1 and 2.

Class IA, IB, and IC drugs reduce movement of sodium ions into the cell during phase 0.

Class III drugs prolong phase 3, which increases repolarization and refractoriness.

Class II drugs inhibit adrenergic stimulation of cardiac tissue by depressing phase 4 spontaneous depolarization and slowing sinoatrial node impulses.

Class is in session

Four classes of antiarrhythmic drugs exist: I, II, III, and IV. Class I is further subdivided into class IA, IB, and IC. Class IA alters the myocardial cell membrane; class IB blocks the rapid influx of sodium ions; and class IC slows conduction. (See "Guide to common antiarrhythmic drugs," pages 327 to 328.) Several antiarrhythmic drugs aren't included in the four classes. These drugs include adenosine and atropine. Epinephrine and vasopressin are also considered antiarrhythmic drugs. For class II antiarrhythmics, see "Beta-adrenergic blockers," page 155. For class IV antiarrhythmics, see "Calcium channel blockers," page 161.

I.V. antiarrhythmics used during ACLS include adenosine, amiodarone hydrochloride, atropine sulfate, ibutilide fumarate, lidocaine, procainamide hydrochloride, and sotalol. Keep in mind

Memory jogger

To remember the main differences among class IA, class IB, and class IC antiarrhythmics, just think of their names:

Class IA: Alters the myocardial cell membrane

Class IB: Blocks the rapid influx of sodium ions

Class IC: Slows Conduction.

that antiarrhythmics may have a more powerful effect when used in combination.

Adenosine

Adenosine (Adenocard) is classified as a miscellaneous antiarrhythmic. A naturally occurring nucleoside, it's used to diagnose and treat paroxysmal supraventricular tachyarrhythmia (PSVT). Adenosine may also be considered for use with regular, monomorphic wide-complex tachycardia (with a pulse) as a diagnostic maneuver. It acts on the AV node to slow conduction and inhibit reentry pathways.

How to give it

Give 6 mg I.V. by rapid bolus injection (over 1 to 3 seconds), followed by a rapid flush with 20 mL of normal saline solution. If the arrhythmia isn't disrupted in 1 to 2 minutes, give 12 mg I.V. If necessary, you may give a third dose of 12 mg I.V. Remember, transient arrhythmias or asystole may occur after a rapid I.V. push.

What can happen

Adverse reactions to adenosine include hypotension, transient bradycardia, ventricular arrhythmias, flushing, chest pain, lightheadedness, nausea, and a metallic taste. However, because the half-life of adenosine is less than 10 seconds, adverse effects usually dissipate rapidly and are self-limiting.

What to consider

• Monitor the patient's heart rate and rhythm and blood pressure response to the drug.
• Don't give adenosine to patients with second- or third-degree heart block unless the patient has a pacemaker.
• Don't give to patients with asthma.
• Use adenosine cautiously with other medications:
  – with carbamazepine (Tegretol)—Higher degrees of heart block may occur with concurrent use
  – with dipyridamole—A smaller dosage may be needed because the drug may potentiate the effects of adenosine
  – with methylxanthines: These drugs antagonize the effects of adenosine.
• Caffeine may antagonize the effects of adenosine; a higher dosage may be needed or the patient may not respond at all.

Key points

Adenosine
• Acts on the atrioventricular node to slow conduction and inhibit reentry pathways
• Indications: first-line drug for paroxysmal supraventricular tachyarrhythmia
• 6 mg I.V. by rapid bolus injection (over 1 to 3 seconds)
• 12 mg I.V. if arrhythmia isn't eliminated in 1 to 2 minutes (a third dose of 12 mg I.V. may be given if necessary)
• Has a short half-life: Must be given as a very rapid I.V. push

Amiodarone hydrochloride

Amiodarone (Nexterone) is a ventricular and supraventricular antiarrhythmic used to treat recurrent VF, unstable VT, supraventricular arrhythmias, or rapid atrial fibrillation. It's recommended as the first-line drug for shock-refractory VF or pulseless VT.

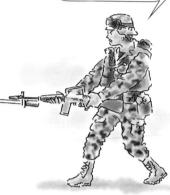

For shock-refractory VF or pulseless VT, amiodarone is the first line of defense.

Take a load off

Amiodarone has mixed class IC and III antiarrhythmic effects, but it's considered a class III drug. It increases the action potential duration (repolarization inhibition) and has alpha- and beta-adrenergic blocking properties. With prolonged therapy, amiodarone slows conduction through the AV node and prolongs the refractory period. Its vasodilating effect decreases cardiac workload and myocardial oxygen consumption. It also affects sodium, potassium, and calcium channels.

How to give it

Here's how to administer amiodarone:
• For cardiac arrest—Give 300 mg by I.V. push or I.O.; repeat with 150 mg I.V. push or I.O. in 3 to 5 minutes; dilute in 20 to 30 mL D_5W.
• For wide complex tachycardia (life-threatening ventricular arrhythmias)—Give a rapid I.V. infusion of 150 mg over the first 10 minutes (15 mg/minute) and repeat every 10 minutes as needed; follow with a slow infusion of 360 mg I.V. over 6 hours (1 mg/minute).
• Maintenance infusion—Give 540 mg I.V. over 18 hours (0.5 mg/minute).
• Maximum cumulative dose—Give 2.2 g I.V. over 24 hours.
  Remember that amiodarone I.V. infusions exceeding 2 hours must be administered in glass or polyolefin bottles containing D_5W.

What can happen

Adverse reactions to amiodarone include bradycardia, hypotension, heart failure, arrhythmias, heart block, or sinus arrest. Such adverse reactions are more prevalent with high doses but usually resolve within about 4 months after drug therapy stops. Additional adverse reactions include pulmonary fibrosis, hepatotoxicity, hyperthyroidism, photosensitivity and skin discoloration, and corneal microdeposits.

Key points

Amidarone hydrochloride
• First-line drug for shock refractory ventricular fibrillation (VF) or pulseless ventricular tachycardia (VT)
• Antiarrhythmic that increases the action potential duration
• Indications: recurrent VF, unstable VT, supraventricular arrhythmias, atrial fibrillation, angina, and hypertrophic cardiomyopathy
• For cardiac arrest give 300 mg I.V. push or I.O.; repeat with 150 mg I.V. push or I.O. in 3 to 5 minutes

(continued)

What to consider

- Watch the patient for hypersensitivity reactions to amiodarone.
- Monitor the patient's heart rate and rhythm and blood pressure response to the drug and monitor the ECG for QT prolongation.
- Don't give amiodarone to patients with severe sinoatrial (SA) node disease resulting in preexisting bradycardia, syncope caused by bradycardia or, unless a pacemaker is present, second- or third-degree AV block.
- When used with beta-adrenergic blockers or calcium channel blockers, amiodarone may cause sinus bradycardia, sinus arrest, and AV block; use together cautiously.
- Remember that amiodarone can't be removed by dialysis.
- The half-life of amiodarone is up to 40 days.

Atropine sulfate

Atropine is classified as a miscellaneous antiarrhythmic. It's used to treat symptomatic bradycardia and bradyarrhythmia (junctional or escape rhythm). It's no longer recommended to treat asystole or bradycardic PEA.

Rate increase

Atropine is an anticholinergic (parasympatholytic) that blocks the effects of acetylcholine on the SA and AV nodes, thereby increasing SA and AV node conduction velocity. It also increases the sinus node discharge rate and decreases the effective refractory period of the AV node. The result is increased heart rate. (See *How atropine speeds the heart rate*, page 142.)

How to give it

Here's how to administer atropine:
- To treat bradycardia—Give 0.5 mg I.V. every 3 to 5 minutes as needed, not to exceed a total dose of 3 mg. Shorter dosing interval of 3 minutes and a higher dose may be used in severe clinical condition.

Remember that effects on the patient's heart rate peak within 2 to 4 minutes after I.V. administration.

What can happen

Tachycardia may occur after higher doses of atropine. Signs of atropine overdose reflect excessive cardiovascular and CNS stimulation; treat with physostigmine (Antilirium).

Key points

Amidarone hydrochloride (continued)

- For wide complex tachycardia (stable): give rapid infusion of 150 mg I.V. over first 10 minutes (15 mg/minute) and repeat every 10 minutes as needed; slow infusion of 360 mg I.V. over 6 hours (1 mg/minute) may be given
- Maintenance infusion is 540 mg I.V. over 18 hours (0.5 mg/minute)
- Maximum cumulative dose is 2.2 g I.V. per 24 hours
- Drug half-life is up to 40 days

Atropine is great for increasing my rate!

Now I get it!

How atropine speeds the heart rate

When acetylcholine is released, the vagus nerve stimulates the sinoatrial (SA) and atrioventricular (AV) nodes, which inhibits electrical conduction. This slows the heart rate. The cholinergic blocker atropine competes with acetylcholine for binding with cholinergic receptors on SA and AV nodal cells. By blocking the effects of acetylcholine, atropine speeds the heart rate.

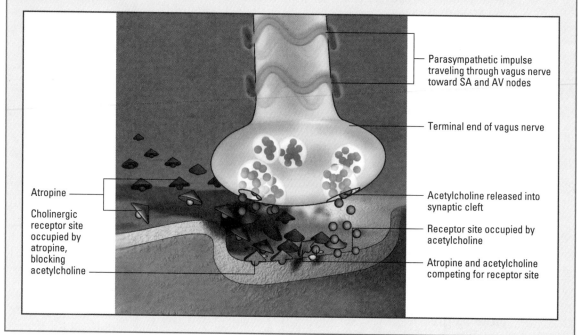

Parasympathetic impulse traveling through vagus nerve toward SA and AV nodes

Terminal end of vagus nerve

Atropine

Cholinergic receptor site occupied by atropine, blocking acetylcholine

Acetylcholine released into synaptic cleft

Receptor site occupied by acetylcholine

Atropine and acetylcholine competing for receptor site

What to consider

- Transplanted hearts lack vagal nerve innervation so atropine won't be effective.
- Monitor the patient's heart rate and rhythm with drug administration.
- Avoid using atropine for hypothermic bradycardia.
- I.V. administration of less than 0.5 mg may cause paradoxical slowing of the heart rate.
- Use atropine with caution in patients with myocardial ischemia and hypoxia because it increases myocardial oxygen demand.

Key points

Atropine sulfate
- Blocks the effects of acetylcholine on the sinoatrial (SA) and atrioventricular (AV) nodes, thereby increasing SA and AV node conduction velocity

(continued)

• Don't give atropine with other anticholinergics or with drugs that have anticholinergic effects.
• Atropine is ineffective for infranodal (type II) AV block and new third-degree AV block with wide QRS complexes because paradoxical slowing may occur.

Ibutilide fumarate

Ibutilide (Corvert) is used for supraventricular arrhythmias. It's most effective for the conversion of new-onset atrial fibrillation or atrial flutter. Ibutilide prolongs the action potential in isolated cardiac myocytes and increases atrial and ventricular refractoriness, namely class III electrophysiologic effects.

How to give it

Here's how to administer ibutilide:
• For adults weighing 132 lb (60 kg) or more—Give a 1 mg I.V. infusion over 10 minutes, diluted or undiluted; a second dose may be repeated after 10 minutes.
• For adults weighing less than 132 lb—Give a 0.01-mg/kg I.V. infusion over 10 minutes; a second dose may be given after 10 minutes.

What can happen

Adverse reactions to ibutilide include AV block, bradycardia, bundle-branch block, hypotension, monomorphic and polymorphic VT, palpitations, prolonged QT interval, and ventricular extrasystoles. Polymorphic VT, including torsades de pointes, develops in 2% to 5% of patients after ibutilide is administered. Additionally, ibutilide may worsen ventricular arrhythmias.

What to consider

• Monitor the patient's ECG continuously during drug administration and for at least 4 hours afterward or until QT interval returns to baseline.
• Make sure that a cardiac monitor, defibrillator, and emergency medication to treat sustained VT or VF are available.
• Don't give class IA and class III antiarrhythmics within 4 hours of administering the ibutilide infusion because they can cause prolonged refractoriness.
• Don't give drugs that prolong the QT interval, phenothiazines, tricyclic and tetracyclic antidepressants, or certain

Always monitor the patient's ECG continuously while giving ibutilide and for at least 4 hours after the drug is administered.

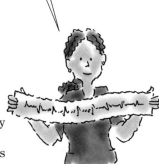

antihistamines, such as H1-receptor antagonists, with ibutilide because they may cause arrhythmias.
• Patients with atrial fibrillation that lasts more than 2 to 3 days must be adequately anticoagulated, generally for at least 2 weeks, before ibutilide is administered.

Lidocaine

Lidocaine is a ventricular antiarrhythmic used for cardiac arrest caused by VF or VT, stable VT, wide-complex tachycardia of an uncertain type, or wide-complex PSVT if amiodarone is unavailable. It seems to act preferentially on diseased or ischemic myocardial tissue.

Super suppressant

As a class IB antiarrhythmic, lidocaine suppresses automaticity and shortens the effective refractory period and action potential duration of the His-Purkinje fibers. It also suppresses spontaneous ventricular depolarization during diastole. By exerting its effects on the conduction system, it inhibits reentry mechanisms and halts ventricular arrhythmias.

How to give it

Here's how to administer lidocaine:
• For cardiac arrest—Give a 1 to 1.5 mg/kg I.V. push or I.O. dose initially; in refractory VF, you may give an additional 0.5 to 0.75 mg/kg by I.V. push or I.O. and repeat in 5 to 10 minutes. The maximum total dosage is 3 mg/kg. A single dose of 1.5 mg/kg by I.V. push may suffice as treatment in cardiac arrest.
• For perfusing arrhythmia with stable VT, wide-complex tachycardia of uncertain type, or significant ectopy—Give 0.5 to 0.75 mg/kg up to 1.5 mg/kg by I.V. push; repeat 0.5 to 0.75 mg/kg every 5 to 10 minutes. The maximum total dosage is 3 mg/kg.
• Maintenance infusion—Give 1 to 4 mg/minute I.V. (20 to 50 mcg/kg/minute).
    Remember to use an infusion pump to precisely monitor the lidocaine infusion. Never exceed the infusion rate of 4 mg/minute. A faster rate greatly increases the risk of toxicity.

What can happen

Adverse reactions to lidocaine include hypotension, bradycardia, AV block, confusion, dizziness, restlessness, paresthesia, tinnitus, and agitation. Effects of lidocaine overdose include signs and symptoms of CNS toxicity, such as seizures or respiratory depression, and cardiovascular toxicity resulting in cardiovascular collapse and cardiac arrest.

What to consider

- Monitor the patient's heart rate and rhythm.
- Watch the patient for signs of excessive cardiac conductivity depression (such as sinus node dysfunction, PR-interval prolongation, QRS-interval widening, and appearance or exacerbation of arrhythmias). If they occur, reduce the dosage or stop the drug.
- Don't give lidocaine to patients with hypersensitivity to amide-type local anesthetics, Stokes-Adams syndrome, Wolff-Parkinson-White (WPW) syndrome, and severe degrees of SA, AV, or intraventricular block in the absence of a pacemaker.
- Use caution when giving lidocaine with beta-adrenergic blockers or cimetidine because these drugs may cause lidocaine toxicity from reduced hepatic clearance. Other antiarrhythmics (such as phenytoin, procainamide, propranolol, and quinidine) may also cause additive or antagonist effects and additive toxicity when given with lidocaine.

> If you notice signs of excessive cardiac conductivity depression when administering lidocaine, reduce the dosage or stop giving the drug altogether.

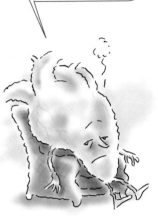

Procainamide hydrochloride

Procainamide is a ventricular and supraventricular antiarrhythmic. It's used for several arrhythmias, including PSVT, stable wide-complex tachycardias, and atrial fibrillation with a rapid ventricular rate in WPW syndrome. Procainamide is also recommended for VF or pulseless VT that recurs after periods of non-VF rhythms during cardiac arrest. In all instances, procainamide must be given as a slow I.V. infusion.

Depress...

As a class IA antiarrhythmic, procainamide depresses the upstroke velocity of the action potential (phase 0 of the depolarization cycle). It's considered a myocardial depressant because it decreases myocardial excitability and conduction velocity and may depress myocardial contractility. Procainamide also acts as an anticholinergic, which may modify direct myocardial effects. In therapeutic doses, the drug reduces conduction velocity in the atria, ventricles, and His-Purkinje system.

Key points

Procainamide hydrochloride
- The need for slow I.V. influsion minimizes the drug's usefulness in advanced cardiac life support situations
- Depresses phase 0 of the action potential: decreases myocardial excitability and conduction velocity and may depress myocardial contractility; also possesses anticholinergic activity that may modify direct myocardial effects

(continued)

...Prolong...

Procainamide also prolongs the PR and QT intervals. It controls atrial tachyarrhythmias by prolonging the effective refractory period and increasing the action potential duration in the atria, ventricles, and His-Purkinje system; the tissue remains refractory even after returning to resting membrane potential.

...Shorten

Procainamide shortens the effective refractory period of the AV node. The drug's anticholinergic action may also increase AV node conductivity. Suppression of automaticity in the His-Purkinje system and ectopic pacemakers accounts for the effectiveness of procainamide in treating ventricular premature beats.

How to give it

Give a slow I.V. infusion at 20 mg/minute with a maximum total dosage of 17 mg/kg for cardiac arrest and arrhythmia suppression or a total dose of 12 mg/kg with renal or cardiac dysfunction. Give 1 to 4 mg/minute as a maintenance infusion. Remember to use an infusion pump to precisely monitor the infusion. If the patient has cardiac or renal dysfunction, reduce the maintenance infusion to 1 to 2 mg/minute.

What can happen

Adverse reactions to procainamide include dizziness, heart block, hypotension, liver failure, agranulocytosis, and lupus erythematosus-like syndrome. Drug toxicity may cause severe hypotension, widening QRS complex, junctional tachycardia, intraventricular conduction delay, VF, oliguria, and confusion.

What to consider

• Monitor the patient's heart rate and rhythm and blood pressure response to the drug.
• Watch the patient for prolonged QT and QRS intervals (50% or greater widening), heart block, or increased arrhythmias. If these appear, stop the drug and monitor the patient closely.
• Don't give procainamide to patients with hypersensitivity to procaine and related drugs, second-, or third-degree AV block in the absence of a pacemaker, myasthenia gravis, systemic lupus erythematosus, or torsades de pointes.
• Use caution when giving procainamide with antihypertensives because these drugs may cause additive hypotensive effects. Other antiarrhythmics may cause additive or antagonistic cardiac effects and possible additive toxic effects.

Key points

Procainamide hydrochloride (continued)
• Indications: wide variety of arrhythmias
• For cardiac arrest and arrhythmia suppression: 20 mg/minute I.V. infusion with a maximum total dose of 17 mg/kg; doses of up to 50 mg/minute I.V. may be used
• Maintenance infusion: 1 to 4 mg/minute

Always give procainamide as a slow I.V. infusion.

Sotalol

Sotalol (Betapace) is a beta-adrenergic blocker used as an antiarrhythmic. It's used for documented, life-threatening ventricular arrhythmias and supraventricular arrhythmias in patients without structural heart disease.

Sotalol depresses the sinus heart rate and slows AV conduction. It increases AV nodal refractoriness and prolongs the refractory period of atrial and ventricular muscle and AV accessory pathways in anterograde and retrograde directions. It also decreases cardiac output and lowers systolic and diastolic blood pressure.

How to give it

Be sure to follow your facility's protocol. For life-threatening ventricular arrhythmias, clinical studies support giving 1.5 mg/kg I.V. over 5 minutes. This can be followed with 75 mg I.V. over 5 hours twice daily, and titrated after 3 days up to 150 mg I.V. twice daily.

What can happen

Adverse reactions to sotalol include bradycardia, chest pain, dizziness, palpitations, and QT prolongation.

What to consider

- Monitor the patient's heart rate and rhythm.
- Watch the patient for QT interval prolongation and observe him carefully until QT intervals are normal. If the QT interval is 500 msec or greater, reduce dosage, reduce rate of infusion, or discontinue drug.
- Don't give sotalol to patients with poor perfusion because of its significant negative inotropic effects. It's also contraindicated in patients with severe sinus node dysfunction, sinus bradycardia, second- and third-degree AV block in the absence of a pacemaker, congenital or acquired long QT syndrome, cardiogenic shock, uncontrolled heart failure, or bronchial asthma.
- Use caution when giving sotalol with calcium channel antagonists because of the risk of enhanced myocardial depression. Additionally, use sotalol cautiously with drugs that prolong the QT interval (procainamide, phenothiazines, tricyclic antidepressants).
- Sotalol may cause increased blood glucose levels and mask symptoms of hypoglycemia in patients with diabetes.
- Adjust dosing interval based on creatinine clearance.

Key points

Sotalol
- Depresses sinus heart rate, slows atrioventricular (AV) conduction, increases AV nodal refractoriness, and prolongs the refractory period of atrial and ventricular muscle and AV accessory pathways in anterograde and retrograde directions
- Indications: life-threatening ventricular arrhythmias
- 1 to 1.5 mg/kg, then infuse at a rate of 10 mg/minute (I.V. administration not approved for use in the United States)

Anticoagulants

Unfractionated heparin (UFH) and its derivatives (low-molecular-weight heparin [LMWH]) are anticoagulant drugs used in cardiac patients to prevent clot formation. These drugs are used as adjuvant therapy with fibrinolytic agents and in combination with aspirin to treat patients with acute coronary syndrome (ACS).

Heparin and heparin derivatives

UFH is prepared commercially from animal tissue. Because heparin doesn't affect clotting factor synthesis, it can't dissolve clots that have already formed. LMWH, such as enoxaparin (Lovenox), is derived by decomposing UFH into simpler compounds.

Clots need not apply

Heparin potentiates the effects of antithrombin, which inhibits the conversion of fibrinogen to fibrin. It also inhibits the action of factors IX, X, XI, and XII. Heparin inactivates the fibrin-stabilizing factor, preventing the formation of a stable fibrin clot.

How to give it

Here's how to administer UFH:
* For ST-segment elevation MI—Give an initial I.V. bolus of 60 units/kg; then 12 units/kg/hour by I.V. infusion.
* For non-ST-segment elevation MI—Give an initial I.V. bolus of 60 to 70 units/kg; then 12 units/kg/hour by I.V. infusion.

Remember to follow your facility's policy for heparin protocol. Adjust the dosage to maintain the partial thromboplastin time (PTT) $1\frac{1}{2}$ to 2 times the control values for 48 hours or until angiography; for activated coagulation time, use 2 to 3 times the control. (The target range for PTT after the first 24 hours is between 50 and 70 seconds but may vary by laboratory.)

To reverse heparin, give 1% solution of protamine sulfate by slow infusion. Remember, hemodialysis doesn't remove heparin.

Here's how to administer LMWH:
* For ST-segment elevation MI as an adjuvant therapy with fibrinolytics—Give enoxaparin 30 mg by I.V. bolus and then 1 mg/kg subcutaneously every 12 hours.
* For non-ST-segment elevation MI—Give enoxaparin 1 mg/kg subcutaneously every 12 hours; the first dose may be preceded by a 30-mg I.V. bolus.

Key points

Herparin
* Potentiates the effects of antithrombin, which inhibits conversion of fibrinogen to fibrin
* Also inhibits the action of factors IX, X, XI, and XII; inactivates fibrin-stablizing factor and prevents formation of a stable fibrin clot
* Indications: adjuvant therapy in acute myocardial infarction and fibrnolytic therapy
* For ST-segment elevation MI: Initial bolus of 60 units/kg, then 12 units/kg/hour I.V. infusion
* Adjust dosage to maintain partial thromboplastin time $1\frac{1}{2}$ to 2 times the control values for 48 hours or until angiography
* For non-ST-segment elevation MI: Initial bolus dose of 60 units/kg; then 12 units/kg/hour I.V. infusion

Remember to adjust the dosage for patients with a creatinine clearance of less than 30 mL/minute. Follow the prescriber's orders and use cautiously in patients with renal insufficiency.

What can happen

Adverse reactions to UFH and LMWH include bleeding, bruising, hematoma formation, skin irritation, and thrombocytopenia. When used with antihistamines and cardiac glycosides, the anticoagulant effects of heparin may be diminished.

What to consider

• Monitor platelet count and coagulation tests frequently, such as PTT, prothrombin time, and activated coagulation time.
• Monitor the patient for signs of bleeding, which may be difficult to detect. Monitor hematocrit (HCT) frequently and check stools for occult blood to detect asymptomatic bleeding. Inspect venipuncture and wound sites and the skin regularly for bleeding.
• Use heparin cautiously in patients with hemorrhaging (or who are at risk for it) or GI conditions, such as ulcerative colitis, because severe hemorrhage, acute thrombocytopenia, and new thrombus formation (white clot syndrome) may occur.
• These drugs are contraindicated in patients with a platelet count of less than 100,000/mm^3 (SI, 100×10^9/L) or in patients with heparin-induced thrombocytopenia.
• When these drugs are used with aspirin, dipyridamole (Persantine), other NSAIDs, or indomethacin (Indocin), impaired platelet aggregation and a possible increased risk of bleeding may occur.
• Heparin is incompatible with alteplase, amiodarone, diazepam, diltiazem, dobutamine, furosemide, morphine sulfate, phenytoin sodium, quinidine gluconate, solutions with a phosphate buffer, sodium carbonate, or sodium oxalate.

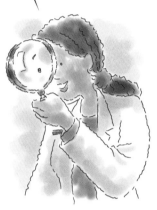

When giving heparin, remember to monitor the patient's platelet count, coagulation tests, and HCT and watch for signs of bleeding, which may be difficult to detect.

Antiplatelet drugs

Antiplatelet drugs block the final common pathway of platelet aggregation, improving the prognosis of patients with ST-segment depression and ischemia. They're also used as adjuncts to percutaneous coronary intervention (PCI). The antiplatelet drugs used during ACLS and in the immediate post–resuscitative period to treat patients with ACS include aspirin, the glycoprotein (GP) IIb/IIIa inhibitors (abciximab, eptifibatide, and tirofiban), and the thienopyridines (clopidogrel and prasugrel).

Awesome analgesic

Aspirin is a nonopioid analgesic with antipyretic, anti-inflammatory, and antiplatelet effects. It's used for all patients with ACS, especially reperfusion candidates, and for anyone with signs of ischemic pain (chest pain described as pressure, heavy weight, squeezing, or crushing). Early administration of aspirin, either in the out-of-hospital setting or emergency department, has decreased mortality in patients with suspected ACS.

Uninhibited inhibitors

GP IIb/IIIa inhibitors are used to treat ACS without ST-segment elevation. These drugs inhibit the integrin GP IIb/IIIa receptor in the membrane of platelets, preventing platelet aggregation and thrombus growth. Be aware of bleeding precautions and other general precautions when using glycoproteins. (See *Bleeding precautions for glycoproteins.*)

Thienopyridines reduce platelet aggregation through a different mechanism than aspirin. They are used in ACS and have been shown to reduce mortality and morbidity in non-STEMI and STEMI.

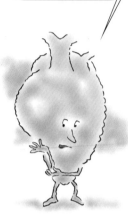

Aspirin is given to all patients with ACS or signs of ischemic pain.

Aspirin

Aspirin works as an analgesic by affecting the hypothalamus (central action) and blocking the generation of pain impulses (peripheral action). As an anti-inflammatory, aspirin is believed to inhibit prostaglandin synthesis.

At low doses, aspirin appears to impede clotting by blocking prostaglandin synthetase action, preventing formation of the platelet-aggregating substance thromboxane A_2. This interference with platelet activity is irreversible and can prolong bleeding time. At high doses (1,000 mg), aspirin interferes with prostacyclin production, a potent vasoconstrictor and inhibitor of platelet aggregation, possibly negating its anti-clotting properties.

How to give it

Give 162 to 325 mg orally (preferably chewable), or 300 mg rectally if the patient can't take it orally, as soon as possible.

What can happen

Adverse reactions to aspirin include heartburn, GI distress, GI bleeding, occult bleeding, bruising, and tinnitus.

Bleeding precautions for glycoproteins

The patient given glycoprotein IIb/IIIa inhibitors may experience bleeding at the arterial access site for cardiac catheterization or internal bleeding involving the GI, genitourinary, or retroperitoneal areas. Follow these precautions when administering glycoproteins:
• Before infusion, measure platelet count, prothrombin time, activated clotting time, and partial thromboplastin time to identify preexisting hemostatic abnormalities.
• Monitor the platelet count before treatment, 2 to 4 hours after treatment, and 24 hours after treatment or before discharge.
• Administer the drug in a separate I.V. line. (Don't add other drugs to infusion solution.)
• Keep emergency medications available in case of anaphylaxis.
• Monitor the patient closely for bleeding.
• Discontinue heparin at least 4 hours before sheath removal.
• Minimize or avoid (if possible) arterial and venous punctures and I.M. injections.
• Avoid invasive procedures (if possible), such as nasotracheal intubation or the insertion of urinary catheters and nasogastric tubes,
• Avoid the use of constrictive devices, such as automatic blood pressure cuffs and tourniquets.
• Remember that antiplatelet drugs, heparin, nonsteroidal anti-inflammatory drugs, thrombolytics, and other anticoagulants may increase the risk of bleeding.

Key points

Aspirin
• At low doses, impedes clotting by blocking prostaglandin synthetase action, preventing formation of platelet-aggregating substance thromboxane A_2
• Indications: acute coronary syndrome and ischemic pain
• 162 to 325 mg P.O. (preferably chewable), or rectally if patient can't take P.O., as soon as possible

What to consider

• Don't give aspirin to patients with bleeding disorders or NSAID-induced sensitivity reactions.
• Use aspirin cautiously in patients with GI lesions, impaired renal function, hypoprothrombinemia, vitamin K deficiency, thrombotic thrombocytopenic purpura, or hepatic impairment.
• Use caution when giving aspirin with other GI irritants, such as antibiotics, corticosteroids, and other NSAIDs, because they may potentiate the adverse GI effects of aspirin.
• Anticoagulants and thrombolytics may potentiate the platelet-inhibiting effects of aspirin.
• Enteric-coated products are absorbed slowly and aren't suitable for acute therapy.

Abciximab

Abciximab (ReoPro) binds to the GP IIb/IIIa receptor of human platelets and inhibits platelet aggregation. Abciximab is used to treat patients with medically managed unstable angina or non-STEMI. It's also used for planned PCI within 24 hours.

How to give it

Here's how to administer abciximab:
- For ACS with PCI—Give an I.V. bolus of 0.25 mg/kg 10 to 60 minutes before the start of the procedure and then give a continuous I.V. infusion of 0.125 mcg/kg/minute; the maximum dosage is 10 mcg/minute for 12 hours.
- For ACS with planned PCI within 24 hours—Give an I.V. bolus of 0.25 mg/kg and then give an I.V. infusion of 10 mcg/minute for 18 to 24 hours, concluding 1 hour after PCI.

Remember to withdraw the necessary amount of abciximab for the bolus injection through a sterile, nonpyrogenic, low-protein-binding 0.2- or 0.22-millipore filter into a syringe. If opaque particles are present, discard the solution and obtain a new vial.

For a continuous I.V. infusion, inject abciximab into sterile normal saline solution or D_5W, as ordered, and infuse through a continuous infusion pump equipped with an in-line filter. Discard the unused portion at the end of the 12-hour infusion.

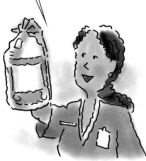

Abciximab is intended for use with aspirin and heparin.

What can happen

Adverse reactions to abciximab include bleeding, thrombocytopenia, bradycardia, and hypotension.

What to consider

- Abciximab is intended for use with aspirin and heparin.
- Monitor the patient closely for bleeding at the arterial access sites and for internal bleeding involving the GI or genitourinary (GU) tract or retroperitoneal sites.
- Platelet function recovers in about 48 hours but abciximab remains in the patient's circulation for up to 10 days in a platelet-bound state.

Clopidogrel

Clopidogrel (Plavix) is a thienopyridine that inhibits platelet function by binding to the adenosine diphosphate (ADP) receptors on platelets. It's used for patients up to age 75 with non-STEMI or STEMI (in addition to standard treatment, including fibrinolysis), for patients with suspected ACS who can't take aspirin, and for patients with recent stroke.

How to give it

For patients younger than age 75 with suspected ACS, non-STEMI, or STEMI, give a loading dose of 300 to 600 mg P.O. followed by

75 mg. P.O. daily. For patients unable to take aspirin, give a loading dose of 300 mg. P.O. For patients with stroke, give 75 mg P.O. daily.

What can happen

Major adverse reactions to clopidogrel include bleeding (which may be life-threatening), thrombotic thrombocytopenic purpura, anemia, bradycardia, atrial fibrillation, hypertension, and hypotension.

What to consider

• Clopidogrel should be withheld for 5 days before coronary artery bypass graft (CABG) or other major surgery because its effects last the life of the platelet cells.
• Carefully monitor patients for bleeding.
• Monitor patients for signs and symptoms of thrombotic thrombocytopenic purpura (thrombocytopenia, hemolytic anemia, neurologic changes, renal impairment, and fever).
• Patients who are genetically poor metabolizers of clopidogrel may have higher rates of cardiovascular events. Genetic tests can identify these patients and can be used to plan alternative treatment.

Eptifibatide

Eptifibatide (Integrilin) functions as a platelet aggregation inhibitor. It's used to treat patients with medically managed unstable angina or non-STEMI. It's also used during PCI.

How to give it

Here's how to administer eptifibatide:
• For ACS—Give an I.V. bolus of 180 mcg/kg and then give an I.V. infusion of 2 mcg/kg/minute for up to 72 hours.
• For PCI—Give an I.V. bolus of 180 mcg/kg over 1 to 2 minutes and then begin an I.V. infusion of 2 mcg/kg/minute for 18 to 24 hours. The bolus may be repeated 10 minutes after the initial bolus is given.

Eptifibatide may be administered in the same I.V. line as alteplase, atropine, dobutamine, heparin, lidocaine, meperidine (Demerol), metoprolol (Lopressor), midazolam, morphine, nitroglycerin, verapamil (Calan), normal saline solution, or dextrose 5% in normal saline solution. The main infusion may also contain up to 60 mEq/L of potassium chloride. However, don't administer eptifibatide in an I.V. line with furosemide.

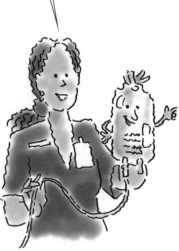

Don't give eptifibatide I.V. with furosemide.

What can happen

Adverse reactions to eptifibatide include bleeding, thrombocytopenia, and hypotension.

What to consider

- Eptifibatide is intended for use with heparin and aspirin.
- Monitor the patient closely for bleeding.
- Platelet function recovers within 4 to 8 hours after discontinuing eptifibatide.
- If the patient is undergoing coronary artery bypass graft surgery, stop the infusion before surgery.

Prasugrel

Prasugrel (Effient) is a thienopyridine that inhibits platelet function by binding to the ADP receptors on platelets. It's used in place of clopidogrel after angiography in patients with non-STEMI or STEMI who aren't at high risk for bleeding. It shouldn't be given to STEMI patients treated with fibrinolytics, to non-STEMI patients before angiography, to patients age 75 and older, or to patients with a history of transient ischemic attack or stroke.

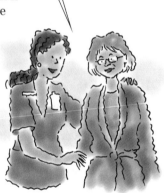

Don't give prasugrel to patients age 75 and older.

How to give it

For patients who weigh 132 lb (60 kg) or more and are managed with PCI, give a loading dose of 60 mg P.O. followed by a maintenance dose of 10 mg P.O. daily. For patients weighing less than 132 lb, consider reducing dosage to 5 mg P.O. daily.

What can happen

Adverse reactions include bleeding (which may be life-threatening), anemia, bradycardia, atrial fibrillation, hypertension, and hypotension.

What to consider

- Prasugrel should be withheld for 7 days before CABG or other major surgery because its effects last the life of the platelet cells.
- Don't use prasugrel in patients with active bleeding. Carefully monitor patients for signs of bleeding. Suspect bleeding in patients with hypotension.
- If possible, manage bleeding without discontinuing prasugrel. Discontinuing the drug, particularly in the first few weeks after ACS, increases the risk of more cardiovascular events.

Tirofiban

Tirofiban (Aggrastat) functions as a platelet aggregation inhibitor. It's used to treat patients with medically managed unstable angina or non-ST-segment elevation MI. It's also used during PCI.

How to give it

Give 0.4 mcg/kg/minute I.V. for 30 minutes for ACS or PCI and then give an I.V. infusion at 0.1 mcg/kg/minute for at least 12 to 24 hours after PCI. Remember that you can administer heparin and tirofiban through the same I.V. catheter.

What can happen

Adverse reactions to tirofiban include bradycardia, coronary artery dissection, bleeding, and thrombocytopenia.

What to consider

• Monitor the patient's hemoglobin level, HCT, and platelet count before starting tirofiban, 6 hours following the loading dose, and at least daily during therapy.
• Tirofiban is intended for use with aspirin and heparin.
• Monitor the patient closely for bleeding.
• Platelet function recovers within 4 to 8 hours after discontinuing tirofiban.

Beta-adrenergic blockers

Used for patients with ACS, including acute MI, suspected MI, and unstable angina in the absence of complications, beta-adrenergic blockers are effective antianginal agents that can reduce morbidity and mortality, nonfatal reinfarction, and recurrent ischemia. Beta-adrenergic blockers are also used as second-line agents (after adenosine, diltiazem, and digoxin) for conversion to normal sinus rhythm or to slow ventricular response (or both) in SVTs, such as PSVT, atrial fibrillation, or atrial flutter.

Angina busters

These drugs help treat chronic stable angina by decreasing myocardial contractility and heart rate (negative inotropic and chronotropic effect), thus reducing myocardial oxygen consumption. The mechanism of action in patients with MI is unknown. However, beta-adrenergic blockers do reduce the frequency of PVCs, chest pain, and enzyme level elevation. (For precautions that apply to

Key points

Beta-adrenergic blockers
Used in patients with acute coronary syndromes to:
• reduce morbidity and mortality
• treat and manage angina
• reduce the incidence of nonfatal reinfarction
• slow ventricular response and convert to sinus rhythm.

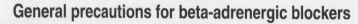

General precautions for beta-adrenergic blockers

Observe these general precautions when you administer beta-adrenergic blockers:
• Severe hypotension can occur if given I.V. with I.V. calcium channel blocking agents, such as verapamil or diltiazem.
• Avoid use in patients with severe bronchospastic diseases, severe heart failure, or severe abnormalities in conduction.
• Myocardial depression may occur.
• Beta-adrenergic blockers are contraindicated in the presence of severe bradycardia, systolic blood pressure less than 100 mm Hg, severe left-sided heart failure, hypoperfusion, or second- or third-degree atrioventricular block.
• Beta-adrenergic blockers may require altered dosage requirements in stable patients with diabetes.
• Signs and symptoms of overdose include severe hypotension, bradycardia, heart failure, and bronchospasm.

all beta-adrenergic blockers, see *General precautions for beta-adrenergic blockers*.)

Pressure reducer

Beta-adrenergic blockers may reduce blood pressure by adrenergic receptor blockade. This decreases cardiac output by decreasing sympathetic outflow from the CNS and suppressing renin release. (See *Major effects of beta-adrenergic blockers*.)

ACLS guidelines point the way

ACLS guidelines recommend that all patients with ischemic chest pain and ST-segment elevation receive a beta-adrenergic blocker within 12 hours of infarction, unless contraindications exist. Beta-adrenergic blockers are also used for emergency antihypertensive therapy for hemorrhagic and acute ischemic stroke. The beta-adrenergic blockers used during ACLS include atenolol, esmolol, labetalol, metoprolol, and propranolol.

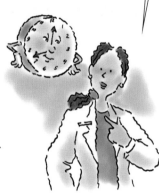

ACLS guidelines recommend that you give a beta-adrenergic blocker within 12 hours of infarction as long as no contraindications are present.

Atenolol

Atenolol (Tenormin) is used as an antihypertensive and antianginal agent. It has been shown to reduce the incidence of VF in post-MI patients who didn't receive fibrinolytic agents and decrease postinfarction ischemia in patients who did receive fibrinolytic therapy.

Major effects of beta-adrenergic blockers

Beta-adrenergic blockers block the action of endogenous catecholamines and other sympathomimetic agents at beta-receptor sites, thus counteracting the stimulating effects of those agents. Pulmonary effects produce constriction of bronchial smooth muscle and peripheral vascular effects produce constriction of peripheral vessels (beta-2 receptor). This illustration depicts the effects of beta-adrenergic blockers on the heart.

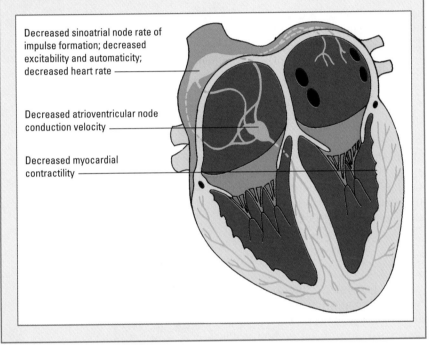

Decreased sinoatrial node rate of impulse formation; decreased excitability and automaticity; decreased heart rate

Decreased atrioventricular node conduction velocity

Decreased myocardial contractility

How to give it

Give 5 mg I.V. over 5 minutes and then another 5 mg I.V. 10 minutes later. If the patient tolerates the I.V. dose after 10 minutes, give 50 mg orally and then continue with 50 mg orally every 12 hours (for a total of 100 mg/day) until discharged.

What can happen

Adverse reactions to atenolol include bradycardia, AV block, hypotension, heart failure, bronchospasm, and light-headedness.

What to consider

• Monitor the patient's heart rate and rhythm.
• Check the patient's apical pulse before giving atenolol. If extremes in the pulse rate occur, withhold the drug and notify the prescriber immediately.
• Report significant lengthening of the PR interval and monitor for AV block.
• Atenolol may mask common signs of shock and hypoglycemia in diabetic patients.
• Use cautiously in patients with reactive airway disease.
• Use caution when giving atenolol with alpha-adrenergic drugs (such as those found in OTC cold remedies), indomethacin, and NSAIDs because these drugs may antagonize the antihypertensive effects of atenolol.

Esmolol hydrochloride

Esmolol (Brevibloc) is a class II antiarrhythmic and ultra-short-acting selective beta-adrenergic blocker used to decrease heart rate, contractility, and blood pressure. It's recommended for the acute treatment of PSVT and rate control in nonpreexcited atrial fibrillation or atrial flutter, ectopic atrial tachycardia, and polymorphic VT due to torsades de pointes.

How to give it

Give 0.5 mg/kg as an I.V. infusion over 1 minute, followed by a continuous 4-minute I.V. infusion of 50 mcg/kg/minute with a maximum infusion of 300 mcg/kg/minute. Titrate the dosage to maintain effect. Esmolol is recommended only for short-term use; discontinue after 48 hours. Don't mix esmolol with other I.V. drugs.

What can happen

Adverse reactions to esmolol include bradycardia, AV block, hypotension, heart failure, bronchospasm, and light-headedness.

What to consider

• Monitor the patient's heart rate and rhythm and blood pressure response to the drug.
• Check the patient's apical pulse before giving esmolol. If extremes in the pulse rate occur, withhold the drug and notify the prescriber immediately.

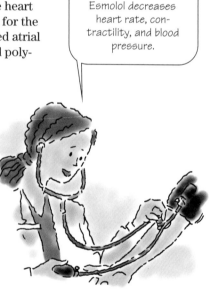

Esmolol decreases heart rate, contractility, and blood pressure.

- Report significant lengthening of the PR interval and monitor for AV block.
- Esmolol may mask common signs of shock and hypoglycemia in diabetic patients.
- Use cautiously in patients with reactive airway disease.
- Remember that the half-life of esmolol is 2 to 9 minutes.
- Morphine may increase esmolol blood levels.
- If the patient's heart rate becomes stable, replace esmolol with alternative (longer-acting) antiarrhythmics such as propranolol.
- Esmolol may increase serum digoxin levels by 10% to 20% with patients taking digoxin.
- Up to 50% of patients treated with esmolol develop hypotension, which can be reversed within 30 minutes by decreasing the dosage or, if needed, by stopping the infusion.
- When used with catecholamine-depleting drugs, esmolol may cause additive bradycardia and hypotension.

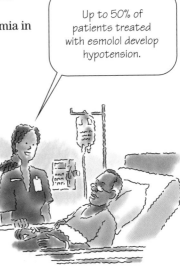

Up to 50% of patients treated with esmolol develop hypotension.

Labetalol hydrochloride

Labetalol is used to treat hypertension. The exact mechanism of how labetalol decreases blood pressure isn't known. However, it may decrease blood pressure by blocking adrenergic receptors and decreasing cardiac output. It's recommended as emergency antihypertensive therapy for hemorrhagic and acute ischemic stroke.

How to give it

Give a 10 mg I.V. push over 1 to 2 minutes; repeat injections of 10 to 20 mg every 10 minutes to a maximum dosage of 150 mg I.V. As an alternative, give an initial I.V. bolus dose and then start an I.V. infusion of 2 to 8 mg/minute until you obtain a satisfactory response.

What can happen

Adverse reactions to labetalol include bradycardia, AV block, ventricular arrhythmias, hypotension, heart failure, bronchospasm, and light-headedness.

What to consider

- Monitor the patient's heart rate and rhythm and blood pressure response to the drug.
- Check the patient's apical pulse before giving labetalol. If extremes in the pulse rate occur, withhold the drug and notify the prescriber immediately.

- Report significant lengthening of the PR interval and monitor for AV block.
- Labetalol may mask common signs of shock and hypoglycemia in diabetic patients.
- Use cautiously in patients with reactive airway disease.

Metoprolol tartrate

Metoprolol (Lopressor) is used to treat hypertension and as an adjunctive treatment for acute MI to reduce the incidence of VF. The exact mechanism of how metoprolol decreases blood pressure isn't known; however, it may decrease blood pressure by blocking adrenergic receptors and decreasing cardiac output.

How to give it

Give a slow I.V. dose of 5 mg at 5-minute intervals for a total dosage of 15 mg. Fifteen minutes following the last I.V. dose, give 50 mg orally every 6 hours.

What can happen

Adverse reactions to metoprolol include bradycardia, AV block, hypotension, heart failure, bronchospasm, and light-headedness.

What to consider

- Monitor the patient's heart rate and rhythm and blood pressure response to the drug.
- Check the patient's apical pulse before giving metoprolol. If extremes in the pulse rate occur, withhold the drug and notify the prescriber immediately.
- Report significant lengthening of the PR interval and monitor for AV block.
- Metoprolol may mask signs of hypoglycemia in diabetic patients.
- Use cautiously in patients with reactive airway disease.
- Use metoprolol cautiously with adrenergic agonists.
- Don't give metoprolol to patients with sinus bradycardia, second- or third-degree AV block, cardiogenic shock, or overt cardiac failure when treating hypertension or angina.

Propranolol hydrochloride

Propranolol (Inderal) is used to treat hypertension, angina, and arrhythmias and as an adjunctive treatment for MI to reduce the incidence of VF. The exact mechanism of how propranolol decreases blood pressure isn't known; however, it may decrease blood pressure by blocking adrenergic receptors and decreasing cardiac output.

How to give it

Give 0.1 mg/kg by slow I.V. push, divided into three equal doses at 2- to 3-minute intervals, not to exceed 1 mg/minute. Transfer to oral therapy as soon as possible.

What can happen

Adverse reactions to propranolol include bradycardia, AV block, hypotension, heart failure, bronchospasm, and light-headedness.

What to consider

- Monitor the patient's heart rate and rhythm.
- Check the patient's apical pulse before giving propranolol. If bradycardia occurs, withhold the drug and notify the prescriber immediately.
- Report significant lengthening of the PR interval and monitor for AV block.
- Propranolol may mask signs of hypoglycemia in diabetic patients.
- Use cautiously in patients with reactive airway disease.
- Monitor blood pressure for hypotension.
- Don't give propranolol to patients with bronchial asthma, sinus bradycardia, heart block greater than first degree, cardiogenic shock, or heart failure (unless the failure is caused by a tachycardia that can be treated with propranolol).
- Use caution when giving propranolol with epinephrine because severe vasoconstriction may occur.

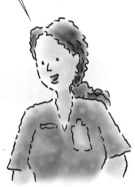

Always give propranolol by slow I.V. push.

Calcium channel blockers

In oral forms, calcium channel blockers are used to prevent angina that doesn't respond to other antianginal agents. I.V. calcium channel blockers are used to control the ventricular rate in atrial fibrillation and atrial flutter. They reduce electrical impulse formation in cardiac pacemaker cells and can convert reentry arrhythmias. (For precautions that apply to all calcium channel blockers, see *General precautions for calcium channel blockers*, page 162.)

General precautions for calcium channel blockers

Adverse reactions to calcium channel blockers include hypotension, arrhythmias, and heart failure. Follow these general precautions when you administer calcium channel blockers:
• Don't use for wide complex tachycardias of uncertain origin or for poison- or drug-induced tachycardia.
• Avoid use in patients with Wolff-Parkinson-White syndrome plus rapid atrial fibrillation or flutter, sick sinus syndrome, or atrioventricular block without a pacemaker.
• Avoid use in patients receiving oral beta-adrenergic blockers.
• Don't give I.V. with I.V. beta-adrenergic blockers because severe hypotension may result.

Demand decrease

Calcium channel blockers work by decreasing myocardial oxygen demand, the force of myocardial contractility, and afterload. They also increase the oxygen supply to the myocardium by dilating the coronary arteries. (See *How calcium channel blockers work*.) The calcium channel blockers used during ACLS include diltiazem and verapamil.

Diltiazem hydrochloride

Diltiazem (Cardizem) is used to treat angina, control the ventricular rate in atrial fibrillation and atrial flutter, and after adenosine to treat refractory reentry SVT in patients with narrow QRS complex and adequate blood pressure. By impeding the slow inward influx of calcium at the AV node, it decreases conduction velocity and increases the refractory period, thereby decreasing the impulses transmitted to the ventricles in atrial fibrillation or atrial flutter. Ventricular rate then decreases.

In patients with Prinzmetal's angina, it inhibits coronary artery spasm, increasing myocardial oxygen delivery.

Dilation = decrease

Diltiazem works by dilating systemic arteries. This dilation decreases total peripheral resistance and afterload, slightly reduces blood pressure, and increases the cardiac index when given in high doses. Afterload reduction and the resulting decrease in myocardial oxygen consumption account for its effectiveness in controlling chronic stable angina.

Diltiazem also decreases myocardial oxygen demand and cardiac workload by reducing heart rate, relieving coronary artery

You look like you could use some diltiazem. Try it! You'll be dilated and feeling less pain in no time.

Now I get it!

How calcium channel blockers work

Calcium channel blockers increase the myocardial oxygen supply and slow the heart rate. By blocking the slow calcium channel, they inhibit the influx of extracellular calcium ions across both myocardial and smooth muscle membranes. Calcium channel blockers achieve this blockade without changing serum calcium concentrations.

Who are you calling normal?

Under normal conditions, a protein complex prevents muscle contraction by keeping actin and myosin (the contractile proteins) apart. Actin and myosin must interact for a muscle to contract. When the muscle cell is stimulated, calcium ions enter the cell. This influx of calcium releases more calcium from the sarcoplasmic reticulum inside the muscle cell.

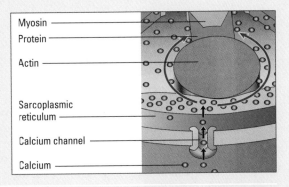

Myosin
Protein
Actin
Sarcoplasmic reticulum
Calcium channel
Calcium

A binding proposition

When enough calcium is released, it binds with the protein complex. The actin and myosin can then interact and the muscle contracts.

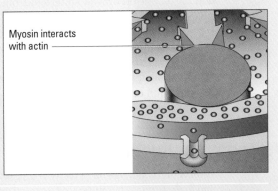

Myosin interacts with actin

An ounce of prevention

Calcium channel blockers prevent calcium transport across the cell membrane, thereby preventing calcium release from the sarcoplasmic reticulum. This causes the cardiac muscle and the smooth muscle of the coronary arteries to dilate.

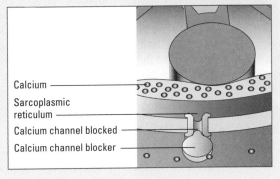

Calcium
Sarcoplasmic reticulum
Calcium channel blocked
Calcium channel blocker

spasm (through coronary artery vasodilation), and dilating peripheral vessels. These effects serve to relieve ischemia and pain.

How to give it

Give 0.25 mg/kg I.V. over 2 minutes. After 15 minutes, you may give another 0.35 mg/kg I.V. over 2 minutes. Give 5 to 15 mg/hour I.V., titrated to the patient's heart rate, as a maintenance infusion. Sublingual nitroglycerin may be administered with diltiazem, as needed, if the patient has acute angina symptoms.

What can happen

Adverse reactions to diltiazem include bradycardia, AV block, hypotension, dizziness, edema, heart failure, and acute hepatic injury.

What to consider

• Monitor the patient's heart rate and rhythm and blood pressure response to the drug.
• Don't give diltiazem to patients with severe left ventricular dysfunction, cardiogenic shock, second- or third-degree AV block (except in the presence of a functioning pacemaker), atrial fibrillation, atrial flutter, or sick sinus syndrome in the presence of WPW syndrome.
• Don't give I.V. diltiazem to patients receiving I.V. beta-adrenergic blockers or to patients with VT or other wide-complex tachycardia.
• Use reduced doses for patients with severely compromised cardiac function or for those receiving beta-adrenergic blockers.
• Diltiazem may increase serum levels of digoxin.

Verapamil hydrochloride

Verapamil (Calan) is used to treat angina, hypertension, and arrhythmias. It's indicated as an alternative drug (after adenosine) to terminate PSVT with narrow QRS complex, adequate blood pressure, and preserved left ventricular function. Verapamil controls ventricular response with atrial fibrillation, atrial flutter, or multifocal atrial tachycardia. Its primary effect is on the AV node; slowed conduction reduces the ventricular rate in atrial tachyarrhythmias and blocks reentry paths in paroxysmal supraventricular arrhythmias.

This drug's got it under control

Verapamil manages unstable and chronic stable angina by reducing afterload, thereby decreasing oxygen consumption. It also decreases myocardial oxygen demand and cardiac workload by

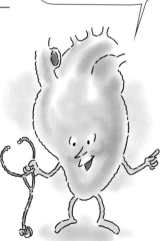

The primary effect of verapamil is on the AV node.

exerting a negative inotropic effect: reducing heart rate, relieving coronary artery spasm (via coronary artery vasodilation), and dilating peripheral vessels. Verapamil reduces blood pressure mainly by dilating peripheral vessels. Its negative inotropic effect blocks reflex mechanisms that lead to increased blood pressure.

How to give it

Give an I.V. bolus of 2.5 to 5 mg over 2 minutes with a second dose of 5 to 10 mg, if needed, in 15 to 30 minutes. The maximum dosage is 20 mg. For elderly patients, remember to administer I.V. doses over at least 3 minutes to minimize the risk of adverse reactions.

What can happen

Adverse reactions to verapamil include bradycardia, AV block, ventricular arrhythmias, hypotension, dizziness, edema, and heart failure.

What to consider

- Monitor the patient's heart rate and rhythm and blood pressure response to the drug.
- Don't give verapamil to patients with severe left ventricular dysfunction, cardiogenic shock, second- or third-degree AV block (except in the presence of a functioning pacemaker), atrial fibrillation, atrial flutter, or sick sinus syndrome in the presence of WPW syndrome.
- Don't give I.V. verapamil to patients receiving I.V. beta-adrenergic blockers or to patients with VT or other wide-complex tachycardia.
- Use reduced doses for patients with severely compromised cardiac function or for those receiving beta-adrenergic blockers.

Diuretics

Diuretics are used to promote the excretion of water and electrolytes by the kidneys. These drugs are used to treat hypertension as well as other cardiovascular conditions, such as edema, heart failure, and pulmonary edema. Frequently used diuretics include furosemide and mannitol.

Furosemide

A highly potent loop diuretic, furosemide (Lasix) is also an antihypertensive. It's used as adjunctive therapy for acute pulmonary edema in patients with systolic blood pressure greater than 90 to 100 mm Hg without signs and symptoms of shock. Furosemide is also used in hypertensive emergencies and in cases of increased intracranial pressure (ICP).

In the loop

Furosemide inhibits sodium and chloride reabsorption in the proximal part of the ascending loop of Henle, promoting sodium, water, chloride, and potassium excretion. Its antihypertensive effect may result from renal and peripheral vasodilation, a temporary increase in the glomerular filtration rate, and a decrease in peripheral vascular resistance.

How to give it

Give a slow I.V. infusion of 0.5 to 1 mg/kg over 1 to 2 minutes; if there's no response, increase to 2 mg/kg I.V. and give slowly over 1 to 2 minutes. If high-dose furosemide therapy is needed, administer the drug as a controlled infusion not exceeding 4 mg/minute. Remember to dilute furosemide in D_5W, normal saline solution, or lactated Ringer's solution and use the infusion within 24 hours.

What can happen

Adverse reactions to furosemide include dizziness, ototoxicity, hypotension, volume depletion and dehydration, hypokalemia, agranulocytosis, and leukopenia. Signs and symptoms of furosemide overdose include profound electrolyte and volume depletion, which may precipitate circulatory collapse. When given with antihypertensives, furosemide may increase the risk of hypotension.

What to consider

- Monitor the patient's weight, heart rate and rhythm, and blood pressure response to the drug.
- Closely monitor electrolyte levels and accurately assess fluid balance.
- Furosemide may decrease hypoglycemic effects in patients with diabetes.
- Use caution when giving NSAIDs with furosemide because they may inhibit the diuretic response.
- Cardiac glycosides and lithium may increase the risk of toxicity when given with furosemide because of furosemide-induced hypokalemia.

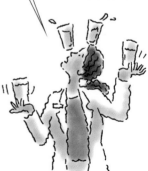

When using diuretics, remember to monitor electrolyte levels and assess fluid balance.

Mannitol

Mannitol (Osmitrol) is an osmotic diuretic used to reduce increased ICP during neurologic emergencies. It may also be used to prevent acute renal failure.

Mannitol increases the osmotic pressure of glomerular filtrate. This inhibits tubular reabsorption of water and electrolytes, promoting diuresis and the urinary elimination of certain drugs. Reduced ICP occurs because the drug elevates plasma osmolality, enhancing the flow of water into extracellular fluid.

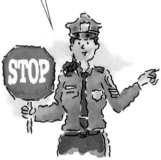

Stop right there! Never use solutions with undissolved crystals.

How to give it

Give 0.5 to 1 g/kg I.V. over 5 to 10 minutes for increased ICP; additional doses of 0.25 to 2 g/kg I.V. may be given every 4 to 6 hours. Remember to always administer mannitol by I.V. line with an in-line filter. If the mannitol solution crystallizes (a common occurrence at low temperatures), place the crystallized solution in a hot water bath, shake vigorously to dissolve the crystals, and cool to body temperature before use. Don't use solutions with undissolved crystals.

What can happen

Adverse reactions to mannitol include dizziness, seizures, tachycardia, angina-like chest pain, dehydration, hypotension, hypertension, and thrombophlebitis.

What to consider

• Monitor the patient's serum and urine sodium and potassium levels daily.
• Don't give mannitol to patients with severe pulmonary congestion, pulmonary edema, severe heart failure, severe dehydration, metabolic edema, progressive renal disease or dysfunction, or active intracranial bleeding except during craniotomy.
• Use mannitol with extreme caution in patients with compromised renal function because fluid overload may result; monitor vital signs (including central venous pressure) hourly as well as intake and output, weight, renal function, and fluid balance.
• Mannitol may enhance the possibility of digoxin toxicity.

Electrolytes and buffers

Electrolytes and buffering agents are used for electrolyte replacement therapy. Calcium chloride, magnesium sulfate, and sodium bicarbonate are the drugs most frequently used in ACLS.

Calcium chloride

Calcium chloride is a calcium supplement used for patients experiencing electrolyte imbalances. It's indicated for known or suspected hyperkalemia (as in renal failure) and in hypocalcemia. It serves as an antidote for calcium channel blocker or beta-adrenergic blocker overdose. It may also be given prophylactically before I.V. calcium channel blockers to prevent hypotension but isn't used routinely in cardiac arrest.

Calcium chloride is essential for maintaining the functional integrity of the nervous, muscular, and skeletal systems as well as for maintaining cell membrane and capillary permeability.

How to give it

Here's how to administer calcium chloride:
- Prophylaxis for I.V. calcium channel blockers—Give 500 to 1,000 mg/kg (5 to 10 mL of a 10% solution) by slow I.V. push and repeat, as needed.
- For hyperkalemia and calcium channel blocker overdose—Give 500 to 1,000 mg/kg (5 to 10 mL of a 10% solution) by slow I.V. push.

Only give calcium chloride by I.V. line, slowly through a small-bore needle into a large vein. Severe necrosis and sloughing of tissue may occur after extravasation.

Calcium gluconate is less irritating to veins and tissue than calcium chloride. Crash carts usually contain gluconate and chloride; be sure to double-check which form is ordered.

What can happen

Adverse reactions to calcium chloride include hypercalcemia when large doses of calcium chloride are given to patients with chronic kidney disease. Acute hypercalcemia syndrome is characterized by a markedly elevated plasma calcium level, lethargy, weakness, nausea and vomiting, and coma; it may lead to sudden death.

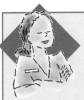

Peak technique

Checking for Trousseau's and Chvostek's signs

Here's how to check for Trousseau's and Chvostek's signs, which aid in the diagnosis of tetany associated with hypocalcemia.

Trousseau's sign

To check for Trousseau's sign, apply a blood pressure cuff to the patient's upper arm and inflate it to a pressure 20 mm Hg above the systolic pressure. Trousseau's sign (carpal spasm) may appear after 1 to 4 minutes. The patient will experience an adducted thumb, flexed wrist and metacarpophalangeal joints, and extended interphalangeal joints (with fingers together) indicating tetany, a major sign of hypocalcemia.

Chvostek's sign

You can induce Chvostek's sign by tapping the patient's facial nerve adjacent to his ear. A brief contraction of the upper lip, nose, or side of the face indicates Chvostek's sign.

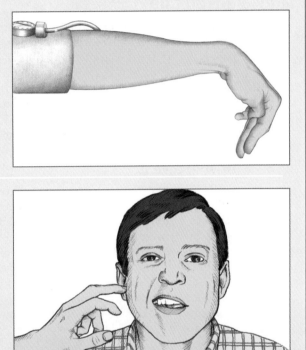

What to consider

• Initially, assess the patient with hypocalcemia for Trousseau's and Chvostek's signs periodically to check for tetany. (See *Checking for Trousseau's and Chvostek's signs.*)

• Monitor the patient for symptoms of hypercalcemia (nausea, vomiting, lethargy, headache, mental confusion, anorexia). Remember to report symptoms immediately.

• Don't use calcium chloride routinely for cardiac arrhythmias.

• Administer calcium chloride very cautiously, if at all, to patients receiving digoxin because of the increased risk of digoxin toxicity.

- Don't mix calcium chloride with sodium bicarbonate.
- Use caution when giving calcium chloride and magnesium together because calcium decreases the amount of bioavailable magnesium.
- Calcium chloride may antagonize the therapeutic effects of calcium channel blockers such as verapamil.

Magnesium sulfate

Magnesium sulfate is a mineral and electrolyte used in cardiac arrest only when torsades de pointes is suspected or hypomagnesemia is present. It isn't likely to be effective in terminating irregular polymorphic VT in patients with a normal QT interval. It may also be used for life-threatening ventricular arrhythmias due to digoxin toxicity.

Magnesium sulfate depresses the CNS and respiratory system. It acts peripherally, causing vasodilation. Moderate doses result in flushing and sweating, while high doses may lead to hypotension.

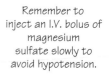

Remember to inject an I.V. bolus of magnesium sulfate slowly to avoid hypotension.

How to give it

Here's how to administer magnesium sulfate:
- For cardiac arrest (hypomagnesia or torsades de pointes)—Give 1 to 2 g (2 to 4 mL of 50% solution) diluted in 10 mL of D_5W by I.V. or I.O. over 5 to 20 minutes.
- For torsades de pointes without cardiac arrest or acute MI with hypomagnesemia—Give a loading dose of 1 to 2 g I.V. in 50 to 100 mL of D_5W over 5 to 60 minutes; follow with 0.5 to 1 g/hour I.V. If indicated, titrate to control torsades de pointes.

Remember, in I.V. bolus form, magnesium sulfate must be injected slowly to avoid hypotension.

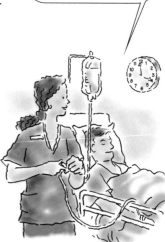

What can happen

Adverse reactions to magnesium sulfate include hypotension, circulatory collapse, depressed cardiac function, and respiratory paralysis.

What to consider

- Use caution when giving magnesium sulfate with cardiac glycosides because it may exacerbate arrhythmias.
- Magnesium sulfate coadministered with I.V. calcium can cause changes in cardiac conduction in patients taking digoxin and may lead to heart block; avoid concomitant use.

Sodium bicarbonate

Sodium bicarbonate is an alkalinizing agent used as a systemic hydrogen ion buffer to treat metabolic acidosis. It restores the buffering capacity of the body and neutralizes excess acid. (See *When to use sodium bicarbonate.*)

Dissociative property

Sodium bicarbonate dissociates to provide bicarbonate ions. Excess bicarbonate (bicarbonate not needed to buffer hydrogen ions) causes systemic alkalinization and, when excreted, urinary alkalinization as well.

How to give it

Give an I.V. bolus of 1 mEq/kg (depending on arterial blood gas [ABG] values, if rapidly available). Calculate the dosage based on bicarbonate concentration.

What can happen

Adverse reactions to sodium bicarbonate include clinical signs of sodium overdose: depressed consciousness and obtundation from hypernatremia, tetany from hypocalcemia, arrhythmias from hypokalemia, and seizures from alkalosis.

What to consider

- Monitor the patient's vital signs and fluid and electrolyte levels closely.
- Remember that adequate ventilation and cardiopulmonary resuscitation are the first-line buffering agents in cardiac arrest.

When to use sodium bicarbonate

Use sodium bicarbonate to treat:
- hyperkalemia
- known preexisting bicarbonate-responsive acidosis (diabetic ketoacidosis)
- overdose from drugs, such as tricyclic antidepressants, cocaine, and diphenhydramine (Benadryl)
- aspirin or other overdose (alkalizes urine).

It's also used for prolonged resuscitation with effective ventilation. However, sodium bicarbonate isn't useful or effective for treating hypercarbic acidosis (a condition that can result from cardiac arrest and cardiopulmonary resuscitation without intubation). It isn't recommended for routine use for patients in cardiac arrest.

- Sodium bicarbonate isn't recommended for routine use during cardiac arrest.
- Don't give calcium salts with sodium bicarbonate because they may cause precipitate.
- Sodium bicarbonate is incompatible with dobutamine, dopamine, epinephrine, and norepinephrine.

Fibrinolytics

Fibrinolytics are thrombolytic enzymes that promote the enzyme plasmin, which in turn dissolves fibrin and fibrous strands that bind clots. They're used for acute MI in adults with:

- ST-segment elevation (greater than or equal to 1 mm in two or more leads)
- evidence of new left bundle-branch block on the ECG and a history and symptoms strongly suspicious of myocardial injury
- onset of acute MI symptoms of less than 12 hours and PCI isn't available within 90 minutes of first medical contact.

Note that certain conditions contraindicate the use of fibrinolytics. (See *Contraindications and precautions for fibrinolytics used in ST-segment elevation MI.*) The fibrinolytics used during ACLS include alteplase, reteplase, and tenecteplase.

Alteplase

Alteplase (recombinant alteplase [Activase] tissue plasminogen activator) is a thrombolytic enzyme used to treat acute MI. In addition, alteplase is the only thrombolytic agent approved for the treatment of acute ischemic stroke. Although alteplase can be given within 12 hours of acute MI simptoms, it can only be given within 3 hours of known onset of acute stroke.

Conversion catalyst

Alteplase exerts thrombolytic action because of an enzyme that catalyzes the conversion of tissue plasminogen to plasmin in the presence of fibrin. This fibrin specificity produces local fibrinolysis in the area of recent clot formation, with limited systemic proteolysis. In patients with acute MI, this allows for reperfusion of ischemic cardiac muscle and improved left ventricular function with a decreased risk of heart failure.

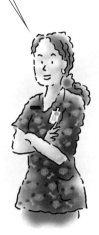

Alteplase is the only thrombolytic approved to treat acute ischemic stroke.

Contraindications and precautions for fibrinolytics used in ST-segment elevation MI

The American Heart Association has provided criteria that must be met before a patient with ST-segment elevation myocardial infarction (MI) may be considered for fibrinolytic therapy.

Criteria that must *not* be present
- Active bleeding
- Known structural cerebral vascular lesion (arteriovenous malformation) or malignancy
- Ischemic stroke within 3 months except for acute ischemic stroke within 3 hours
- Significant closed head trauma or facial trauma within 3 months
- History of intracranial hemorrhage
- Suspected aortic dissection

Criteria that shouldn't be present
- Severe, uncontrolled hypertension at the time of treatment or history of poorly controlled hypertension
- Active peptic ulcer
- Major surgery or serious trauma within 21 days, or more than 10 minutes of CPR

- Pregnancy
- Lumbar puncture performed within 7 days
- Recent noncompressible arterial puncture
- Internal bleeding within past 2 to 4 weeks
- Current medications include anticoagulants

Special precautions
- Monitor the patient for adverse reactions, including cerebral hemorrhage; hypotension; arrhythmias; severe, spontaneous bleeding (cerebral, retroperitoneal, genitourinary, GI); and bleeding at puncture sites.
- Avoid I.M. injections, venipuncture, and arterial puncture during therapy; use pressure dressings or ice packs on recent puncture sites to prevent bleeding. If arterial puncture is needed, select a site on the arm and apply pressure for 30 minutes afterward.

Source: 2010 American Heart Association Guidelines for Cardiopulmonary Resuscitation and Emergency Cardiovascular Care. © 2010, American Heart Association.

How to give it

Here's how to administer alteplase:
- For acute MI with ST-segment elevation—Give an accelerated infusion over 1 1/2 hours. Give an initial I.V. bolus of 15 mg I.V. and then administer 0.75 mg/kg I.V. over the next 30 minutes (dosage not to exceed 50 mg) and 0.5 mg/kg over the next 60 minutes (dosage not to exceed 35 mg). The total dosage shouldn't exceed 100 mg.
- For acute ischemic stroke—Infuse 0.9 mg/kg (maximum dose of 90 mg) I.V. over 60 minutes; give 10% of the total dosage as an initial I.V. bolus over 1 minute and give the remaining dose over the next 60 minutes.

Remember to prepare the alteplase solution for injection using sterile water, not bacteriostatic water. Alteplase may be further diluted with an injection of normal saline solution or D_5W to yield a concentration of 0.5 mg/mL. When preparing a dose from a 50-mg vial, use an 18G needle for preparing the solution—aim the water stream at the lyophilized cake. Expect a slight foaming to occur and don't use if a vacuum isn't present. When preparing a dose from a 100-mg vial, use a transfer device for reconstitution and remember that the 100-mg vial doesn't have a vacuum. Reconstituted or diluted solutions are stable for up to 8 hours at room temperature.

ASAP is the key

Expect to begin alteplase infusions as soon as possible after the onset of MI symptoms. Administer alteplase within 3 hours after the onset of stroke symptoms but only after excluding intracranial hemorrhage by computed tomography scan or another diagnostic imaging method.

What can happen

Adverse reactions to alteplase include hypotension; arrhythmias; bleeding, including GI bleeding, bleeding at puncture sites, and cerebral hemorrhage; and hypersensitivity reactions.

What to consider

• Monitor the patient's ECG for reperfusion arrhythmias.
• Monitor coagulation studies and assess the patient for bleeding. Avoid I.M. injections, invasive procedures, and nonessential handling of the patient.
• Heparin is usually administered during or after alteplase injection as part of the treatment regimen for acute MI or pulmonary embolism.
• Don't mix alteplase with other drugs.
• Treatment with alteplase should be performed only in facilities that can provide appropriate evaluation and management of intracranial hemorrhage.
• Don't give anticoagulant or antiplatelet therapy for 24 hours when alteplase is used for acute ischemic stroke.
• Drugs that antagonize platelet function (abciximab and dipyridamole) may increase the risk of bleeding if given before, during, or after alteplase therapy; avoid concomitant use.
• Discontinue the alteplase infusion immediately if signs or symptoms of bleeding occur and notify the prescriber.

Key points

Alteplase
• Produces local fibrinolysis in the area of recent clot formation, with limited systemic proteolysis
• Indications: acute myocardial infarction (MI) and acute ischemic stroke
• In acute MI accelerated infusion: over 1 ½ to 2 hours; give 15 mg I.V. bolus initially, then administer 0.75 mg/kg I.V. over the next 30 minutes (not to exceed 50 mg), and 0.5 mg/kg over the next 60 minutes (not to exceed 35 mg); total dose shouldn't exceed 100 mg
• For acute ischemic stroke: give 0.9 mg/kg over 60 minutes; 10% of the total dose should be given as an I.V. bolus over the first minute

Reteplase

Reteplase (recombinant, Retavase) is used to treat acute MI. It enhances cleavage of plasminogen to generate plasmin, which leads to fibrinolysis.

How to give it

Give reteplase as an I.V. double-bolus injection. First, give 10 units over 2 minutes; 30 minutes later, give a second dose of 10 units over 2 minutes. Remember to flush the I.V. line with normal saline solution before and after each bolus.

What can happen

Adverse reactions to reteplase include hypotension; arrhythmias; bleeding, including GI bleeding, bleeding at puncture sites, and cerebral hemorrhage; and hypersensitivity reactions.

What to consider

- Monitor the patient's ECG for reperfusion arrhythmias.
- Monitor coagulation studies and assess the patient for bleeding. Avoid I.M. injections, invasive procedures, and nonessential handling of the patient.
- Use caution when giving heparin, oral anticoagulants, or platelet inhibitors (abciximab, aspirin, or dipyridamole) with reteplase because these drugs may increase the risk of bleeding.
- Reteplase may alter coagulation studies.
- Potency is expressed in units specific for reteplase and isn't comparable to other thrombolytic drugs.
- Heparin and reteplase are incompatible in a solution.

Tenecteplase

Tenecteplase (TNKase) is used to treat acute MI. It's as effective as conventional fibrinolytics but differs in that it's given in a single-dose injection. Tenecteplase promotes plasmin activity to produce fibrinolysis. It targets established clots and, therefore, doesn't impair the natural clotting process throughout the body.

How to give it

Give as a 30- to 50-mg I.V. bolus injection over 5 seconds. Dosage is based on the patient's weight with a maximum total do age of 50 mg.

What can happen

Adverse reactions to tenecteplase include arrhythmias; hypotension; bleeding, including GI bleeding, bleeding at puncture sites, and cerebral hemorrhage; and hypersensitivity reactions.

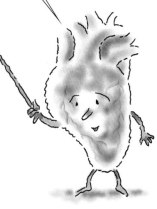

TNKase is as effective as conventional fibrinolytics but differs in that it's given in a single-dose injection.

What to consider

- Monitor the patient's ECG for reperfusion arrhythmias.
- Monitor coagulation studies and assess the patient for bleeding. (Tenecteplase may alter coagulation studies.) Avoid I.M. injections, invasive procedures, and nonessential handling of the patient.
- Use caution when giving heparin, oral anticoagulants, or platelet inhibitors (abciximab, aspirin, or dipyridamole) with reteplase because these drugs may increase the risk of bleeding. (Discontinue concomitant heparin and antiplatelet therapy if bleeding occurs.)

Inotropics

Inotropic agents, which include the subcategories of chronotropics and dromotropics, influence the force of muscular contractions.

Positives and negatives are all positive

Inotropics are typically used in treating heart failure and have either positive or negative effects. For example, positive dromotropic agents influence the conductivity of cardiac muscle and action of cardiac nerves while negative dromotropic agents slow the electrical impulse conduction through the nodal pathway (AV node). Inotropics include digoxin and inamrinone.

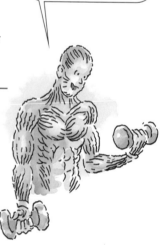

46, 47...Inotropics influence the force of muscular contractions... 48, 49, 50. Whew!

Digoxin

Digoxin (Lanoxin) is an inotropic and antiarrhythmic used in heart failure, atrial fibrillation, atrial flutter, and PSVT. It depresses the SA node and increases the refractory period of the AV node. It also indirectly increases intracellular calcium by inhibiting sodium-potassium activated adenosine triphosphatase.

How to give it

Give a loading dose of 10 to 12 mcg/kg (ideal body weight) I.V. or in divided doses over 24 hours. Follow with a maintenance dose determined by the patient's body weight and renal function. Don't mix digoxin with other drugs or give in the same I.V. line.

What can happen

Adverse reactions to digoxin include an increased risk of arrhythmias, confusion, irritability, and vision changes (blurred vision, yellow-green halos around visual images).

What to consider

- Monitor the patient's heart rate and rhythm. Excessive slowing of the pulse rate (60 beats/minute or less) may be a sign of digoxin toxicity. Withhold the drug and notify the prescriber.
- Before giving a loading dose, obtain baseline data (heart rate, rhythm, blood pressure, and electrolyte levels).
- The therapeutic serum level of digoxin is 0.5 to 2 ng/mL based on the patient's body weight and response to the drug.
- Avoid electrical cardioversion with digoxin unless the patient's condition is life-threatening; if necessary, use a lower current setting (10 to 20 joules).
- Don't give digoxin with dobutamine.
- Don't give digoxin with calcium salts because severe arrhythmias caused by the effects on cardiac contractility and excitability may occur.
- Don't give digoxin to patients with digoxin toxicity, AV block, profound sinus bradycardia, VT, atrial and junctional tachycardia, or PVCs.
- Use caution when giving digoxin with amiodarone, captopril, diltiazem, nifedipine (Procardia), quinidine, spironolactone (Aldactone), and verapamil because these drugs increase digoxin levels.
- Digoxin immune Fab can be used to treat digoxin toxicity.

Inamrinone lactate

Inamrinone is used for the short-term management of severe heart failure. It produces inotropic action by increasing cellular levels of cAMP. Inamrinone produces vasodilation through a direct relaxant effect on vascular smooth muscle.

How to give it

Give an I.V. bolus of 0.75 mg/kg over 2 to 3 minutes (give loading dose over 10 to 15 minutes with left ventricular dysfunction), followed by a maintenance infusion of 5 to 15 mcg/kg/minute I.V.; titrate to desired effect. Dosage depends on clinical response, including assessment of PAWP and cardiac output.

Remember not to dilute inamrinone with solutions containing dextrose. Also, don't administer furosemide and inamrinone through the same I.V. line because precipitation occurs.

What can happen

Adverse reactions to inamrinone include myocardial ischemia, arrhythmias, and thrombocytopenia. Additionally, excessive hypotension may occur with concomitant use of disopyramide.

> ### Key points
>
> **Inamrinone lactate**
> - Produces inotropic action by increasing cellular levels of cyclic adenosine monophosphate; produces vasodilation through a direct relaxant effect on vascular smooth muscle
> - Indications: short-term management of heart failure
> - I.V. bolus of 0.75 mg/kg over 10 to 15 minutes, followed by a maintenance infusion of 5 to 15 mcg/kg/ minute; titrate to clinical effect

What to consider

• Inamrinone is prescribed primarily for patients who haven't responded to cardiac glycosides, diuretics, and other inotropic drugs.
• Use hemodynamic monitoring to monitor the patient's heart rate, rhythm, function, and fluid balance.
• Monitor the patient's platelet level. If it falls below 150,000/mm³ (SI, 150×10^9/L), notify the prescriber for a dosage adjustment.

Nitrates

Nitrates are used to prevent or relieve angina and to reduce high blood pressure. (See *How antianginal agents relieve angina.*) The most commonly used nitrate is nitroglycerin.

Nitroglycerin

Nitroglycerin functions as an antianginal agent and vasodilator. It's used to treat suspected ischemic pain during the initial 24 to 48 hours in patients with acute MI complicated by heart failure, large anterior wall infarction, persistent or recurrent ischemia, hypertension, recurrent angina, persistent pulmonary congestion, or hypertensive urgency.

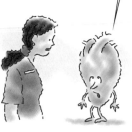

Nitroglycerin gives troubled hearts a boost. Come to think of it, I could use some of that!

To the rescue

Nitroglycerin relaxes the vascular smooth muscle of the venous and arterial beds, resulting in decreased myocardial oxygen consumption. It dilates coronary vessels, leading to the redistribution of blood flow to ischemic tissue.

Because peripheral vasodilation decreases venous return to the heart (preload), nitroglycerin also helps to treat pulmonary edema and heart failure. Arterial vasodilation decreases arterial impedance (afterload), thereby decreasing left ventricular workload and aiding the failing heart.

How to give it

Here's how to administer nitroglycerin:
• I.V. bolus (emergency route of choice)—Give an I.V. infusion at 10 mcg/minute increased by 10 mcg/minute every 5 to 10 minutes until the desired hemodynamic or clinical response occurs. Administration as an I.V. infusion requires special nonabsorbent tubing because regular plastic tubing may absorb up to 80% of the drug. Prepare the infusion in a glass bottle or container.

Key points

Nitroglycerin
• Antianginal and vasodilator
• Indications: ischermic pain, myocardial infarction, hypertension, angina, pulmonary congestion
• I.V. infusion at 10 mcg/minute increased by 10 mcg/minute untill desired response occurs
• Sublingual route: 1 tablet (0.30 to 0.4 mg) and repeat every 5 minutes
• Aeroso spray: 0.5 to 1 second at 5-minute intervals, which provides 0.4 mg per dose

Now I get it!

How antianginal agents relieve angina

Angina occurs when the coronary arteries—the heart's primary source of oxygen—supply insufficient oxygen to the myocardium. This increases the heart's workload, which in turn increases heart rate, preload (blood volume in ventricles at end of diastole), afterload (pressure in arteries leading from ventricles), and force of myocardial contractility. The antianginal agents (nitrates, beta-adrenergic blockers, and calcium channel blockers) relieve angina by decreasing one or more of these four factors. This illustration summarizes how antianginal agents affect the cardiovascular system.

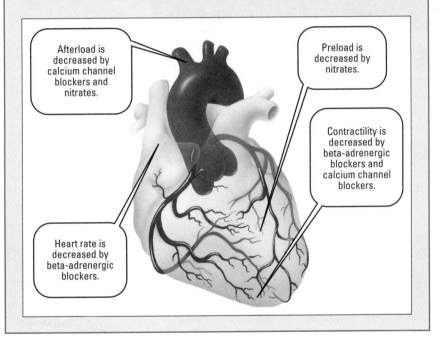

Afterload is decreased by calcium channel blockers and nitrates.

Preload is decreased by nitrates.

Contractility is decreased by beta-adrenergic blockers and calcium channel blockers.

Heart rate is decreased by beta-adrenergic blockers.

- Sublingual route—Give 1 tablet (0.3 to 0.4 mg); repeat every 5 minutes up to a total of three doses.
- Aerosol spray—Give a 0.5 to 1 second spray at 5-minute intervals (provides 0.4 mg per dose). The maximum dose is three sprays within 15 minutes.

What can happen

Adverse reactions to nitroglycerin include hypotension and headache. Drug toxicity may cause hypotension, persistent throbbing headache, palpitations, flushing of the skin, nausea and vomiting, bradycardia, heart block, tissue hypoxia, metabolic acidosis, and circulatory collapse; circulatory collapse or asphyxia may cause death.

What to consider

• In I.V. form, nitroglycerin is contraindicated in patients with cardiac tamponade, restrictive cardiomyopathy, or constrictive pericarditis.
• Use nitroglycerin cautiously in patients with hypotension or volume depletion.

Vasodilating antihypertensive agents

Vasodilating antihypertensive agents include direct vasodilators (typically nitroprusside sodium and I.V. nitroglycerin) and calcium channel blockers (typically verapamil). Direct vasodilators act on arteries, veins, or both and commonly produce adverse reactions related to reflex activation of the SNS. Calcium channel blockers produce arteriolar relaxation, which reduces the mechanical activity of vascular smooth muscle. These drugs are usually used as adjuncts in treating hypertension rather than as primary agents.

Nitroprusside sodium is discussed below. For a discussion of I.V. nitroglycerin, see page 178. For a discussion of verapamil, see page 164.

Nitroprusside sodium

Nitroprusside (Nipride) is a potent vasodilator used to treat hypertensive crisis. It's known to reduce afterload in heart failure, acute pulmonary edema, and acute mitral or aortic valve regurgitation. Nitroprusside acts directly on vascular smooth muscle, causing peripheral vasodilation.

How to give it

Begin an I.V. infusion of 0.1 mcg/kg/minute and titrate upward every 3 to 5 minutes to the desired effect (up to 5 mcg/kg/minute, but dosages up to 10 mcg/kg may be needed). Action will occur within 1 to 2 minutes.

Prepare nitroprusside using D_5W. Foil-wrap the I.V. solution (but not the tubing) because of light sensitivity. Fresh solutions have a faint brownish tint; discard after 24 hours.

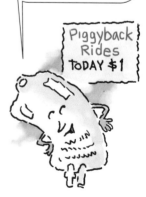

Nitroprusside is best given piggyback through a peripheral line with no other drugs.

Piggyback Rides TODAY $1

Remember to use an infusion pump when giving nitroprusside. Nitroprusside is best run piggyback through a peripheral line with no other drugs. Don't adjust the rate of the main I.V. line while the drug is running because even small boluses can cause severe hypotension. Ideally, the patient should have an arterial line to continuously monitor blood pressure.

What can happen

Nitroprusside may cause cyanide toxicity, which can produce profound hypotension, metabolic acidosis, dyspnea, ataxia, and vomiting.

What to consider

- Check serum thiocyanate levels every 72 hours (levels above 100 mg/mL are associated with cyanide toxicity).
- Don't give epinephrine with nitroprusside because this causes increased blood pressure.
- Use caution when giving other antihypertensives with nitroprusside because these drugs may potentiate its effects.
- If symptoms of cyanide toxicity occur, stop the infusion and reevaluate therapy.

Antidotes

Antidotes are used to reverse the effects of medications or situations in which the patient's life might be in danger. Among these are digoxin immune Fab, flumazenil, glucagon, and naloxone.

Digoxin immune Fab

Digoxin immune Fab (Digibind) is an antibody fragment that prevents or reverses the toxic effects of cardiac glycosides. It's used for potentially life-threatening digoxin toxicity (life-threatening arrhythmias and hyperkalemia with a plasma level greater than 5 mEq/L).

A binding agreement

With digoxin immune Fab, specific antigen-binding fragments bind with free digoxin intravascularly or in extracellular spaces, making them unavailable for binding at their sites of action.

Key points

Nitroprusside sodium
- A potent vasodilator indicated for hypertensive crisis
- Known to reduce afterload in heart failure, acute pulmonary edema, and acute mitral or aortic valve regurgitation
- Acts directly on vascular smooth muscle, causing peripheral vasodilation
- For hypertension, begin at 0.1 mcg/kg/minute and titrate upward every 3 to 5 minutes to desired effect (up to 5 mcg/kg/minute)
- Can cause cyanide toxicity; check serum thiocyanate levels every 72 hours; levels above 100 μg/ml are associated with cyanide toxicity, which can produce profound hypotension, metabolic acidosis, dyspnea, ataxia, and vomiting; if such symptoms occur, stop infusion and reevaluate therapy

How to give it

Here's how to administer digoxin immune Fab:
• For adults—Give a dose based on the ingested amount or serum level of digoxin.
• If cardiac arrest is imminent—Give rapidly by direct I.V. injection into the vein or use an I.V. line containing a free-flowing, compatible solution, using a 0.22-micron filter needle.

What can happen

Adverse reactions to digoxin immune Fab include heart failure, decreased cardiac output, hypokalemia, and rapid ventricular rate in patients with atrial fibrillation.

What to consider

• Digoxin levels greater than 2.5 ng/mL may be toxic. Ingestion of more than 10 mg of digoxin (in adults) or 4 mg (in children) at one time may cause cardiac arrest; therefore, use Digibind.
• Obtain serum digoxin levels 8 hours after the last dose to ensure accuracy.
• Closely monitor the patient's serum potassium level during and after drug administration.

Flumazenil

Flumazenil (Romazicon) is a benzodiazepine antagonist. It's used to treat the respiratory depression and sedative effects caused by pure benzodiazepine overdose. Flumazenil competitively inhibits the actions of benzodiazepines on the gamma-aminobutyric acid–benzodiazepine receptor complex.

How to give it

The initial dosage is 0.2 mg I.V. over 15 seconds. If the patient doesn't reach the desired level of consciousness, give 0.3 mg I.V. over 30 seconds. If the patient is still not responding adequately, give 0.5 mg I.V. over 30 seconds; repeat 0.5-mg doses at 1-minute intervals until a cumulative dosage of 3 mg has been given. On rare occasions, a total dose of 5 mg may be necessary.

Sedation that persists after 5 minutes when a total of 5 mg has been given is unlikely to be caused by benzodiazepines. (See *Contraindications and precautions for flumazenil.*) If the patient becomes sedated again, the dosage may be repeated after 20 minutes; however, no more than 1 mg should be given at any one time.

Contraindications and precautions for flumazenil

Flumazenil is contraindicated in patients who:
• have been given a benzodiazepine for a potentially life-threatening condition (such as to control intracranial pressure or status epilepticus)
• show signs of serious cyclic antidepressant overdose
• are at risk for mixed overdose (especially in cases when seizures are likely to occur).
    Use flumazenil with caution in patients who:
• are at high risk for developing seizures
• are withdrawing from sedative-hypnotics
• are displaying some signs of seizure activity (such as myoclonus)
• may be at risk for unrecognized benzodiazepine dependence
• are experiencing alcohol or other drug dependencies because of the increased risk of benzodiazepine tolerance
• have a head injury.

Before administering flumazenil, review the drug's contraindications.

Caution

What can happen

Adverse reactions to flumazenil include resedation, which may occur because the duration of flumazenil action is shorter than that of all benzodiazepines; agitation; dizziness; seizures; flushing; tachycardia; and hypertension.

What to consider

• Make sure the patient has a secure airway and I.V. access before administering flumazenil. Also make sure to wake him gradually.
• Monitor the patient closely for resedation after reversal of benzodiazepine effects. The duration of monitoring depends on the specific drug being reversed; for example, monitor the patient after long-acting benzodiazepines, such as diazepam (Valium), or after high doses of short-acting benzodiazepines such as midazolam.
• Monitor the patient's cardiac and respiratory status during drug use.
• Monitor for withdrawal symptoms after administering flumazenil to a patient with long-term benzodiazepine use.

Glucagon

Glucagon reverses low blood glucose levels. It's used as an adjuvant treatment of the toxic effects of calcium channel blockers or beta-adrenergic blockers. Glucagon promotes hepatic glycogenolysis and gluconeogenesis, raising serum glucose levels. It also relaxes GI smooth muscle and produces a positive inotropic and chronotropic myocardial effect.

How to give it

Give 1 mg I.V. over 2 to 5 minutes for treatment of hypoglycemia. For treatment of toxic effects of calcium channel blockers or beta-adrenergic blockers, give an initial I.V. dose of 3 mg to 10 mg over 3 to 5 minutes, followed by an infusion at 3 to 5 mg/hour, as needed. Remember that glucagon is incompatible with normal saline solution and other solutions with a pH of 3.0 to 9.5 because it may cause precipitation.

What can happen

• Adverse reactions to glucagon include vomiting and hypotension.

What to consider

• If a patient with hypoglycemia doesn't respond to glucagon, give I.V. dextrose.
• Glucagon may fail to relieve coma because of markedly depleted hepatic stores of glycogen or irreversible brain damage caused by prolonged hypoglycemia.
• Glucagon has been used as a cardiac stimulant in managing toxicity resulting from the use of beta-adrenergic blockers, quinidine, and tricyclic antidepressants.

Naloxone hydrochloride

Naloxone is used as an antidote for respiratory and neurologic depression caused by opioid intoxication. In patients who have received an opioid agonist or other analgesic with opioid-like effects, naloxone antagonizes most of the effects, especially respiratory depression, sedation, and hypotension. The precise mechanism of action is unknown, but it's thought to involve competitive antagonism of more than one opiate receptor in the CNS.

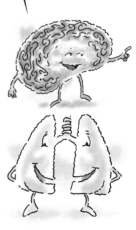

Naloxone is used to reverse the respiratory and neurologic depression caused by opioid intoxication.

How to give it

Give 0.04 to 0.4 mg I.V. repeated every 2 to 3 minutes as needed; higher doses may be used for complete opioid reversal, and up to 10 mg can be administered over a short period (less than 10 minutes). For suspected opioid-addicted patients and postoperative opioid depression, use smaller doses and titrate the dosage until ventilations are adequate. Naloxone can be diluted in D_5W or normal saline solution; use within 24 hours after mixing for continuous infusion.

What can happen

Adverse reactions to naloxone include tachycardia, hypertension (with higher-than-recommended doses), hypotension, VF, and cardiac arrest.

What to consider

• Because the duration of activity with naloxone is shorter than that of most opioids, continued monitoring and repeated doses are usually necessary to manage acute opioid overdose in a non-addicted patient. A continuous infusion may be indicated.
• Don't give naloxone with cardiotoxic drugs because they may cause potentially serious cardiovascular effects, including ventricular arrhythmias.
• Withdrawal symptoms may occur in opioid-dependent patients with higher-than-recommended doses of naloxone.
• Naloxone isn't effective in treating respiratory depression caused by nonopioid drugs.

Quick quiz

1.   The patient's cardiac monitor reveals short runs of VT. He becomes symptomatic, and a bolus of amiodarone is ordered followed by a continuous infusion. What amount should you expect to administer?
   A.   300 mg followed by a 1 mg/minute continuous infusion for 6 hours
   B.   300 mg followed by a 0.5 mg/minute continuous infusion for 6 hours
   C.   150 mg followed by a 1 mg/minute continuous infusion for 6 hours
   D.   150 mg followed by a 0.5 mg/minute continuous infusion for 6 hours

Answer: C. For wide-complex tachycardia, give a rapid infusion of 150 mg I.V. over the first 10 minutes (15 mg/minute) followed by a slow infusion of 360 mg I.V. over 6 hours (1 mg/minute). A maintenance infusion of 540 mg I.V. over 18 hours (0.5 mg/minute) may then be given.

> ### Key points
>
> **Medication tips**
> • Most emergency medications are given I.V.
> • Elderly patients and patients with decreased renal or liver function may need smaller dosages.
> • Atropine is no longer indicated for the treatment of asystole and pulseless electrical activity.
> • The first-line medications used most commonly in adult acute cardiac life support include epinephrine, vasopressin, atropine, amiodarone, sotalol, procainamide, adenosine, beta-adrenergic blockers, and calcium channel blockers.

2.   When administering amiodarone, you should monitor for
which ECG abnormality?
   A.   Inverted P waves
   B.   Prolonged QT interval
   C.   Narrowed QRS complex
   D.   Shortened PR interval

Answer: B. During amiodarone therapy, the QT interval may be
prolonged.

3.   Indications for the administration of atropine sulfate include:
   A.   symptomatic bradycardia and bradyarrhythmias.
   B.   VF and atrial fibrillation.
   C.   asystole and atrial fibrillation.
   D.   third-degree heart block, PEA, and VT.

Answer: A. Atropine is an antiarrhythmic indicated for symptomatic
bradycardia and bradyarrhythmias (junctional or escape rhythm).

4.   The use of which medication may precipitate torsades de
pointes?
   A.   procainamide
   B.   diltiazem
   C.   atenolol
   D.   atropine

Answer: A. Procainamide can precipitate torsades de pointes
secondary to its prolonging effect on the QT interval.

5.   Sodium bicarbonate is used to treat:
   A.   hypokalemia.
   B.   hypercarbic acidosis.
   C.   metabolic alkalosis.
   D.   diabetic ketoacidosis.

Answer: D. Indications for sodium bicarbonate use include treatment of known preexisting bicarbonate-responsive acidosis (diabetic ketoacidosis), hyperkalemia, or overdose from drugs, such
as tricyclic antidepressants, cocaine, and aspirin. It's also used for
prolonged resuscitation with effective ventilation.

Scoring

☆☆☆ If you answered all five questions correctly, wow! Pharmacologi-
        cally speaking, you're down with these drugs.

☆☆   If you answered four questions correctly, hooray! Your knowledge
        is impressive.

☆   If you answered fewer than four questions correctly, give it
        another try! Just a small dose of review will prepare you for a
        perfect score next time.

I.V. access and invasive techniques

Just the facts

In this chapter, you'll learn:

♦ basics of I.V. access

♦ use of basic venipuncture devices

♦ techniques for gaining peripheral and central I.V. access

♦ blood sampling techniques and use of infusion pumps

♦ techniques for emergency invasive procedures.

I.V. access basics

An I.V line is necessary to gain peripheral or central access to the patient's venous circulation. An I.V. line is inserted to:
• administer drugs and fluids
• administer blood and blood products
• obtain blood for laboratory tests
• provide for insertion of a catheter into the central circulation for hemodynamic monitoring and electrical pacing.

Choosing an access site

During resuscitation attempts, obtain venous access at the site of the largest vein available that doesn't require interrupting resuscitation (such as the antecubital or femoral vein).

Choose wisely, my son

The site you choose for I.V. access is based on the patient's needs and condition. Factors include:
• availability and condition of adequate peripheral veins
• volume of fluid required and time available to administer fluids
• type of fluid to be administered
• purpose and duration of I.V. therapy.

Veins used in I.V. therapy

This illustration shows the veins commonly used for peripheral I.V. and central venous therapy.

Internal jugular

External jugular

Left subclavian

Superior vena cava

Cephalic

Basilic

Median cubital

Median cephalic

Median antebrachial

Accessory cephalic

Dorsal venous arch

Metacarpal

Digital

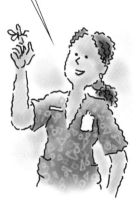

Remember that the most prominent veins may not be the best veins to use.

Here are some suggestions for selecting a vein:

• Keep in mind that the most prominent veins aren't necessarily the best veins; they may be sclerotic from previous use.

• Optimally, select a vein in the nondominant arm or hand.

• Avoid selecting a vein in an edematous or impaired arm, if possible.

• Never select a vein in the arm closest to an area that's surgically compromised, such as veins compromised by a mastectomy or by placement of dialysis access.

- For subsequent venipunctures, select sites above the previously used or injured vein.
- Always rotate access sites. (See *Veins used in I.V. therapy.*)

I.V. safety

Regardless of the site you choose, you must take precautions to ensure safety for yourself and your patient. These include:
- using standard precautions
- cleaning the site using an antiseptic solution
- disposing of needles appropriately
- changing the I.V. site every 3 days or according to your facility's policy
- evaluating the site for infiltration, extravasation, or thrombosis.

It's also important to change I.V. lines placed in the patient outside the hospital setting within 24 hours, if possible. Because these I.V. lines aren't usually inserted under ideal circumstances, they're more likely to cause infection or complications.

Memory jogger

In selecting the best site for venipuncture, remember the acronym **VIP**:

Vein

Infusion

Patient.

For the vein, consider its location, condition, and physical path along the extremity.

For the infusion, consider its purpose and duration.

For the patient, consider his degree of cooperation and compliance, along with his preference. Also consider patient history.

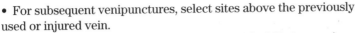

Basic venipuncture devices

Two major types of venipuncture devices exist: over-the-needle catheters and winged steel needle sets. Which catheter you choose is based on what type of I.V administration is needed or what equipment is available. Over-the-needle catheters are preferred for long-term therapy (such as in a hospital stay) and winged steel needles may be preferred for short-term therapy such as administering medication for a procedure. (See *Comparing basic venous access devices*, page 190.)

Over-the-needle catheters

The over-the-needle catheter can be used for long-term therapy and is often useful for an active or agitated patient.

Advantages of the over-the-needle catheter include:
- Inadvertent puncture of the vein is less likely than with a winged steel needle set.
- Patients are more comfortable.
- Its radiopaque thread makes location easy.
- The syringe attached to some units permits an easy check of blood return and prevents air from entering the vessel on insertion.
- An activity-restricting device, such as an arm board, is rarely required.

Comparing basic venous access devices

These illustrations show the differences between an over-the-needle catheter and a winged steel needle set.

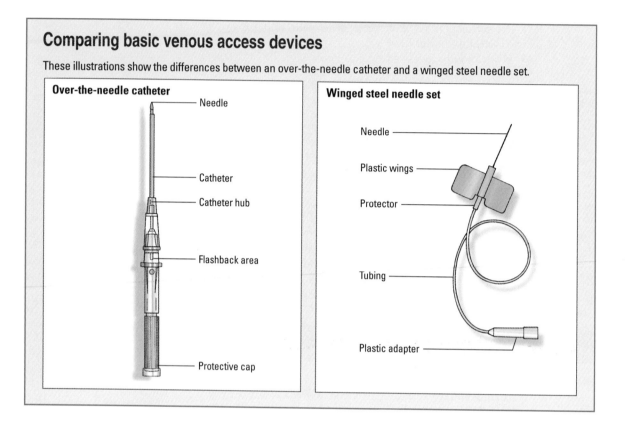

Over-the-needle catheter

- Needle
- Catheter
- Catheter hub
- Flashback area
- Protective cap

Winged steel needle set

- Needle
- Plastic wings
- Protector
- Tubing
- Plastic adapter

One disadvantage of the over-the-needle catheter is that it requires expertise to insert. In addition, extra care is needed to ensure that both the needle and catheter are inserted into the vein.

Winged steel needle sets

The winged steel needle set is used for short-term I.V. therapy in a cooperative adult patient. It's also used for therapy of any duration for an elderly patient with fragile or sclerotic veins.

Advantages of the winged steel needle set include:
- It's the easiest intravascular device to insert because the needle is thin-walled and extremely sharp.
- It's ideal for I.V. push drugs, short-term therapy, or single-dose administration.
- It's available with a catheter that can be left in place such as an over-the-needle catheter.

The disadvantage of the winged steel needle set is that infiltration can easily occur if a rigid needle winged infusion device is used.

Establishing peripheral I.V. lines

Peripheral venipuncture sites—located on the dorsal and ventral surfaces of the upper extremities—include the antecubital, metacarpal (hand), cephalic, basilic, and median veins. The leg veins shouldn't be used routinely because of increased risk of thrombophlebitis, ulcers, and infection. The selection of the site depends on the type of solution to be infused; the frequency and duration of the infusion; the patency and location of accessible veins; and the patient's age, size, and condition. The external jugular vein may also be used for rapid access in an emergency. (See *Comparing peripheral venipuncture sites*, pages 192 and 193.)

Advantages of a peripheral I.V. line include:
- It can be inserted rapidly by trained personnel.
- It offers easy access to veins and rapid administration of solutions, blood, and drugs.
- It allows continuous administration of drugs to produce rapid systemic changes.
- It's easy to monitor.

Disadvantages of a peripheral I.V. line include:
- It's an invasive vascular procedure that carries associated risks of bleeding, infiltration, and infection.
- It can't be used indefinitely.
- It's more costly than oral, subcutaneous, or I.M. therapy.

(See *Risks of peripheral I.V. therapy*, pages 194 to 199.)

Upper extremity veins

The largest veins of the arm are generally located in the antecubital fossa. Of these veins, the most commonly selected for I.V. access are the median cephalic and median basilic.

Up the ante for quick I.V. access

The antecubital fossa site is useful when you need to establish rapid I.V. access because its veins are easily accessed. You can also use this site for patients in circulatory collapse or cardiac arrest. The cephalic and basilic veins may also be accessible both above and below the antecubital fossa. If long-term therapy is anticipated, start with the most distal, adequate site possible, such as the dorsal hand veins. Don't use the distal cephalic vein above the thumb and the veins of the inner wrist, to avoid damaging nerves.

> **Key points**
>
> **Peripheral I.V. lines**
> - Sites varied; may provide easy, rapid access
> - May be inserted by trained personnel
> - Easily removed
> - Access site may be inappropriate for adminstration of some medications
> - Not appropriate for administration of hypertonic or irritating solutions
> - May be easily dislodged

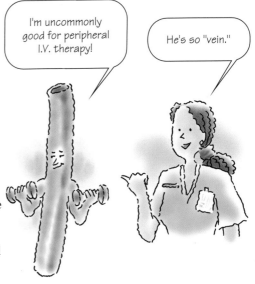

I'm uncommonly good for peripheral I.V. therapy!

He's so "vein."

Comparing peripheral venipuncture sites

This chart includes some of the major advantages and disadvantages of several common venipuncture sites.

Site	Advantages	Disadvantages
Digital veins Run along the lateral and dorsal portions of the fingers	• May be used for short-term therapy • May be used when other means aren't available	• Splinting the fingers with a tongue blade is required, which decreases the patient's ability to use his hand • Uncomfortable for the patient • Significant risk of infiltration • Not used if veins in the dorsum of the hand are already used • Not useful for certain medication infusions such as dopamine
Metacarpal veins On the dorsum of the hand; formed by the union of digital veins between the knuckles	• Easily accessible • Lie flat on the back of the hand; more difficult to dislodge • In an adult or large child, bones of the hand act as a splint	• Wrist movement decreased unless a short catheter is used • Painful insertion is likely because of the large number of nerve endings in the hands • Phlebitis is likely at the site • Not useful for certain medication infusions such as dopamine
Accessory cephalic vein Runs along the radial bone as a continuation of metacarpal veins of the thumb	• Large vein excellent for venipuncture • Readily accepts large-gauge needles • Doesn't impair mobility • Doesn't require an arm board in an older child or adult	• Some difficulty positioning catheter flush with skin • Discomfort during movement due to device located at bend of wrist
Cephalic vein Runs along the radial side of the forearm and upper arm	• Large vein excellent for venipuncture • Readily accepts large-gauge needles • Doesn't impair mobility	• Decreased joint movement due to proximity of the device to the elbow • Tendency of vein to roll during insertion
Median antebrachial vein Arises from the palm and runs along the ulnar side of the forearm	• Holds winged needles well • A last resort when no other means are available	• Painful insertion or infiltration damage is possible due to the large number of nerve endings in the area • High risk of infiltration in the area
Basilic vein Runs along the ulnar side of the forearm and upper arm	• Readily accepts large-gauge needles • Straight, strong vein suitable for large-gauge venipuncture devices	• Uncomfortable position for the patient during insertion • Tendency of vein to roll during insertion • Except for antecubital area, the vein usually lies deeper and may be more difficult to visualize

Comparing peripheral venipuncture sites *(continued)*

Site	Advantages	Disadvantages
Antecubital veins Located in the antecubital fossa (median cephalic, on radial side; median basilic, on ulnar side; median cubital, which rises in front of the elbow joint)	• Large veins; facilitate drawing blood • Often visible or palpable in children when other veins won't dilate • May be used in an emergency or as a last resort	• Difficult to splint the elbow area with an arm board • Veins may be small and scarred if blood has been drawn frequently from the site

What you need

- Chlorhexidine solution
- Gloves
- Tourniquet
- I.V. access device with safety shield
- I.V. solution with attached and primed administration set
- I.V. pole
- Sharps container
- Transparent semipermeable dressing
- Catheter securement device or 1" hypoallergenic tape
- I.V. start kit (available in some facilities)

How it's done

- Select the site and place the arm in a dependent position if possible.
- Apply a tourniquet 4 to 6" (10 to 15 cm) above the intended puncture site to dilate the vein.
- Leave the tourniquet in place for no longer than 3 minutes. If you're unable to locate a vein and prepare the site in that time, release the tourniquet and reapply it after the site is prepared.
- Put on clean gloves.
- Clean the site with chlorhexidine solution using a back-and-forth scrubbing motion and allow it to dry.
- If the patient is conscious, ask him to open and close his fist a few times to enhance your visualization of the veins.
- Remove the cover from the access device and make sure the needle is smooth and intact.
- Stabilize the vein by stretching the skin taut below the intended insertion site.

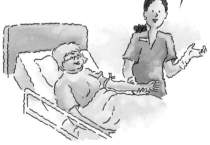

Ask a conscious patient to open and close her fist a few times to help you visualize her veins.

(Text continues on page 200.)

Risks of peripheral I.V. therapy

Peripheral I.V. therapy complications may be local or systemic. This chart lists some common complications along with their signs and symptoms, possible causes, and nursing interventions, including preventive measures.

Signs and symptoms	Possible causes

Local complications

Phlebitis
- Tenderness at and above tip of device
- Erythema at tip of catheter and along vein
- Vein hard on palpation
- Elevated temperature

- Poor blood flow around device
- Friction from catheter movement along vein
- Device left in vein too long or clot in cannula tip
- Solution with high or low pH or high osmolarity

Infiltration
- Swelling at and above I.V. site (may extend along entire limb)
- Discomfort, burning, or pain at site
- Feeling of tightness at site
- Blanching at site
- Continuing fluid infusion even when vein is occluded, although rate may decrease
- Absent blood backflow
- Skin cool to the touch around I.V. site

- Device dislodged from vein or perforated vein

Catheter dislodgment
- Catheter partly backed out of vein
- Infiltrated tissue
- Leaking of I.V. fluid at site

- Loosened tape or tubing snagged in bedclothes, resulting in partial retraction of catheter

Occlusion
- Infusion doesn't flow
- Infusion pump alarm reads "occlusion"
- Discomfort at insertion site

- I.V. flow interrupted
- Intermittent device not flushed regularly
- Blood backup in line
- Hypercoagulable patient
- Line clamped too long

Vein irritation or pain at I.V. site
- Pain during infusion
- Possible blanching if vasospasm occurs
- Red skin over vein during infusion
- Rapidly developing signs of phlebitis

- Solution with high or low pH or high osmolarity, such as 40 mEq/L of potassium chloride, phenytoin, and some antibiotics (vancomycin and nafcillin)

Nursing interventions	Prevention
• Remove device. • Apply warm pack. • Notify the practitioner. • Document the patient's condition and your interventions.	• Restart the infusion using a larger vein for irritating substances or restart with a smaller-gauge device to ensure adequate blood flow. • Secure the device to prevent dislodgment.
• Stop the infusion and remove the device. • Apply warm soaks to aid absorption. • Elevate the limb. • Periodically assess circulation by checking for pulse and capillary refill. • Restart infusion above the infiltration site or in another limb. • Document the patient's condition and your interventions.	• Check the I.V. site frequently (especially when using an I.V. pump). • Don't obscure the area above the site with tape. • Teach the patient to observe the I.V. site and report discomfort, pain, or swelling.
• Remove the catheter.	• Tape the device securely on insertion.
• Use mild flush pressure during injection; don't force. If unsuccessful, remove and reinsert the I.V. device.	• Maintain the I.V. flow rate. • Flush promptly after intermittent piggyback administration. • Have the patient walk with his arm below heart level to reduce risk of blood backup.
• Decrease the flow rate. • Try using an electronic flow device to achieve a steady, regulated flow.	• Dilute solutions before administration. For example, give antibiotics in a 250-mL solution rather than 100 mL. If the drug has a low pH, ask the pharmacist if it can be buffered with sodium bicarbonate. (Refer to your facility's policy.) • If long-term therapy of an irritating drug is planned, ask the practitioner to insert a central I.V. line.

(continued)

Risks of peripheral I.V. therapy *(continued)*

Signs and symptoms	Possible causes
Severed catheter • Leakage from catheter shaft	• Catheter inadvertently cut by scissors • Reinsertion of needle into catheter • Agitated patient
Hematoma • Tenderness at venipuncture site • Bruising around site	• Vein punctured through ventral wall at time of venipuncture • Leakage of blood into tissue
Venous spasm • Pain along vein • Sluggish flow rate when clamp is completely open • Blanched skin over vein	• Severe vein irritation from irritating drugs or fluids • Administration of cold fluids or blood • Very rapid flow rate (with fluids at room temperature)
Thrombosis • Painful, reddened, swollen, hard vein • Sluggish or stopped I.V. flow	• Injury to endothelial cells of vein wall, allowing platelets to adhere and thrombus to form
Thrombophlebitis • Severe discomfort • Reddened, swollen, and hardened vein	• Thrombosis and inflammation
Nerve, tendon, or ligament damage • Extreme pain (similar to electric shock when nerve is punctured) • Numbness and muscle contraction • Delayed effects, including paralysis, numbness, and deformity	• Improper venipuncture technique, resulting in injury to surrounding nerves, tendons, or ligaments • Tight taping or improper splinting with arm board

Nursing interventions	Prevention
• If the broken part is visible, attempt to retrieve it. If unsuccessful, notify the practitioner. • If a portion of the catheter enters the bloodstream, place a tourniquet above the I.V. site to prevent progression of broken portion. Notify the practitioner and the radiology department. • Document the patient's condition and your interventions.	• Don't use scissors around the I.V. site. • Never reinsert a needle into the catheter. • Remove an unsuccessfully inserted catheter and needle together. • Immediately remove a damaged catheter.
• Remove the device. • Apply pressure and cold compresses to the affected area. • Recheck for bleeding. • Document the patient's condition and your interventions.	• Choose a vein that can accommodate the size of the intended venous access device. • Release the tourniquet as soon as you achieve successful insertion.
• Apply warm soaks over the vein and surrounding area. • Slow the flow rate.	• Use a blood warmer for blood or packed red blood cells when appropriate.
• Remove the device; restart the infusion in the opposite limb if possible. • Apply warm soaks. • Watch for I.V. therapy-related infection (thrombi provide an excellent environment for bacterial growth). • Notify the practitioner.	• Use proper venipuncture techniques to reduce injury to the vein.
• Remove the device; restart the infusion in the opposite limb if possible. • Apply warm soaks. • Watch for I.V. therapy-related infection (thrombi provide an excellent environment for bacterial growth). • Notify the practitioner.	• Check the site frequently. Remove the device at the first sign of redness and tenderness.
• Stop the procedure and notify the practitioner.	• Know where the superficial nerves are and avoid placing an I.V. catheter close to their location. • Don't repeatedly penetrate tissues with the venipuncture device. • Don't apply excessive pressure when taping. Don't encircle the limb with tape. • Pad the arm board and, if possible, pad the tape securing the arm board.

(continued)

Risks of peripheral I.V. therapy *(continued)*

Signs and symptoms	Possible causes

Systemic complications

Circulatory overload
- Discomfort
- Jugular vein distention
- Respiratory distress
- Increased blood pressure
- Crackles
- Large positive fluid balance (Intake is greater than output.)

- Roller clamp loosened to allow run-on infusion
- Flow rate too rapid
- Miscalculation of fluid requirements
- Infusion pump failure

Systemic infection (septicemia or bacteremia)
- Fever, chills, and malaise for no apparent reason
- Contaminated I.V. site, usually with no visible signs of infection at site

- Failure to maintain aseptic technique during insertion or site care
- Severe phlebitis, which can set up ideal conditions for organism growth
- Poor securing that permits access device to move, which can introduce organisms into bloodstream
- Prolonged indwelling time of device
- Immunocompromised patient

Air embolism
- Respiratory distress
- Weak pulse
- Increased central venous pressure
- Decreased blood pressure
- Loss of consciousness

- Solution container empties; next container pushes air down line
- Disconnected lines allow air into system
- Failure of I.V. pump in-line air detector

Allergic reaction
- Itching
- Tearing eyes and runny nose
- Bronchospasm, wheezing
- Edema at I.V. site
- Urticarial rash
- Anaphylactic reaction, including flushing, chills, anxiety, agitation, generalized itching, palpitations, paresthesia, throbbing in ears, wheezing, coughing, seizures, and cardiac arrest

- Allergens such as medications

Nursing interventions	Prevention
• Raise the head of bed. • Administer oxygen as needed. • Slow the infusion rate. • Notify the practitioner. • Administer medications (probably furosemide) as ordered.	• Use a pump, volume-control set, or rate minder for elderly or compromised patients. • Recheck your calculations of fluid requirements. • Monitor the infusion frequently.
• Notify the practitioner. • Administer medications as prescribed. • Culture the site and device. • Monitor vital signs.	• Use scrupulous aseptic technique when handling solutions and tubings, inserting the venipuncture device, and discontinuing the infusion. • Secure all connections. • Change the I.V. solutions, tubing, and access device at recommended times.
• Discontinue the infusion. • Place the patient in left lateral Trendelenburg's position to allow air to enter the right atrium. • Administer oxygen. • Notify the practitioner. • Document the patient's condition and your interventions.	• Purge tubing or air completely before infusion. • Use an air-detection device on the pump or an air-eliminating filter proximal to the I.V. site. • Secure connections.
• If reaction occurs, stop the infusion immediately. Maintain I.V. access with a normal saline infusion. • Maintain a patent airway. • Notify the practitioner. • Administer antihistamine, corticosteroid, and antipyretic drugs as ordered. • Give aqueous epinephrine subcutaneously.	• Obtain the patient's allergy history. Be aware of cross-allergies. • Assist with test dosing. • Monitor the patient carefully during the first 15 minutes when administering new drugs.

- With the needle bevel side up, puncture the skin.
- Check the flash-back chamber behind the hub for blood return, signifying that the vein is accessed.
- If using a winged infusion set, advance the needle and hold it in place.
- If using an over-the-needle cannula, advance the catheter and remove the needle.
- Remove the tourniquet.
- Using sterile technique, attach the primed I.V. administration tubing.
- Secure the catheter with tape.
- Dispose of the stylet in a sharps container.
- Clean the area, apply a catheter securement device, and apply a transparent semipermeable dressing.
- Label the site and document the procedure according to your facility's protocol.

What to consider

- Remember that I.V. insertion at the antecubital fossa or dorsal veins may restrict movement in a conscious patient.
- Dorsal hand veins may be short and difficult to stabilize.
- If infiltration occurs, sites below the insertion site may be unusable.
- Accessing any peripheral vein may be difficult if the patient is in circulatory collapse.
- Drugs given peripherally take longer to reach central circulation during cardiac arrest. For this reason, raise the patient's arm after drug administration during cardiopulmonary resuscitation (CPR) and follow administration with a 20-mL bolus of normal saline solution.
- Hypertonic or irritating solutions shouldn't be administered through a peripheral vein.

External jugular vein

The external jugular vein is large and easily accessible. It's used when rapid I.V. access is desired. It's often used for patients in circulatory collapse or cardiac arrest when peripheral insertion in other places isn't attainable. Many facilities restrict cannulation of this site to physicians or advanced practice health care professionals. Know your facility's policy.

What you need

- Chlorhexidine solution
- Clean gloves

- I.V. access device with safety shield
- I.V. solution with attached and primed administration set
- I.V. pole
- Sharps container
- Transparent semipermeable dressing
- Catheter securement device or 1" hypoallergenic tape
- I.V. start kit (available in some facilities)

How it's done

- Position the patient in Trendelenburg's position to enhance your visualization of the vein.
- Turn the patient's head to the opposite side of insertion.
- Perform hand hygiene and put on gloves.
- Clean the site with the chlorhexidine solution and allow to dry.
- Anesthetize the skin if the patient is conscious.
- Remove the cover from the access device and make sure the needle is smooth and intact.
- With the bevel side up, aim the needle toward the ipsilateral (same side) shoulder.
- Stabilize the vein by holding the skin taut right above the clavicle.
- Insert the needle midway between the angle of the jaw and the midclavicular line.
- Check the flash-back chamber behind the hub for blood return, signifying that the vein has been accessed.
- If using an over-the-needle cannula, advance the catheter and remove the needle.
- If using a winged infusion set, advance the needle and hold it in place.
- Using sterile technique, attach the primed I.V. administration tubing.
- Dispose of the stylet in a sharps container.
- Secure the catheter with tape.
- Clean the area, apply a catheter securement device, and apply a transparent semipermeable dressing.
- Label the site and document the procedure according to your facility's protocol.

What to consider

- I.V. insertion into the external jugular vein requires more skill than insertion into other peripheral veins and is usually performed by a practitioner.
- Infiltration of I.V. solutions at this site may affect the patency of the patient's airway.
- Movement of the patient's head may affect the flow of I.V. solutions.

Establishing central I.V. lines

You can use the internal jugular, subclavian, and femoral veins to establish a nontunneled central I.V. access during an emergency or when a patient's peripheral veins are inaccessible. This procedure is usually restricted to physicians or advanced practice health care practitioners. In central venous (CV) therapy, drugs or fluids are infused directly into a major vein. (See *Comparing CV insertion sites.*)

Central I.V. lines are used for:

• infusing large volumes of fluid
• multiple infusions
• long-term I.V. therapy
• drawing blood samples
• measuring central venous pressure (CVP), an important indicator of circulatory function
• administering medications that may be irritating to peripheral veins
• administering hyperalimentation therapy.

> Here I am! Major Super Vein to help you gain central I.V. access.

Comparing CV insertion sites

This chart lists the most common insertion sites for a central venous (CV) catheter and the advantages and disadvantages of each.

Site	Advantages	Disadvantages
Subclavian vein	• Easy and fast access • Easier to keep dressing in place • High flow rate, which reduces the risk of thrombus	• Proximity to the subclavian artery (If artery is punctured during catheter insertion, hemorrhage can result.) • Difficult to control bleeding • Increased risk of pneumothorax
Internal jugular vein	• Short, direct route to superior vena cava • Catheter stability, resulting in less movement with respiration • Decreased risk of pneumothorax	• Proximity to the common carotid artery (If artery is punctured during catheter insertion, uncontrolled hemorrhage, emboli, or impedance to flow can result.) • Difficult to keep the dressing in place • Proximity to the trachea
Femoral vein	• Easy and fast access • No need to interrupt CPR to access • No risk of pneumothorax	• Less direct route • May have increased risk of infection due to location • Proximity to femoral artery and nerve • Site should be changed at first opportunity

The fewer, the better

The main advantage of central I.V. access is that it reduces the need for repeated venipunctures. Fewer venipunctures decrease the patient's anxiety and help to preserve or restore the peripheral veins.

However, using a CV catheter also has disadvantages. A CV catheter:
• requires more time and skill to insert than a peripheral I.V. catheter and is usually inserted by a practitioner
• costs more to maintain than a peripheral I.V. catheter
• carries a risk of pneumothorax during insertion or air embolism postinsertion and an increased risk of infection.

Central I.V. access is contraindicated when the patient has scar tissue in the area or the configuration of his lung apices doesn't lend itself to inserting a central I.V. line. Use caution if central I.V. access will interfere with the patient's surgical site or other therapy or his lifestyle or daily activities. (See *Risks of CV therapy,* pages 204 to 207.)

Key points

Central I.V. lines
• Access important in emergencies or when peripheral access inaccessible or inappropriate
• Usually inserted by physician or specially trained professional
• Allows hemodynamic monitoring
• Complication rate higher than with peripheral access
• Appropriate for hypertonic or irritating solutions, blood samples, and multiple infusions.

Internal jugular vein

The internal jugular vein is lateral and anterior to the common carotid artery. The right side is preferred for I.V. access because the lung and pleura are lower and there's a fairly straight line to the superior vena cava. You don't have to visualize the internal jugular vein to access it.

Hypertonic? Irritating? This vein's for you!

Use the internal jugular vein when peripheral venous access is unsuccessful or you need to measure CVP. It's useful for administering emergency medications and hypertonic or irritating solutions and inserting catheters into the heart and pulmonary circulation.

Fill it up! And check the fluids, please

The internal jugular vein allows direct access to the central circulation. It also allows for rapid administration of large volumes of fluid. In addition, multiple blood samples can be withdrawn through the catheter. Most facilities require using an infusion pump for infusing fluids through a central line.

Remember, you don't have to visualize the internal jugular vein to access it.

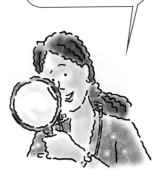

What you need
• Two (14 or 16G)CV catheters (antimicrobial-impregnated, if indicated)
• Central line introducer kit (available in most facilities)
• Sterile gown and gloves
• Sterile towel and large sterile drape
• Masks with shields, cap

Risks of CV therapy

As with any invasive procedure, central venous (CV) therapy can have complications. This chart outlines how to recognize, manage, and prevent these complications.

Signs and symptoms	Possible causes
Pneumothorax, hemothorax, chylothorax, or hydrothorax • Chest pain • Dyspnea • Cyanosis • Decreased breath sounds on affected side • With hemothorax, decreased hemoglobin because of blood pooling • Abnormal chest X-ray	• Lung puncture by catheter during insertion or exchange over a guide wire • Large blood vessel puncture with bleeding inside or outside of the lung • Lymph node puncture with leakage of lymph fluid • Infusion of solution into chest area through infiltrated catheter
Air embolism • Respiratory distress • Weak pulse • Increased CV pressure • Decreased blood pressure • Churning murmur over precordium • Change in level of consciousness	• Intake of air into CV system during catheter insertion or tubing changes; inadvertent opening, cutting, or breaking of catheter • Inadvertent disconnection of tubing
Thrombosis • Edema at or below puncture site • Ipsilateral swelling of arm, neck, and face • Fever spike, malaise • Tachycardia • Pain	• Sluggish flow rate • Hematopoietic status of the patient • Repeated or long-term use of same vein • Preexisting cardiovascular disease • Irritation of vein lining during insertion
Local infection • Redness, warmth, tenderness, and swelling at insertion or exit site • Possible exudate of purulent material • Local rash or pustules • Fever, chills, malaise • Pain	• Failure to maintain aseptic technique during catheter insertion or care or dressing changes • Wet or soiled dressing remaining on site • Immunosuppression • Irritated suture line

Nursing interventions	Prevention
• Notify the practitioner and stop the infusion. • Remove the catheter or assist with its removal, as ordered. • Administer oxygen, as ordered. • Set up for and assist with chest tube insertion. • Document your interventions.	• Position the patient's head down, with a towel roll between his scapulae, to dilate and expose the internal jugular or subclavian vein as much as possible during catheter insertion. • Assess for early signs of fluid infiltration, such as swelling in the shoulder, neck, chest, and arm area. • Ensure immobilization of the patient with adequate preparation for the procedure and restraint during the procedure; active patients may need to be sedated or taken to the operating room for CV catheter insertion. • Minimize patient activity after insertion, especially if a peripheral CV catheter is used. • Confirm CV catheter placement by X-ray.
• Clamp the catheter immediately. • Turn the patient on his left side with his head down so air can enter the right atrium. Maintain this position for 20 to 30 minutes or as ordered by the practitioner. • Don't have the patient perform Valsalva's maneuver. (A large intake of air will worsen the situation.) • Administer oxygen. • Notify the practitioner. • Document your interventions.	• Purge all air from the tubing before hookup. • Teach the patient to perform Valsalva's maneuver during catheter insertion and tubing changes. • Use an infusion-control device with air detection capability. • Use luer-lock tubing, tape connections, or use locking devices for all connections. • Use air-eliminating filters.
• Stop the infusion. • Notify the practitioner, who may remove the catheter. • Possibly, infuse a thrombolytic to dissolve the clot. • Verify thrombosis with diagnostic studies. • Don't use the limb on the affected side for subsequent venipuncture. • Document your interventions.	• Verify that the catheter tip is in the superior vena cava before use.
• Monitor the patient's temperature frequently. • Culture the site if drainage is present. • Redress aseptically. • Treat systemically, as ordered, with antibiotics or antifungals. • Notify the practitioner, who may remove the catheter and send the tip for culture. • Document your interventions.	• Maintain strict aseptic technique. Use cap, gloves, masks, and gowns when appropriate. • Adhere to dressing change protocols. • Change a wet or soiled dressing immediately. • Change the dressing more frequently if the catheter is located in the femoral area or near a tracheostomy. • Complete tracheostomy care after catheter care.

(continued)

Risks of CV therapy *(continued)*	
Signs and symptoms	Possible causes
Systemic infection • Fever, chills without other apparent reason • Leukocytosis • Nausea, vomiting • Malaise • Elevated urine glucose level	• Contaminated catheter • Failure to maintain aseptic technique during solution hookup • Frequent opening of catheter or long-term use of single I.V. access • Immunosuppression

- Skin preparation kit with chlorhexidine sponges
- Alcohol pads
- 3 mL syringe with 25G needle
- 1% or 2% injectable lidocaine
- Suture material
- Three 10-mL syringes filled with normal saline solution
- Catheter securement device or sterile tape
- Transparent semipermeable dressing

How it's done

- Explain the procedure to the patient and obtain consent as required. (In an emergency situation, steps in the procedure may need to be altered.)
- Confirm the patient's identity and perform a "time-out" verification process according to the facility's policy if possible.
- Perform hand hygiene.
- Place the patient in Trendelenburg's position to dilate the vein and reduce the risk of air embolism.
- Turn the patient's head in the opposite direction to make the site more accessible and to prevent site contamination from airborne pathogens.
- After establishing a sterile field on a table, open the catheter and central line insertion tray. Make sure to label all medications, medication containers, and other solutions on and off the sterile field.
- Put on a cap, mask, sterile gown, and gloves.

Nursing interventions	Prevention
• Draw central and peripheral blood cultures; if the same organism is present, the catheter is the primary source of sepsis and should be removed. • Treat the patient with an antibiotic regimen, as ordered. • Culture the tip of the catheter if removed. • Assess for other sources of infection. • Monitor the patient's vital signs closely. • Document your interventions.	• Examine the infusate for cloudiness and turbidity before infusing, and check the fluid container for leaks. • Monitor the urine glucose level in patients receiving total parenteral nutrition; if greater than 2+, suspect early sepsis. • Use strict sterile technique for hookup and disconnection of fluids. • Use a 0.2-micron filter. • The catheter may be changed frequently to decrease the chance of infection. • Keep the system closed as much as possible.

• Clean the area with the chlorhexidine sponge using a side-to-side motion for 30 seconds; allow the area to dry.
• The practitioner puts on a cap, mask, sterile gown, and gloves and then anesthetizes the area with 1% or 2% lidocaine.
• The practitioner locates the suprasternal notch and moves laterally until the clavicular head of the sternomastoid muscle is located. The carotid artery is identified by its pulse. The internal jugular vein runs lateral to the carotid artery.
• The practitioner inserts the needle with the bevel side up at the apex of the triangle formed by the two heads of the sternomastoid muscle and the clavicle. (See *The central approach*, page 208.)
• Negative pressure is maintained on the syringe as the needle is advanced. The vein is normally ¾ to 1½" (2 to 4 cm) deep.
• After the vein is accessed and before the caps are attached, the conscious patient is asked to perform Valsalva's maneuver, which increases the intrathoracic pressure, reducing the possibility of an air embolus. (See *Performing Valsalva's maneuver*, page 209.)
• After a blood return is visualized in the catheter, all ports are flushed with normal saline solution and the catheter is sutured in place.
• A chest X-ray is obtained to confirm placement of the line in the superior vena cava.
• After using an antimicrobial solution to remove any blood, secure the catheter and apply a dressing according to the facility's policy. Label the dressing with the date, time, and your initials.
• Remove your gloves, perform hand hygiene, and document the procedure.

Peak technique

The central approach

To perform the central approach for accessing the internal jugular vein, the practitioner:
* Places the patient in a supine position with his head turned toward the left side.
* Stands at the patient's head and locates the vessel.
* With the needle bevel side up, inserts it into the internal jugular vein.

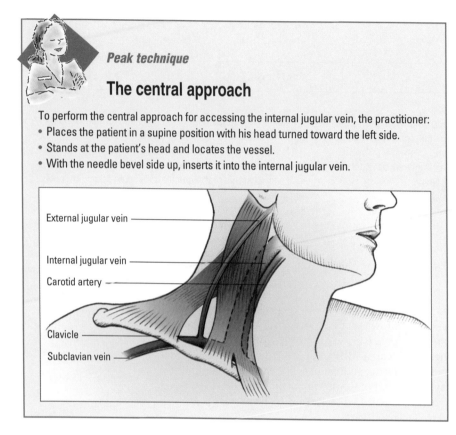

External jugular vein

Internal jugular vein

Carotid artery

Clavicle

Subclavian vein

What to consider

* Accessing the internal jugular vein requires more skill than accessing peripheral veins and is usually performed by a practitioner.
* You many need to interrupt CPR to access the internal jugular vein.
* Nearby structures (carotid artery, apical pleura, lymphatic ducts, and nerves) can be damaged.
* Using the internal jugular vein carries a higher risk of complications than peripheral I.V. access.

Subclavian vein

The subclavian vein lies beneath the clavicle. It's frequently used for I.V. access when peripheral venous access is unsuccessful. Generally, the subclavian is the preferred site, although during an emergency the internal jugular or common femoral vein may be easier and quicker to access.

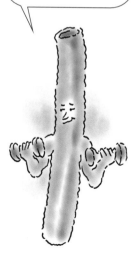

Nothing succeeds like access

The subclavian vein offers the opportunity to measure CV pressure. It's also indicated for administering hypertonic or irritating solutions and for inserting catheters into the heart and pulmonary circulation. More neck movement is possible with this site than with the internal jugular site.

What you need

- Two (14 or 16G) CV catheters (antimicrobial-impregnated if indicated)
- Central line kit (available in most facilities)
- Sterile gown and gloves
- Sterile towel and large sterile drape
- Masks with shields, cap
- Skin preparation kit with chlorhexidine sponges
- Alcohol pads
- 3-mL syringe with 25G needle
- 1% or 2% injectable lidocaine
- Suture material
- Three 10-mL syringes filled with normal saline solution
- Catheter securement device or sterile tape
- Transparent semipermeable dressing
- Rolled bath towel

How it's done

- Explain the procedure to the patient and obtain consent as required. (In an emergency situation, steps in the procedure may need to be altered.)
- Confirm the patient's identity and perform a "time-out" verification process according to the facility's policy if possible.
- Perform hand hygiene.
- Place the patient in Trendelenburg's position to dilate the vein and reduce the risk of air embolism.
- Place a rolled towel under the patient's opposite shoulder to extend his neck, making anatomic landmarks more visible.
- Turn the patient's head in the opposite direction to make the site more accessible and to prevent site contamination from airborne pathogens.
- After establishing a sterile field on a table, open the catheter and central line insertion tray. Make sure to label all medications, medication containers, and other solutions on and off the sterile field.
- Put on a cap, mask, sterile gown, and gloves.
- Clean the area with the chlorhexidine sponge using a side-to-side motion for 30 seconds; allow the area to dry.
- The practitioner puts on a cap, mask, sterile gown, and gloves and then anesthetizes the area with 1% or 2% lidocaine.

Performing Valsalva's maneuver

Use Valsalva's maneuver as a diagnostic tool for patients with suspected heart abnormalities or as a treatment measure for patients with an abnormal heart rhythm.

How it's done

To perform Valsalva's maneuver, instruct your patient to:
• forcibly exhale while keeping his mouth and nose closed, and bear down (as if having a bowel movement)
• blow against an aneroid pressure measuring device (manometer) and maintain a pressure of 40 mm Hg for 30 seconds.

What happens

Performing Valsalva's maneuver causes specific changes in blood pressure and the rate and volume of blood returning to the heart. Characteristic heart sounds that indicate a heart abnormality can be auscultated during the maneuver. When performed by patients with a rapid heart rate, the maneuver may cause the heart to correct its rhythm and slow its rate.

What to consider

Valsalva's maneuver shouldn't be performed by patients who have:
• severe coronary artery disease
• experienced a recent heart attack
• a severe reduction in blood volume.
    Possible complications include:
• dizziness or syncope
• detachment of blood clots
• abnormal ventricular rhythm
• cardiac arrest.

• The practitioner locates the suprasternal notch and moves laterally until the clavicular head of the sternomastoid muscle is located. The carotid artery is identified by its pulse. The internal jugular vein runs lateral to the carotid artery.
• The practitioner inserts the needle with the bevel side inferior to the clavicle at the deltopectoral groove.
• Negative pressure is maintained on the syringe as the needle is advanced. A guide wire is introduced and the catheter is threaded over the guidewire.
• After the vein is accessed and before the caps are attached, the conscious patient is asked to perform Valsalva's maneuver, which increases the intrathoracic pressure, reducing the possibility of an air embolus. (See *Performing Valsalva's maneuver.*)
• After a blood return is visualized in the catheter, all ports are flushed with normal saline solution and the catheter is sutured in place.
• A chest X-ray is obtained to confirm placement of the line in the superior vena cava.
• After using an antimicrobial solution to remove dried blood, secure the catheter and apply a dressing according to the facility's policy. Label the dressing with the date, time, and your initials.
• Remove your gloves, perform hand hygiene, and document the procedure.

What to consider

- Accessing the subclavian vein requires more skill than is needed to access peripheral veins. (This procedure is performed by a practitioner.)
- You may need to interrupt CPR to access the subclavian vein.
- Nearby structures (carotid artery, apical pleura, lymphatic ducts, and nerves) can be damaged.
- Using the subclavian vein carries a higher risk of complications than peripheral access.
- Using the subclavian vein carries a higher risk of pleural puncture than the internal jugular vein.
- Hematomas may not be readily visible and aren't easily compressible.

Femoral vein

The femoral vein lies medial to the femoral artery below the inguinal ligament. Use the femoral vein only as a temporary access when you need rapid I.V. access, primarily for patients in circulatory collapse or cardiac arrest.

It's a wonderful site

You don't need to interrupt CPR when accessing the femoral vein. Also, you may easily access the femoral vein when peripheral veins have collapsed. In addition, a long catheter can be passed through this site above the diaphragm to access the central circulation.

What you need

- Two (14 or 16G) CV catheters (antimicrobial-impregnated if indicated)
- Central line introducer kit (available in most facilities)
- Sterile gown and gloves
- Sterile towel and large sterile drape
- Masks with shields, cap
- Skin preparation kit with chlorhexidine sponges
- Alcohol pads
- 3-mL syringe with 25G needle
- 1% or 2% injectable lidocaine
- Suture material
- I.V. solution with attached and primed administration set
- Infusion pump
- Three 10-mL syringes filled with normal saline solution
- Transparent semipermeable dressing

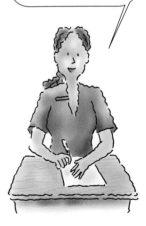

The femoral vein is used to gain rapid I.V. access for patients in circulatory collapse or cardiac arrest.

How it's done

• Explain the procedure to the patient and obtain consent as required. (In an emergency situation, steps in the procedure may need to be altered.)
• Confirm the patient's identity and perform a "time-out" verification process according to the facility's policy if possible.
• Place the patient in a supine position with his hip on the desired side in a neutral or slightly externally rotated position.
• After establishing a sterile field on a table, open the catheter and central line insertion tray. Make sure to label all medications, medication containers, and other solutions on and off the sterile field.
• Put on a cap, mask, sterile gown, and gloves.
• Clean the area with the chlorhexidine sponge using a side-to-side motion for 30 seconds; allow the area to dry.
• The practitioner puts on a cap, mask, sterile gown, and gloves and then anesthetizes the area with 1% or 2% lidocaine.
• The practitioner locates the femoral artery by palpating the femoral artery pulse; the femoral vein will lie just medial to the pulsation.
• The practitioner attachs a 10-mL syringe to the needle. The needle is aligned with the vein and is pointed toward the patient's head.
• The needle is inserted with the bevel up at a 45-degree angle to the skin.
• Negative pressure is maintained on the syringe until blood appears.
• The needle is lowered to be more parallel with the patient's leg and the catheter is advanced.
• Either connect the I.V. solution or cap and flush the line with normal saline solution.
• The catheter may be secured with a suture.
• After using an antimicrobial solution to remove any blood, secure the catheter and apply a dressing according to your facility's policy. Label the dressing with the date, time, and your initials.
• Remove your gloves, perform hand hygiene, and document the procedure.

What to consider

• Complications include excess bleeding (especially if the artery was traumatized), pseudoaneurysm, significant hematoma, arteriovenous fistula, venous thromboembolism, and leg ischemia.
• More skill is required to access the femoral vein. (This procedure is performed by a practitioner.)
• The femoral vein may be difficult to locate if the femoral artery pulse isn't palpable.
• The femoral artery may not be readily apparent in a patient in cardiac arrest because of low arterial pressure.
• Keeping dressings clean and the catheter secure in this area may be difficult.

Establishing intraosseous access

During emergency situations, when rapid venous access is difficult or impossible, intraosseous (I.O.) access allows the safe and effective short-term delivery of fluids, medications, or blood into the bone marrow for all age groups. Any drug that can be given I.V. can be given by the I.O. route with comparable absorption and effectiveness, and the effects of that drug are more predictable compared to drugs given by endotracheal tube. I.O. access can also be used to obtain blood samples for laboratory analysis. In addition, CPR doesn't have to be interrupted to establish an I.O. infusion.

Unshockable!

In shock, blood is shunted away from the peripheral vessels and to the central circulation, often making peripheral I.V. access difficult or impossible. In contrast, the highly vascular, noncompressible intraosseous space within bone remains unchanged during shock. In I.O. access, the venous sinusoids within the bone provide access to the circulation during emergency treatment. During cardiac arrest, establishing an I.O. access may be quicker than establishing either central or peripheral venous access.

I.O. infusion is commonly undertaken at the anterior surface of the tibia. Alternative sites include the iliac crest, spinous process and, rarely, the upper anterior portion of the sternum. Only personnel trained in this procedure should perform it. Usually, a nurse assists. (See *Understanding intraosseous infusion*, page 214.)

I.O. infusion is contraindicated in patients with osteogenesis imperfecta, osteoporosis, and ipsilateral fracture because of the potential for subcutaneous extravasation. I.O. infusion is also contraindicated through an area of cellulitis or an infected burn because of the increased risk of infection.

What you need

- Bone marrow biopsy needle or specially designed I.O. infusion needle (cannula and obturator) or bone injection device
- Antiseptic pads
- Antiseptic ointment
- Sterile gauze pads
- Sterile gloves
- Sterile drape
- Syringe with flush solution
- I.V. fluids and tubing
- 1% or 2% lidocaine
- 3- to 5-mL syringe

Understanding intraosseous infusion

During intraosseous infusion, the bone marrow serves as a noncollapsible vein; thus, fluid infused into the narrow cavity rapidly enters the circulation by way of an extensive network of venous sinusoids. Here, the needle is shown positioned in the patient's tibia.

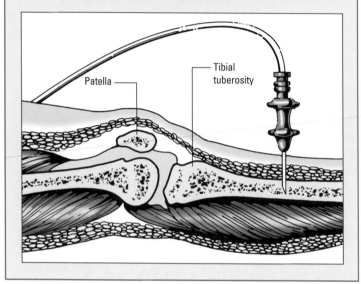

Patella

Tibial tuberosity

- Tape
- Sterile occlusive dressing
- Sterile marker and sterile labels
- Sedative, if prescribed

How it's done

- If possible, confirm the patient's identity using two patient identifiers according to your facility's policy. (In an emergency, you may need to alter steps in the procedure.)
- If the patient is conscious, explain the procedure to allay his fears and promote his cooperation. If time permits, ensure that the patient understands the procedure and a consent form has been signed.
- Tell the patient which bone site will be infused. Inform him that he will receive a local anesthetic (check for allergies) and will feel pressure from needle insertion.
- Perform hand hygiene.
- Administer a sedative, if prescribed, before the procedure following safe medication administration practices.
- Position the patient based on the selected puncture site.
- Perform hand hygiene again and put on sterile gloves.

• Using sterile technique, the practitioner cleans the puncture site with an antiseptic pad and allows it to dry. He then covers the area with a sterile drape.
• Using sterile technique, hand the practitioner the 3- or 5-mL syringe with 1% lidocaine so that he can anesthetize the infusion site.
• The practitioner inserts the infusion needle through the skin and into the bone at an angle of 10 to 15 degrees from vertical. He advances it with a forward and backward rotary motion through the periosteum until the needle penetrates the marrow cavity. Or, he uses the bone injection device to deliver the needle. The needle should "give" suddenly as it enters the marrow and should stand erect when released.
• The practitioner removes the obturator from the needle and attaches a 5-mL syringe. He aspirates some bone marrow to confirm needle placement.
• The practitioner replaces this syringe with the syringe containing the flush solution and flushes the cannula to confirm needle placement and clear the cannula of clots or bone particles.
• The practitioner removes the syringe of flush solution and attaches I.V. tubing to the cannula to allow infusion of medications and I.V. fluids.
• Clean the infusion site with antiseptic pads; then secure the site with tape and a sterile gauze dressing.
• Monitor the patient's vital signs and check the infusion site for bleeding and extravasation.
• Remove and discard your gloves, perform hand hygiene, and document the procedure according to the facility's policy.

What to consider

• I.O. infusion should be discontinued as soon as conventional vascular access is established (within 2 to 4 hours, if possible, and no more than 24 hours). Prolonged infusion significantly increases the risk of infection.
• After the needle has been removed, apply firm pressure to the site for 5 minutes and place antiseptic ointment and a sterile occlusive dressing over the injection site.
• I.O. flow rates are determined by needle size and flow through the bone marrow. Fluids should flow freely if needle placement is correct and infusion pumps should be used.
• Possible complications of I.O. infusion include extravasation of fluid into subcutaneous tissue resulting from incorrect needle placement, subperiosteal effusion resulting from failure of fluid to enter the marrow space, and clotting in the needle resulting from delayed infusion or failure to flush the needle after placement. Other complications include subcutaneous abscess, osteomyelitis (rarely), and epiphyseal injury.

Position the patient for an I.O. infusion based on the selected puncture site.

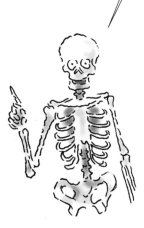

Key points

Intraosseous infusions
• During emergencies, intraosseous (I.O.) infusions may be quicker to start than peripheral or central line infusions.
• I.O. access can be used to obtain blood samples.
• I.O. infusions can be used for any I.V. medications, fluids, or blood products.
• I.O. infusions provide more predictable dosing than drug doses through an endotracheal tube.
• An I.O. access can be used only for 24 hours.

Invasive techniques

Emergency invasive techniques, such as pericardiocentesis and needle thoracostomy, are sometimes needed to restore cardiac function or treat cardiac arrest. A practitioner should perform these procedures, with the nurse assisting. While there are risks to invasive techniques, the ultimate advantage is that the procedure may save the patient's life, therefore outweighing the risk of complications that may occur.

Pericardiocentesis

Pericardiocentesis is the aspiration of fluid or blood with a needle from the pericardial sac surrounding the heart. It's indicated to relieve cardiac tamponade (fluid or blood in the pericardial sac) or to obtain fluid for diagnostic studies. (See *Cardiac tamponade.*) Pericardiocentesis is contraindicated in cardiac tamponade without evidence of hemodynamic instability; surgical treatment is safer.

Complications of pericardiocentesis include:
* cardiac arrhythmias
* puncture of the heart or its vessels
* inadvertent introduction of air into the heart chambers
* hemothorax
* pneumothorax
* hemorrhage from myocardial or coronary artery puncture or laceration.

What you need

* Electrocardiogram monitor, pulse oximeter
* Resuscitative equipment
* Sterile alligator clip connected to V_1 lead
* Sterile 14G, 16G, and 18G 4″ or 5″ cardiac needles
* 50-mL syringe with luer lock tip and three-way stop cock
* Antiseptic solution (2% chlorhexidine-based)
* Syringe with 1% or 2% lidocaine for anesthesia
* Sterile gloves and gown
* Sterile drapes
* Caps, masks with shields
* Sterile 4″ × 4″ dressing and gauze pads
* Tape
* Sterile marker, labels, and specimen container

How it's done

* Conduct the pre-procedure verification process. Confirm the patient's identity using two patient identifiers according to the facility's policy.

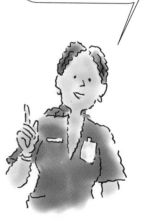

An invasive technique is used to restore your patient's cardiac function or prevent cardiac arrest.

Cardiac tamponade

Pericardiocentesis is typically used to treat cardiac tamponade, a condition in which fluid or blood fills the pericardial sac causing a decrease in ventricular filling.

Causes
- Trauma, cardiac surgery
- Infection
- Neoplastic disease
- Myocardial infarction or rupture
- Uremia
- Collagen-vascular disease
- Cardiopulmonary resuscitation
- Radiation or drug reactions
- Perforation of the heart or its vessels by a vascular catheter

Signs and symptoms
- Hypotension (due to decreased ventricular filling and decreased contractility of the heart)
- Jugular vein distention
- Muffled heart sounds
- Pulsus paradoxus (a decline greater than 10 mm Hg in systolic pressure with normal inspiration)
- Dyspnea or cyanosis
- Signs of shock
- Decreasing voltage of electrocardiogram complexes

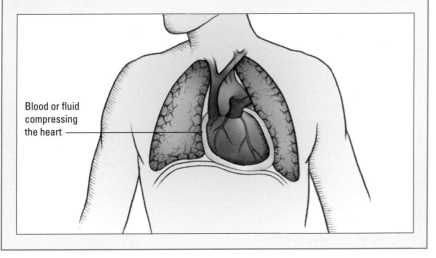

Blood or fluid compressing the heart

- Give an I.V. bolus of normal saline solution to transiently increase filling pressures while preparing to perform pericardiocentesis, if appropriate.
- Explain the procedure to the patient
- Create a sterile field on a table. Label all medications, medication containers, and other solutions on and off the sterile field.
- Place the patient in a supine position or elevate his head 60 degrees and attach cardiac monitoring leads.
- Perform hand hygiene (this applies to both the practitioner and the nurse) and put on caps, masks, sterile gowns and gloves.
- Conduct a "time-out."

- Clean the area (left fifth intercostal space) with antiseptic solution.
- Anesthetize the area with 1% lidocaine.
- The practitioner attaches the 50-mL syringe to one end of the 3-way stop cock and the cardiac needle to the other. The V_1 lead of the electrocardiogram may be attached to the hub of the aspirating needle using the alligator clips.
- The practitioner slowly inserts the needle perpendicular to the patient's chest into the pericardial sac and aspirates the fluid. (Removing as little as 5 to 10 mL of fluid can improve cardiac performance.) (See *Aspirating pericardial fluid.*)
- Remove the needle after the pericardial fluid is withdrawn and send the fluid to the laboratory for analysis. Apply pressure to the site with sterile gauze pads for 3 to 5 minutes.
- Place a sterile dressing over the site and tape it securely.
- Remove personal protective equipment, perform hand hygiene, and obtain a post procedure chest X-ray.
- Document the procedure.

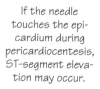

If the needle touches the epicardium during pericardiocentesis, ST-segment elevation may occur.

What to consider

- Continually monitor the patient's cardiac rhythm, vital signs, and oxygen saturation level during the procedure. If the needle touches the epicardium, ST-segment elevation may occur.
- Removal of fluid from the pericardial sac should produce immediate improvement in the patient's symptoms. Grossly bloody fluid aspirate may indicate inadvertent puncture of a cardiac chamber.
- Blood obtained from the pericardial space won't clot. (Blood is defibrinated from agitation during myocardial contraction; in addition, this blood will have a lower hematocrit than venous blood.)
- Be alert to the possibility that emergency thoracostomy may be needed. Prepare the patient for surgery if necessary.

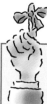

Caution

Needle thoracostomy

Needle thoracostomy may be necessary during a cardiac arrest to treat tension pneumothorax (caused by air entering the pleural space) by removing air from the pleural space, relieving pressure on the lungs, heart, trachea, and great vessels. When tension pneumothorax occurs, needle thoracostomy must be performed as soon as possible to improve oxygenation, ventilation, and cardiac output and stabilize the patient until a chest tube is inserted.

Give me a sign

Signs and symptoms of tension pneumothorax include:
- dyspnea, tachypnea, absent breath sounds on the affected side
- chest pain, tachycardia
- jugular vein distention
- deviated trachea (away from the affected side)

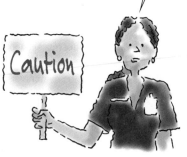

Memory jogger

Use the acronym **ACT** to remember the signs and symptoms of tension pneumothorax so that you can "act" fast to protect your patient:

Acute respiratory distress

Chest wall motion that's asymmetrical

Tracheal shifting.

- initial hypertension, followed by hypotension
- hyperresonance on injured side
- increasing difficulty when using a bag-mask device to manually ventilate an intubated patient.

Damage control

Complications of needle thoracostomy include damage to vessels or nerves or pleural infection. If the patient has suffered only simple pneumothorax, needle thoracostomy converts it to open pneumothorax. If the patient had no pneumothorax, needle thoracostomy produces pneumothorax.

What you need

- Antiseptic solution
- 14G catheter with a one-way valve
- Sterile gloves
- 4 × 4 gauze dressing, tape

Peak technique

Aspirating pericardial fluid

To perform pericardiocentesis, the practitioner inserts a needle with a syringe through the chest wall into the pericardial sac (as shown below). Electrocardiogram (ECG) monitoring, with a leadwire attached to the needle and electrodes placed on the limbs (right arm [RA], left arm [LA], and left leg [LL]), helps ensure proper placement and avoid damage to the heart.

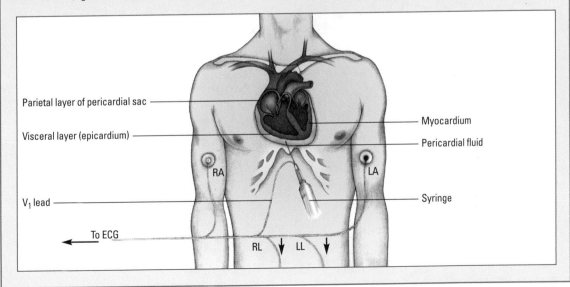

How it's done

- Confirm the patient's identity using two patient identifiers according to the facility's policy.
- Explain the procedure to the patient. Tell him he may feel some discomfort and a sensation of pressure when the needle is inserted.
- Obtain baseline vital signs and assess respiratory function.
- You may give a sedative as ordered.
- Perform hand hygiene and put on personal protective equipment.
- Elevate the head of the bed and expose the patient's entire chest.
- Conduct a " time-out" before starting the procedure.
- Remind the patient not to cough, breathe deeply, or move suddenly during the procedure to avoid puncture of the visceral pleura or lung.
- Using sterile technique, put on sterile gloves, open the equipment, and clean the site.

Peak technique

Landmarks for needle thoracostomy

Needle thoracostomy is an emergency procedure performed when the patient has hemothorax or pneumothorax. Typically, an expert practitioner accesses the second intercostal space if pneumothorax is suspected and the fifth intercostal space if hemothorax is suspected.

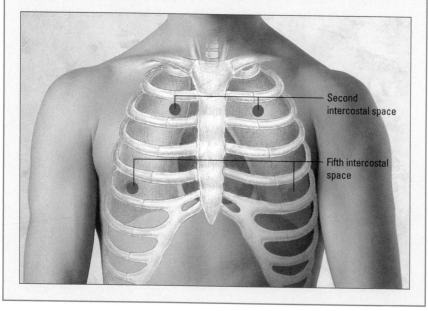

• The practitioner inserts the needle into the second intercostal space in the midclavicular line, just above the top of the third rib on the injured side; alternatively, he may insert the needle into the fifth intercostal space in the midaxillary line on the injured side. (See *Landmarks for needle thoracostomy.*)
• When the pleural space is entered, you'll hear the air escape.
• The needle is removed and the one-way valve is attached to the catheter. The valve prevents air from entering the pleural space and allows air inside the pleural space to escape.
• The catheter may be left in place until a chest tube is inserted.
• Secure the flutter valve with the 4 × 4 gauze dressing and tape.
• Remove personal protective equipment, perform hand hygiene, and document the procedure.

What to consider
• Monitor the patient's vital signs, cardiac rhythm, and oxygenation saturation during the procedure.
• Provide supplemental oxygen.
• Prepare the patient for chest tube insertion.

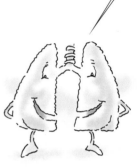

Remember to monitor your patient's oxygen saturation during needle thoracostomy.

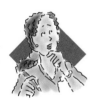

Quick quiz

1. A local complication of I.V. therapy is:
    A. phlebitis.
    B. sepsis.
    C. air embolism.
    D. catheter-fragment embolism.

Answer: A. Phlebitis is a local complication of I.V. therapy. The other options are considered systemic complications.

2. You're performing CPR on a patient with a peripheral I.V. line in the antecubital vein. Which intervention would best help get medications to the central circulation?
    A. Increase the rate of chest compressions for 1 to 2 minutes after drug administration.
    B. Give a 20-mL bolus of normal saline solution and raise the arm.
    C. Give all I.V. medications over 1 to 2 seconds.
    D. Pause respirations during I.V. medication administration.

Answer: B. Medications administered peripherally take a longer time to reach the central circulation than those given through a central vein. To assist drugs in reaching the central circulation sooner, give a 20-mL bolus of normal saline solution and raise the arm after medication administration.

3.   After inserting a subclavian line, it's necessary to obtain a chest X-ray to:
    A.   confirm correct placement.
    B.   identify hematomas.
    C.   rule out air embolism.
    D.   check for fluid overload.

Answer: A. A chest X-ray can confirm that the subclavian line catheter tip is in the superior vena cava. If the catheter tip is in the right atrium or ventricle instead, it may cause cardiac arrhythmias or perforation. A chest X-ray is also ordered to check for pneumothorax—a complication of CV therapy.

4.   The preferred peripheral access site for a patient in cardiac arrest is the:
    A.   external jugular vein.
    B.   most distal site (usually the hand).
    C.   antecubital fossa.
    D.   saphenous vein.

Answer: C. During cardiac arrest, peripheral veins in the upper extremities are preferred. The largest and easiest to access are typically those in the antecubital fossa.

5.   Immediate treatment for cardiac tamponade involves:
    A.   pericardiocentesis.
    B.   emergency thoracotomy.
    C.   needle thoracostomy.
    D.   emergency pericardial window.

Answer: A. The immediate, life-saving treatment for cardiac tamponade is pericardiocentesis. Surgery may be necessary after the procedure to fully correct the condition.

Scoring

⭐⭐⭐ If you answered all five questions correctly, spectacular! You've accessed a perfect score.

⭐⭐ If you answered four questions correctly, way to go! You're in a very therapeutic range.

⭐ If you answered fewer than four questions correctly, nice effort! After a quick review, you'll be "pumped" for a perfect score next time.

Treatment algorithms

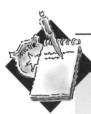

Just the facts

In this chapter, you'll learn:

♦ basic use of algorithms

♦ appropriate use of the adult cardiac arrest algorithm

♦ applications of the algorithms for pulseless arrest, brady-cardia, tachycardia, and acute coronary syndromes.

Understanding algorithms

Algorithms are memory aids that quickly summarize the key information you need to know when treating patients in emergencies. Algorithms are helpful, concise tools to use when studying for the advanced cardiac life support (ACLS) course. When used properly, an algorithm can point you quickly to an assessment (observation) or intervention (action) step and serve as an initial treatment approach for a broad range of patients.

Remember the golden rule

Keep these points in mind when using algorithms:
• They tend to oversimplify the complex processes of assessment and intervention.
• They aren't standards of care in a legal sense; therefore, they can't replace clinical understanding.

Remember that in any patient care situation, the rule is always to treat the patient, not the algorithm. Aim to remain flexible because the patient may require care not covered by an algorithm. Never let an algorithm limit your treatment of the patient.

Multitasking matters

Although algorithms appear sequential, they aren't. Most resuscitations require multiple, simultaneous assessments and interventions. It isn't unusual to "jump" between several algorithms during a cardiac arrest, depending on the patient's rhythm, vital

Classification of intervention recommendations

The American Heart Association and the American College of Cardiology have issued an evidence-based classification of recommendations for treatment interventions. The classification is as follows:

- Class I—The action has a benefit that greatly outweighs its risk.
- Class IIa—The action has more of a benefit than a risk and is reasonable to perform.
- Class IIb—The action has a slightly better benefit or is equal to the risk and may be considered.
- Class III—The action has more of a risk than a benefit and shouldn't be performed.

Source: *2010 American Heart Association Guidelines for Cardiopulmonary Resuscitation and Emergency Cardiovascular Care.* © 2010, American Heart Association.

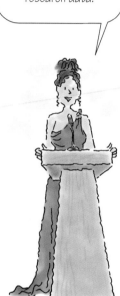

It isn't just a matter of class. Treatment recommendations are based on current research data.

signs, level of consciousness (LOC), and response to treatment. For this reason, treatment recommendations are based on current research findings. The ultimate goal of treatment is return of spontaneous circulation (ROSC). The American Heart Association (AHA) and the American College of Cardiology issue an evidence-based classification of intervention recommendations based on the risk-benefit ratio. (See *Classification of intervention recommendations.*)

Adult BLS health care providers algorithm

The adult basic life support (BLS) health care providers algorithm begins with a basic step-by-step assessment, which applies to all adult patients and is recommended as the initial step in all ACLS situations. It emphasizes high-quality cardiopulmonary resuscitation (CPR) and early defibrillation. This approach helps keep team members organized and is useful before, during, and after resuscitation. Follow the BLS health care providers algorithm whenever you find a person collapsed. (See *Adult BLS health care providers algorithm.*)

Back to basics

Remember these basic concepts when using the adult BLS health care providers algorithm:

- When a patient is in cardiac arrest, cerebral resuscitation is of utmost importance.

Go with the flow

Adult BLS health care providers algorithm

This algorithm shows the steps to follow when you suspect cardiac arrest in an adult patient.

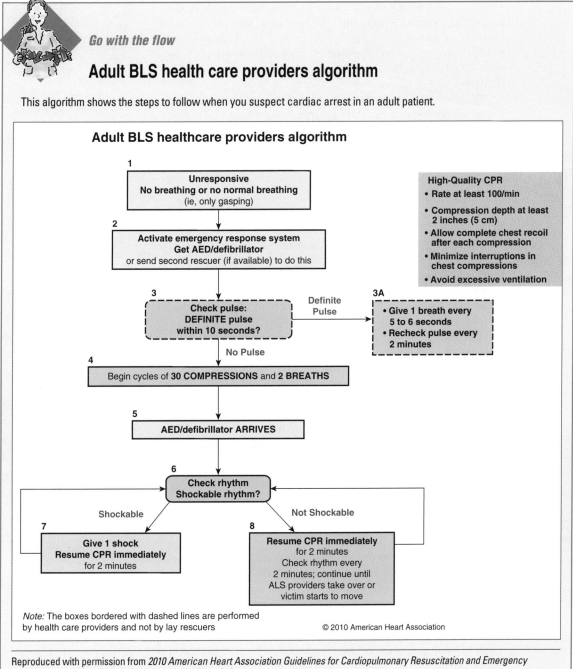

Adult BLS healthcare providers algorithm

1
Unresponsive
No breathing or no normal breathing
(ie, only gasping)

2
Activate emergency response system
Get AED/defibrillator
or send second rescuer (if available) to do this

High-Quality CPR
- Rate at least 100/min
- Compression depth at least 2 inches (5 cm)
- Allow complete chest recoil after each compression
- Minimize interruptions in chest compressions
- Avoid excessive ventilation

3
Check pulse:
DEFINITE pulse
within 10 seconds?

Definite Pulse →

3A
- Give 1 breath every 5 to 6 seconds
- Recheck pulse every 2 minutes

No Pulse

4
Begin cycles of **30 COMPRESSIONS** and **2 BREATHS**

5
AED/defibrillator ARRIVES

6
Check rhythm
Shockable rhythm?

Shockable

Not Shockable

7
Give 1 shock
Resume CPR immediately
for 2 minutes

8
Resume CPR immediately
for 2 minutes
Check rhythm every
2 minutes; continue until
ALS providers take over or
victim starts to move

Note: The boxes bordered with dashed lines are performed
by health care providers and not by lay rescuers

© 2010 American Heart Association

• When caring for a patient, always maintain standard precautions. This requires, at minimum, gloved hands and usually an airway barrier device for CPR.

• After you perform an intervention, reassess the patient to see what effect your action has caused and adjust later actions accordingly.

The adult BLS health care providers algorithm is divided into the initial finding and circulation, airway, breathing, and defibrillation (CABD) assessments and actions.

Initial finding

The initial finding occurs when you suspect a patient has collapsed as a result of cardiac arrest. Although cardiac arrest is a likely cause, people can lose consciousness for many reasons.

When you suspect a patient is unconscious, follow these steps:

• Assess his responsiveness by shaking him and shouting or touching him and shouting, "Are you OK?" Assessing responsiveness is always the first step because a patient may only be sleeping or may have fainted. Also check the patient for no breathing or no normal breathing (gasping).

• If the patient is responsive (he arouses), you should observe him and support his hemodynamic stability. Accessing the emergency medical service (EMS) is still warranted for follow-up because the patient may be responsive but may still require oxygen, an I.V. line, or medications to maintain stability.

• If the patient isn't responsive (doesn't arouse) and breathing isn't normal, assume the patient is in cardiac arrest and activate the EMS immediately. Call "911" or activate the in-hospital "cardiac arrest" emergency response system.

• After you've activated the EMS, begin the CABD sequence of steps.

Circulation

Assess the patient's circulation. Palpate no longer than 10 seconds for a carotid pulse. If a pulse is present, continue rescue breathing by delivering one ventilation every 5 to 6 seconds. Monitor the patient by checking his pulse every 2 minutes and wait for the EMS to arrive.

If you are unable to detect a pulse within 10 seconds, give 30 compressions followed by two ventilations. The compression rate should be at least 100/minute. Push hard and fast. The depth of compressions should be at least 2 inches (5 cm). Allow the chest to recoil after each compression. Continue this for five cycles

---

Key points

Using basic life support skills in C-A-B-D sequence

• Skills apply to all acute cardiac life support situations.

• Skills promote return of spontaneous circulation.

• Establish responsiveness of collapsed patient.

• Circulation: If no pulse, provide effective chest compressions (hard and fast).

• Airway: Open and maintain a patent airway.

• Breathing: Give each breath over 1 second to produce a visible chest rise.

• Defibrillation: Obtain a defibrillator or an automatic external difibrillator, identify shockable rhythm, and defibrillate as soon as possible.

(about 2 minutes) before rechecking for a pulse. When a monitor, automated external defibrillator (AED), or conventional defibrillator is available, attach it to the patient. Minimize interruptions in chest compressions.

Airway

Make sure the patient has a patent airway. To open his airway, open his mouth using the basic CPR head-tilt, chin-lift maneuver. As a health care provider, if you suspect neck injury, use the jaw-thrust maneuver. If the jaw-thrust maneuver doesn't effectively open the airway, use the head-tilt, chin-lift maneuver.

Breathing

If the unresponsive patient has adequate breathing and a pulse, place him in the recovery position because this position helps facilitate breathing. If he has a pulse but adequate breathing isn't present, ventilate the patient with a pocket face mask (preferably with a one-way valve) or bag-mask device at a rate of one breath every 5 to 6 seconds. Each breath should be delivered over 1 second and should produce a visible chest rise. Avoid overventilation. During CPR, use a compression-to-ventilation rate of 30 chest compressions to two ventilations. When an advanced airway is placed, give one ventilation every 6 to 8 seconds.

Defibrillation

Early recognition and rapid defibrillation of ventricular fibrillation (VF) and pulseless ventricular tachycardia (VT) are key to surviving cardiac arrest. After identifying that the patient is unresponsive and pulseless, the lone BLS health care provider rescuer activates the EMS, brings the AED or defibrillator to the patient, and applies it. If a shockable rhythm is identified, the rescuer defibrillates the patient and, if necessary, resumes CPR, beginning with compressions for 2 minutes, and then checks for a shockable rhythm again. The rescuer repeats this cycle until the patient starts to move, or ACLS providers take over. (If a defibrillator rather than an AED is used, defibrillate using 100 to 200 joules of biphasic energy or 360 joules of monophasic energy.) If two or more BLS health care provider rescuers are present, one rescuer initiates CPR, beginning with compressions, while the second rescuer activates the EMS, obtains the AED or defibrillator, and applies it. If a shockable rhythm is identified, the patient is defibrillated immediately and both rescuers resume CPR, beginning with compressions for 2 minutes; then the rhythm is checked again. This cycle is repeated until the patient starts to move or until ACLS providers take over.

Cardiac arrest algorithm

The cardiac arrest algorithm covers the actions you'll need to perform when treating VF, pulseless VT, asystole, and pulseless electrical activity (PEA). Surviving these lethal rhythms depends upon effective BLS, ACLS, and post–cardiac arrest care. (See *Adult cardiac arrest algorithm*.)

VF or pulseless VT

VF is the most common rhythm for a patient in cardiac arrest and rapid defibrillation is key to survival.

First steps

Begin treatment on a collapsed patient by following the BLS health care providers algorithm. If the cardiac arrest is witnessed or when the patient is being monitored by an electrocardiogram (ECG), shout for help, activate the emergency response system, and follow the ACLS adult cardiac arrest algorithm. Provide high-quality CPR with hard and fast compressions of at least 100/minute. Minimize interruptions in compressions whenever possible. Administer oxygen when available. Once a monitor or defibrillator is available, have the second rescuer attach it to the patient and confirm VF or VT.

Defibrillation

Defibrillate the patient with 360 joules if you're using a traditional monophasic defibrillator. (If you're using a biphasic defibrillator, use 120 to 200 joules). If you're using an AED, follow the prompts to shock the patient.

After you shock the patient, resume CPR for five cycles and then check his rhythm. If VF or pulseless VT persists, defibrillate the patient again at 360 joules (or the biphasic equivalent) or as prompted by the AED.

Action potential

Resume CPR, minimize interruptions in compressions, and consider the following actions:
• Place the patient on a cardiac monitor (if he isn't already) to monitor his cardiac rhythm.

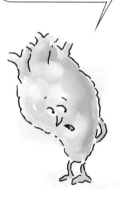

VF is the most common rhythm for a person in cardiac arrest. I sure don't want that!

Go with the flow

Adult cardiac arrest algorithm

This algorithm shows the guidelines for treating an adult in cardiac arrest.

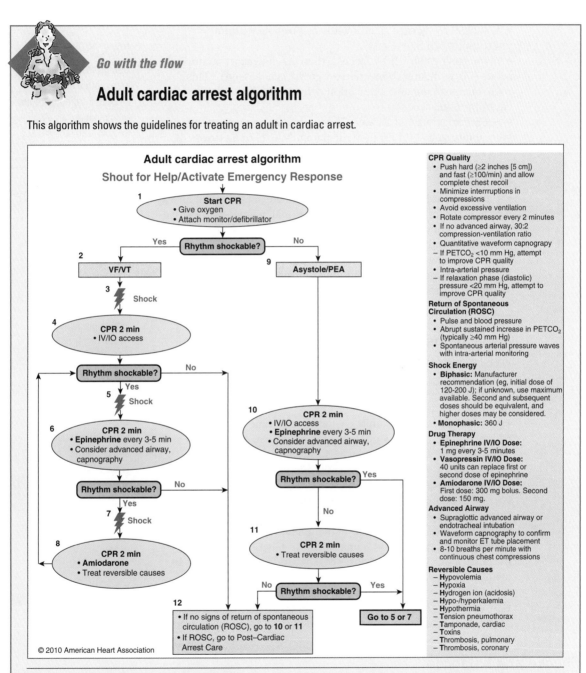

© 2010 American Heart Association

Reproduced with permission from *2010 American Heart Association Guidelines for Cardiopulmonary Resuscitation and Emergency Cardiovascular Care.* © 2010, American Heart Association.

- Establish I.V. access as efficiently as possible without interrupting ACLS.
- If you can't establish I.V. access, then you may start an intraosseous (I.O.) infusion (bone marrow cavity is accessed). (This route enables fluid and medication delivery similar to delivery by central venous access.)
- Secure an advanced airway. Choose an airway that's within your ability to insert based on the patient's level of alertness. If an endotracheal (ET) tube is used to secure the airway, compressions should be interrupted for no more than 10 seconds during insertion.
- If the patient has an advanced airway, make sure that the airway device is appropriately placed and functional; administer positive-pressure ventilation with 100% oxygen through the device, as appropriate. Continuous waveform capnography is recommended for confirmation and monitoring of ET tube placement. Administer oxygen if spontaneous breathing returns.
- Administer medications as indicated and as the patient's condition permits.

Medications

If VF or pulseless VT persists after you defibrillate the patient, administer:

- epinephrine—Give 1 mg by I.V. push or I.O.; repeat every 3 to 5 minutes.
- vasopressin—Give 40 units I.V. or I.O. one time only as an alternative to the first or second dose of epinephrine; epinephrine can be resumed after administering vasopressin.

If VF or VT still persists, consider administering:
- amiodarone (Cordarone), first-line drug—Give 300 mg rapidly I.V. or I.O. diluted in 20 to 30 mL of normal saline solution or dextrose 5% in water (D_5W); if VF recurs, give a second dose of 150 mg by rapid I.V. push or I.O.; maximum cumulative daily dose is 2.2 g.
- lidocaine (if amiodarone is unavailable)—Give 1 to 1.5 mg/kg by I.V. push or I.O. with repeat doses of 0.5 to 0.75 mg/kg over 5 to 10 minutes for a total of 3 mg/kg.
- magnesium sulfate—Give 1 to 2 g I.V. or I.O. diluted in 10 mL of D_5W over 5 to 20 minutes to treat hypomagnesemia or torsades de pointes (associated with a prolonged QT interval)with cardiac arrest.

Checks and balances

Recheck the patient's rhythm on the monitor and recheck his pulse. If VF or VT persists, repeat the "CPR—defibrillation—drug" cycle (continue CPR during drug administration) until a change in rhythm occurs. If you successfully defibrillate the patient,

Key points

Using the adult cardiac arrest algorithm
- Begin cardiopulmonary resuscitation, provide oxygen, and attach monitor/defibrillator.
- Determine rhythm.
- Provide defibrillation of ventricular tachycardia/ fibrillation as soon as possible.
- Establish I.V./I.O. access.
- Administer epinephrine.
- Consider advanced airway placement.
- Administer amiodarone.
- Identify and treat reversible causes of asystole or pulseless electrical activity.
- If return of spontaneous circulation occurs, provide post–cardiac arrest care.

administer an antiarrhythmic by I.V. infusion. (See *Scenario: Adult cardiac arrest*, page 232.)

Asystole

Ventricular asystole usually signals confirmation of death rather than a treatable rhythm. Spontaneous circulation rarely returns after a positive diagnosis of asystole. However, you may mistake fine VF for asystole, or a monitor error may have occurred. For this reason, you must confirm the presence of asystole in two leads.

First steps

As with any possible cardiac arrest situation, begin with the initial assessment. If asystole isn't present, follow the appropriate algorithm for the determined rhythm. If you suspect asystole, ask yourself these questions before attempting resuscitation:
• Does the patient have a pulse or is he awake?
• Does the patient have an objective indicator of "do-not-resuscitate" status, such as a bracelet, written documentation, or family statements?

   If either of these factors is present, don't start resuscitation attempts. If you determine that the asystolic rhythm should be treated, initiate CPR immediately and follow the adult cardiac arrest algorithm. Make sure to identify and treat reversible causes.

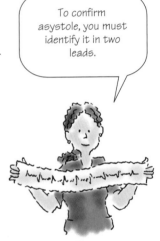

To confirm asystole, you must identify it in two leads.

Defibrillation

Defibrillation isn't performed for asystole because studies have shown that there's no improvement in rhythm change or patient outcome.

Medications

Epinephrine is the only drug of choice for treating asystole. Administer 1 mg by I.V. push or I.O. every 3 to 5 minutes. If asystole persists, consider terminating resuscitative efforts.

   You may substitute vasopressin for epinephrine, but only administer it once. The dose of vasopressin is 40 units by I.V. push or I.O.

Family presence

Surveys suggest that many family members want to be present during resuscitation attempts, but frequently will not ask to be present unless they are encouraged to do so.

Now I get it!

Scenario: Adult cardiac arrest

Mrs. B. is a 68-year-old woman admitted to the hospital with a diagnosis of heart failure. She's presently on a medical-surgical floor, preparing for discharge to home. When the nurse makes morning rounds, she finds Mrs. B. unresponsive. The health care team takes the following actions:

• A "code blue" (for cardiac arrest team) is called from the room and the nurse shouts for help from nearby nurses to bring the emergency cart to the room.

• The carotid artery is palpated in under 10 seconds for a pulse and no pulse is found. Compressions are started as the team applies defibrillator "hands off" pads to the patient's chest.

• The patient's airway is opened and her breathing is assessed.

• Two breaths are given, using a bag-mask device and 100% oxygen. The patient's chest is noted to rise with each ventilation.

• The patient's cardiac rhythm is assessed on the defibrillator monitor; ventricular fibrillation (VF) is diagnosed.

• Cardiopulmonary resuscitation (CPR) has been performed for over 2 minutes and the defibrillator is charged to 200 joules (biphasic defibrillator).

• The team member ready to press the SHOCK button on the defibrillator calls out "Is oxygen off?" and then "All clear." She then confirms that the oxygen source is removed from the patient and no personnel are touching the patient or bed. She presses the SHOCK button.

• The shock is delivered and CPR immediately resumes for five cycles or 2 minutes, at a rate of at least 100 compressions per minute and a compression depth of at least 2 inches.

• The rhythm is reassessed; VF continues and CPR continues.

• Epinephrine 1 mg is given I.V. as CPR continues.

• The defibrillator is recharged to 200 joules.

• The team member ready to press the SHOCK button on the defibrillator calls out "Is oxygen off?" then "All clear." She confirms that the oxygen source is removed from the patient and no personnel are touching the patient or bed. She presses the SHOCK button.

• The shock is delivered and CPR resumes for five cycles.

• The rhythm is reassessed; sinus tachycardia appears.

• The patient's carotid pulse is assessed and is palpable; oxygen saturation is 89% by pulse oximetry.

After defibrillation, perform these steps:

• Obtain the patient's vital signs and oxygen saturation and monitor her cardiac rhythm.

• If indicated, insert an endotracheal tube and manually ventilate the patient with a bag-mask device and 100% oxygen to improve oxygenation.

• Check I.V. access.

• Administer an I.V. infusion of normal saline solution.

• Arrange to immediately transfer the patient to the intensive care unit for further care.

> This cardiac arrest scenario is a classic.

Typically, families are allowed to remain in the resuscitation area during patient care. If the resuscitation efforts aren't successful, this will be the last time that the family sees the patient alive and family members report that being present helps them adjust to the death. Use compassion and be sensitive to the family's cultural and religious beliefs. Follow these steps when delivering bad news to the family:

• If family members weren't present during resuscitation efforts, call them and explain that their relative has been admitted to the emergency department.

• If possible, avoid telling the family over the telephone that the patient has died; rather, tell them that the patient's condition is serious. (If the patient's family is geographically distant, you may need to disclose information concerning the patient's death.)

• Review with the resuscitation team what was done on behalf of the patient.

• Take the family to a private area.

• Sit down with the family members, introduce yourself, and address the patient's closest relative. (Remember to use eye contact and make sure that the family members understand what you're saying.)

• Briefly review the events that occurred during the resuscitation efforts.

• Avoid using phrases such as "passed on" or "no longer with us." Use concrete terms such as "death," "dying," or "died." (For example, "Your family member died without suffering.")

• Allow time for questions, reflection, and discussion.

• Check with the staff caring for the patient's body to make sure that it's an appropriate time to let the family view the body.

• Describe to the family members what they'll see, hear, or smell to prepare them for seeing their loved one, especially if equipment is still connected to the patient's body.

• Let the family know the procedure for contacting the funeral home.

• Have the family sign legal documents required for release of the body, according to your facility's policy.

• Enlist the aid of clergy or social workers to help support the family, if applicable.

> Family members are typically allowed to remain in the resuscitation area.

PEA

PEA isn't a rhythm on its own but it's characterized by some electrical activity with little to no mechanical activity. It exists when there's a rhythm on the monitor but the patient has no detectable pulse. Cardiac ultrasound studies show that the heart may actually be contracting during PEA but is too weak to produce a viable pulse.

First steps

Begin treatment by following the adult cardiac arrest algorithm. The patient with PEA can be resuscitated, and resuscitation is more successful if the underlying cause is rapidly identified and treated.

Treating underlying causes of PEA

After you've started CPR, assessed the patient for VF or pulseless VT, and treated the rhythm accordingly, you must examine and promptly treat the underlying causes of PEA.

    PEA can involve:
- electromechanical dissociation
- idioventricular rhythms
- ventricular escape rhythms.

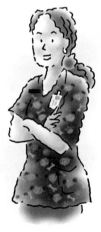

Several drugs can cause PEA, including tricyclic antidepressants and digoxin.

Follow the five H's and T's

The underlying causes of PEA include:
- hypovolemia
- hypoxia
- hydrogen ion acidosis
- hyperkalemia or hypokalemia
- hypothermia
- toxins (drug overdose)
- tamponade (cardiac)
- tension pneumothorax
- thrombosis (coronary)
- thrombosis (pulmonary).

Hypovolemia
Treat hypovolemia with a volume infusion of fluid or blood products, as appropriate. If you note an obvious cause of fluid depletion (such as hemorrhage), attempt the appropriate intervention.

Hypoxia
Hypoxia implies that the patient's airway and breathing aren't secure. Assure proper ET tube or other advanced airway placement by checking the patient's breath sounds after intubation and confirming placement by utilizing continuous waveform capnography, if available. Treat hypoxia with proper ventilation and oxygenation. Don't forget to monitor pulse oximetry.

Hydrogen ion acidosis

Routine use of sodium bicarbonate isn't recommended for patients in cardiac arrest. Give sodium bicarbonate (1 mEq/kg) only in special situations to treat preexisting metabolic acidosis, hyperkalemia, or tricyclic antidepressant overdose. Keep in mind that administering sodium bicarbonate diminishes the chance of successful defibrillation. Provide adequate ventilation and oxygen and restore tissue perfusion and circulation to most effectively treat acidosis resulting from cardiac arrest.

Hyperkalemia or hypokalemia

Treatment of potassium imbalance depends on the severity of the patient's condition. For severe hyperkalemia, give regular insulin I.V. and hypertonic dextrose solution and sodium bicarbonate (1 mEq/kg) to shift potassium into the cells; give furosemide to promote diuresis and potassium excretion. For hypokalemia, administer an I.V. infusion with a potassium supplement at a rate of 10 to 20 mEq/hour. Continually monitor cardiac rhythm.

Hypothermia

Continue resuscitation efforts while attempting to aggressively rewarm the patient. When the patient's body temperature reaches 86° F (30° C), perform full ACLS measures. Institute interventions to prevent additional heat loss.

Toxins (drug overdose)

Commonly, tricyclic antidepressants, beta-adrenergic blockers, calcium channel blockers, and digoxin can cause PEA. Focus on clearing the drug from the patient's system. You may use an antidote to combat the effects of the overdosed drug. Support hemodynamic functioning while initiating other therapies; for example, performing dialysis if the drug can't be cleared by the patient's renal system.

Tamponade (cardiac)

Perform pericardiocentesis to treat cardiac tamponade. This will remove the fluid from the pericardial space, allowing the patient's heart to expand and perform effectively.

Tension pneumothorax

Perform needle thoracostomy to treat tension pneumothorax. This condition may be apparent if there's tracheal deviation and absent breath sounds on one side of the

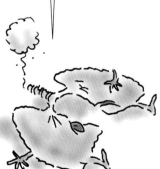

Ugh...Tension pneumothorax can be fatal. Someone get me some oxygen—STAT!

chest. Adequate ventilation and oxygenation is crucial. If not corrected, tension pneumothorax can be fatal.

Thrombosis (coronary)

Coronary thrombosis is considered an acute coronary syndrome (ACS). To treat an ACS, (See *Acute coronary syndromes algorithm,* pages 246).

Thrombosis (pulmonary)

Administer thrombolytics, if indicated. Surgical embolectomy or percutaneous mechanical embolectomy have also been used successfully, even with fibrinolytic therapy. Be sure to continue supportive treatment.

Other treatments

While treating the underlying causes of PEA, you need to simultaneously administer epinephrine and continue CPR.

Epinephrine

Give epinephrine 1 mg by I.V. push or I.O. every 3 to 5 minutes and assess its effect. You may substitute vasopressin for epinephrine. Give vasopressin 40 units I.V. or I.O. to replace the first or second dose of epinephrine.

Adult bradycardia algorithm (with pulse)

Bradycardia is considered a resting heart rate less than 60 beats/ minute. In some patients, a heart rate less than 60 beats/minute may be physiologically normal. Generally, when brandycardia causes signs and symptoms, the ventricular rate is less than 50 beats/minute. (See *Adult bradycardia algorithm [with pulse].*)

Treatment

As with any ACLS patient, begin by following the BLS health care providers algorithm. Always assess the patient for a palpable pulse to provide adequate circulation and an adequate airway and breathing.

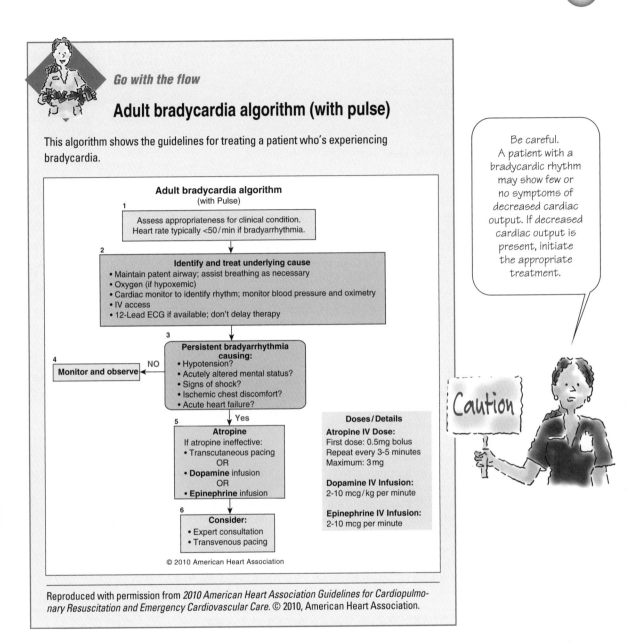

Go with the flow

Adult bradycardia algorithm (with pulse)

This algorithm shows the guidelines for treating a patient who's experiencing bradycardia.

Adult bradycardia algorithm
(with Pulse)

1
Assess appropriateness for clinical condition.
Heart rate typically <50/min if bradyarrhythmia.

2
Identify and treat underlying cause
• Maintain patent airway; assist breathing as necessary
• Oxygen (if hypoxemic)
• Cardiac monitor to identify rhythm; monitor blood pressure and oximetry
• IV access
• 12-Lead ECG if available; don't delay therapy

3
Persistent bradyarrhythmia causing:
• Hypotension?
• Acutely altered mental status?
• Signs of shock?
• Ischemic chest discomfort?
• Acute heart failure?

NO →

4
Monitor and observe

Yes

5
Atropine
If atropine ineffective:
• Transcutaneous pacing
OR
• **Dopamine** infusion
OR
• **Epinephrine** infusion

Doses/Details
Atropine IV Dose:
First dose: 0.5mg bolus
Repeat every 3-5 minutes
Maximum: 3 mg

Dopamine IV Infusion:
2-10 mcg/kg per minute

Epinephrine IV Infusion:
2-10 mcg per minute

6
Consider:
• Expert consultation
• Transvenous pacing

© 2010 American Heart Association

Be careful. A patient with a bradycardic rhythm may show few or no symptoms of decreased cardiac output. If decreased cardiac output is present, initiate the appropriate treatment.

Caution

Reproduced with permission from *2010 American Heart Association Guidelines for Cardiopulmonary Resuscitation and Emergency Cardiovascular Care.* © 2010, American Heart Association.

First steps

In your assessment, look for signs and symptoms associated with bradycardia. Remember that sometimes patients don't experience any ill effects from bradycardia. For example, trained athletes have much slower heart rates and tolerate them without difficulty.

Signs associated with bradycardia may include:
- hypotension, shock
- pulmonary congestion
- increased ventricular activity.
    Symptoms may include:
- chest pain
- shortness of breath
- decreased or altered level of consciousness.

Identify and treat the underlying cause

Implement ECG monitoring, identify the bradycardic rhythm, and look for the underlying cause of the patient's symptoms. Identification of the cause of bradycardia will direct treatment. For example, bradycardia caused by another condition such as hypoxemia will respond to treatment of the hypoxemia (provide adequate ventilation and oxygenation). While attempting to identify the cause of the bradycardia, maintain the patient's airway, provide oxygen and assist with ventilation, and obtain I.V. access if it isn't already present. Monitor vital signs and pulse oximetry. Obtain a 12-lead ECG but don't delay treatment.

Medications

If the bradycardia persists despite treatment of the suspected cause and the patient is hemodynamically unstable, consider administering atropine 0.5 mg by I.V. push every 3 to 5 minutes, for a total of 3 mg. Atropine will decrease vagal tone and increase the heart rate. Assess the patient's response after each dose. Be aware that patients with transplanted hearts don't respond to atropine because their hearts have been denervated. These patients need a transcutaneous pacemaker or a catecholamine infusion.

Other medications to consider include an epinephrine infusion (2 to 10 mcg/minute) or a dopamine infusion (2 to 10 mcg/kg/minute) if a transcutaneous pacemaker isn't available or effective, or isn't tolerated. Expert consultation should be obtained and a transvenous pacemaker may be necessary.

Adult tachycardia algorithm (with pulse)

A heart rate over 100 beats/minute is considered tachycardia. However, tachycardia can stem from many factors but is generally

Key points

Using the adult bradycardia algorithm
- Assess appropriateness for clinical condition.
- In symptomatic patients, heart rate is generally less than 50 beats/minute.
- Identify and treat underlying cause, if possible.
- Administer atropine if needed.
- If atropine is ineffective, use transcutaneous pacing if available.
- Administer dopamine or epinephrine infusion if needed.
- Consider expert consultation and transvenous pacing.

If you detect signs of decompensation, apply a transcutaneous pacemaker to the patient.

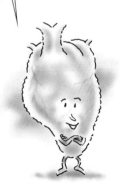

more significant and likely to be caused by an arrhythmia when the ventricular rate is 150 beats/minute or more. Tachycardia may be classified in different ways, based on the appearance of the QRS complex. General classifications include narrow complex tachycardia and wide complex tachycardia.

Narrow complex tachycardia (QRS of less than 0.12 second) includes:

- sinus tachycardia
- atrial fibrillation
- atrial flutter
- AV nodal reentry
- accessory pathway-mediated tachycardia
- atrial tachycardia (ectopic and reentrant)
- multifocal atrial tachycardia
- junctional tachycardia.

Wide complex tachycardia (QRS ≥ 0.12 second) includes:

- ventricular tachycardia
- supraventricular tachycardia with aberrancy
- preexcited tachycardia
- ventricular paced rhythms.

You must diagnose the type of tachycardia that the patient is experiencing and identify if he has impaired cardiac function to treat the rhythm appropriately. (See *Adult tachycardia algorithm [with pulse]*, page 240.)

Treatment

Begin by following the BLS health care providers algorithm and then assess the patient for stability. Be sure to maintain a patent airway with adequate ventilation; provide oxygen as appropriate. Evaluate and identify the cardiac rhythm while monitoring the patient's blood pressure and oximetry. Attempt to identify and treat the underlying cause.

First steps

If the patient is unstable (experiencing chest pain, shortness of breath, altered LOC, low blood pressure), perform synchronized cardioversion or consider giving adenosine if the rythm is regular with a narrow QRS complex. Synchronization (shock that is delivered with the QRS complex) is important so that the energy isn't delivered during the vulnerable period of ventricular repolarization.

Go with the flow

Adult tachycardia algorithm (with pulse)

This algorithm shows the guidelines for treating a patient who's experiencing tachycardia.

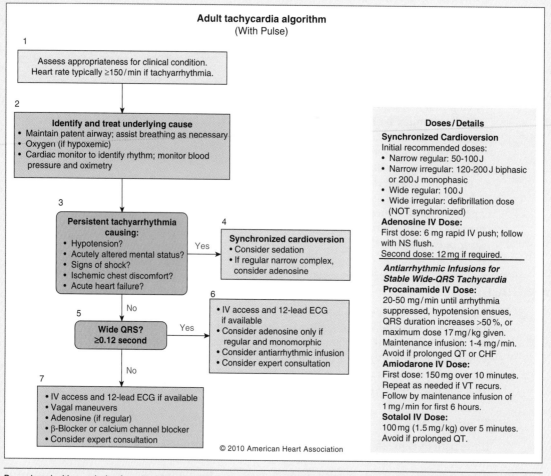

Adult tachycardia algorithm
(With Pulse)

1
Assess appropriateness for clinical condition.
Heart rate typically ≥150/min if tachyarrhythmia.

2
Identify and treat underlying cause
- Maintain patent airway; assist breathing as necessary
- Oxygen (if hypoxemic)
- Cardiac monitor to identify rhythm; monitor blood pressure and oximetry

3
Persistent tachyarrhythmia causing:
- Hypotension?
- Acutely altered mental status?
- Signs of shock?
- Ischemic chest discomfort?
- Acute heart failure?

Yes →

4
Synchronized cardioversion
- Consider sedation
- If regular narrow complex, consider adenosine

No ↓

5
Wide QRS?
≥0.12 second

Yes →

6
- IV access and 12-lead ECG if available
- Consider adenosine only if regular and monomorphic
- Consider antiarrhythmic infusion
- Consider expert consultation

No ↓

7
- IV access and 12-lead ECG if available
- Vagal maneuvers
- Adenosine (if regular)
- β-Blocker or calcium channel blocker
- Consider expert consultation

Doses/Details

Synchronized Cardioversion
Initial recommended doses:
- Narrow regular: 50-100 J
- Narrow irregular: 120-200 J biphasic or 200 J monophasic
- Wide regular: 100 J
- Wide irregular: defibrillation dose (NOT synchronized)

Adenosine IV Dose:
First dose: 6 mg rapid IV push; follow with NS flush.
Second dose: 12 mg if required.

Antiarrhythmic Infusions for Stable Wide-QRS Tachycardia
Procainamide IV Dose:
20-50 mg/min until arrhythmia suppressed, hypotension ensues, QRS duration increases >50%, or maximum dose 17 mg/kg given.
Maintenance infusion: 1-4 mg/min.
Avoid if prolonged QT or CHF
Amiodarone IV Dose:
First dose: 150 mg over 10 minutes.
Repeat as needed if VT recurs.
Follow by maintenance infusion of 1 mg/min for first 6 hours.
Sotalol IV Dose:
100 mg (1.5 mg/kg) over 5 minutes.
Avoid if prolonged QT.

© 2010 American Heart Association

Reproduced with permission from *2010 American Heart Association Guidelines for Cardiopulmonary Resuscitation and Emergency Cardiovascular Care.* © 2010, American Heart Association.

The rhythm difference

If the patient is stable and the QRS complex is 0.12 second or less, a vagal maneuver may be attempted. If the vagal maneuver is unsuccessful, medication may be administered to help convert and slow the rhythm. If the QRS complex is 0.12 second or greater, administer antiarrhythmics by I.V. infusion, to help convert the rhythm, and obtain expert consultation. With all tachyarrhythmic patients, obtain I.V. access and a 12-lead ECG.

Medications

Medication administration is based on the type of tachycardia that the patient is experiencing.

For a tachyarrhythmia that is regular with a QRS complex of 0.12 second or less, consider administering adenosine (Adenocard) 6 mg by rapid I.V push (over 2 seconds or less) followed by a normal saline solution flush. If the rhythm doesn't slow and convert, consider giving adenosine 12 mg by rapid I.V. push. Then consider obtaining expert consultation and possibly administering a calcium channel blocker such as diltiazem (Cardizem) or a beta-adrenergic blocker such as labetalol (Trandate).

For a tachyarrhythmia with a wide QRS complex (0.12 second or greater), consider giving adenosine 6 mg by rapid I.V. push but only if the rhythm is regular and monomorphic. Other antiarrhythmic infusions to consider, with expert consultation, include amiodarone, procainamide, and sotalol: Give amiodarone 150 mg by I.V. bolus over 10 minutes. Repeat bolus if VT recurs. Follow this with an amiodarone maintenance infusion of 1 mg/minute for the first 6 hours. You may give procainamide 20 mg/minute I.V. for a maximum dose of 17 mg/kg (50 mg/minute can be given urgently if necessary), followed by a maintenance infusion of 1 to 4 mg/minute. Or, give sotalol 1 to 1.5 mg/kg according to the facility's policy. Both procainamide and sotalol should be avoided if the patient has a prolonged QT interval.

Key points

Using the adult tachycardia (with pulse) algorithm
- Assess appropriateness for clinical condition.
- Treat underlying causes for tachyarrhythmia, if possible.
- Perform synchronized cardioversion if patient's condition deteriorates.
- Administer adenosine if rhythm is regular and monomorphic.
- Administer antiarrhythmic, beta blocker, or calcium channel blocker as appropriate for identified rhythm.

Acute coronary syndromes algorithm

Acute myocardial infarction (MI), ST-segment elevation MI (STEMI), non-STEMI, and unstable angina are each considered an ACS. Rupture or erosion of plaque—an unstable and lipid-rich substance—initiates nearly all ACSs. This rupture results in platelet adhesions, fibrin clot formation, and activation of thrombin.

A thrombus among us

If a thrombus fully occludes the vessel for a prolonged time, it's known as a STEMI. Most patients with STEMI will develop abnormal Q waves. In this type of MI, there's a greater concentration of thrombin and fibrin and more myocardial damage.

For patients with unstable angina, a thrombus partially occludes a coronary vessel. This thrombus is full of platelets. The partially occluded vessel may have distal microthrombi that cause necrosis in some myocytes. The smaller vessels infarct and the patient has a higher risk of developing MI, which may progress to a non-STEMI.

Set the stage

Three stages occur when a vessel is occluded—ischemia, injury, and infarct.
• Ischemia: Blood flow and oxygen demand are out of balance; ECG changes indicate ST-segment depression or T-wave changes. (Ischemia can be resolved by improving oxygen flow or reducing oxygen needs.)
• Injury: Ischemia is prolonged enough to damage the affected area of the heart; ECG changes usually reveal ST-segment elevation (usually in two or more contiguous leads).
• Infarct: Death of myocardial cells occurs; ECG changes may reveal abnormal Q waves. (Q waves are considered abnormal when they appear greater than or equal to 0.04 second wide and their height is greater than 25% of the R wave height in that lead.)

Damage by degrees

The degree of blockage and the time that the affected vessel remains occluded are major determinants for the type of infarct that occurs. The amount of damage to the myocardium depends on several factors:
• the area of the heart supplied by the affected vessel (see *Viewing the coronary vessels.*)
• the demand for oxygen in the affected area of the heart
• the collateral circulation in the affected area of the heart. (Collateral circulation is an alternate circulation that develops when blood flow to tissue is blocked and rerouted.)

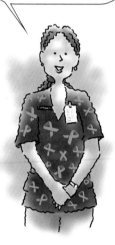

Most patients with ST-segment elevation MI develop abnormal Q waves.

The affected area of the heart, the demand for oxygen, and the collateral circulation all affect the outcome of an MI.

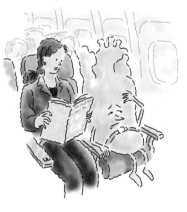

Viewing the coronary vessels

This illustration shows the major coronary vessels that may be affected during myocardial infarction.

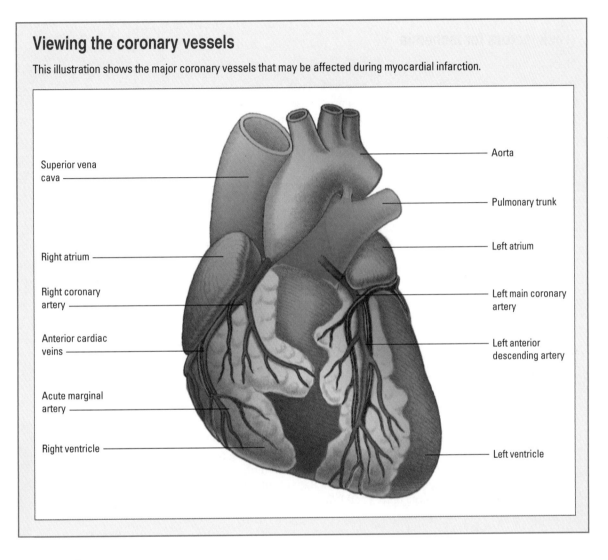

Superior vena cava

Right atrium

Right coronary artery

Anterior cardiac veins

Acute marginal artery

Right ventricle

Aorta

Pulmonary trunk

Left atrium

Left main coronary artery

Left anterior descending artery

Left ventricle

No laughing matter

Patients typically describe these symptoms when experiencing acute ischemia and MI:
• uncomfortable pressure, squeezing, pain, or fullness in the center of the chest lasting several minutes (usually longer than 15 minutes)

Risk factors for ischemia

Patients at risk for ischemia fall into three categories: high, intermediate, and low risk.

High risk

High-risk patients have one or more of the following risk factors:

• previous myocardial infarction
• previous life-threatening episode of arrhythmia
• known coronary artery disease
• major complaint of chest or left arm pain and reproducible pain of past angina
• significant electrocardiogram (ECG) changes (ST-segment changes with chest symptoms or marked T-wave changes)
• elevated troponin or CK-MB.

Intermediate risk

Intermediate-risk patients have one of the following risk factors:

• major complaint of chest or left arm pain
• age older than 70
• male
• history of diabetes
• ECG findings (abnormal ST- or T-wave changes) not new.

Low risk

Low-risk patients have one of the following risk factors:

• possible signs of angina
• reproducible chest pain on palpation
• normal ECG or ECG changes (T-wave inversion).

• pain radiating to the shoulders, neck, arms, or jaws or pain in the back between the shoulder blades (women may complain of abdominal pain)
• fatigue, light-headedness, fainting, sweating, nausea, and shortness of breath, accompanied by a feeling of impending doom.

Unusual or isolated symptoms may be seen more commonly in diabetics, older patients, and women. Patients at risk for ischemia fall into high-, intermediate-, and low-risk categories. (See *Risk factors for ischemia.*)

Treatment

Treatment goals for the patient experiencing an ACS include:
• reducing the amount of myocardial necrosis if the infarction is ongoing
• preventing major adverse cardiac events (nonfatal MI, need for urgent revascularizarion, and death)

- treating life-threatening complications of ACS, such as unstable arrhythmias, cardiogenic shock, pulmonary edema, and mechanical complications from acute AMI.

Prehospital screening, including a 12-lead ECG, should be done by EMS personnel, if possible, to determine if a patient is a candidate for thrombolytic therapy. Thrombolytic therapy should begin immediately (within 30 minutes of first medical contact) if the patient meets the criteria and the EMS personnel are able to administer thrombolytics (depending on the specific licensing criteria of your state or county). Prehospital treatment may also include aspirin and nitrates unless contraindicated. Morphine may be given carefully if chest pain doesn't respond to nitrates.

PCI preference

Administering fibrinolytics or performing percutaneous coronary intervention (PCI), which may decrease or limit the amount of necrosis, is the preferred treatment. Keep in mind that fibrinolytics aren't effective in patients with unstable angina. In many instances, PCI is superior to fibrinolytic administration because the restoration of vessel patency occurs in more than 90% of patients, leading to reduced mortality and reinfarction rates. However, when the first medical contact to balloon time (PCI) may be delayed (more than 90 minutes) and the patient presents within 2 hours of the onset of symptoms, fibrinolytic therapy is indicated.

You can also give glycoprotein IIb/IIIa inhibitors, heparin, and aspirin to treat thrombus because these drugs affect platelet formation and decrease platelet adhesion.

Use the acute coronary syndromes algorithm, which includes ECG changes you may encounter, to quickly classify patients so you can direct treatment appropriately. Base your treatment on ECG findings and the patient's status. (See *Acute coronary syndromes algorithm*, page 246.)

First steps

Begin your assessment immediately. Obtain a 12-lead ECG within the first 10 minutes of your interaction with the patient, if possible, because it's a crucial component in determining if myocardial ischemia is present. After you obtain an ECG, you must interpret the findings, which will direct your treatment plan. Administer oxygen, aspirin, nitroglycerin, and morphine,

Key points

Using the acute coronary syndromes algorithm

- Immediate 12-lead electrocardiogram (ECG) is crucial to treatment.
- Use ECG to identify type of syndrome: STEMI (ST-elevation myocardial infarction) or new left bundle-branch block), unstable angina/non-STEMI (ST depression or dynamic T-wave inversion), normal or nondiagnostic ECG.
- Administer oxygen, aspirin, nitroglycerin, and morphine as indicated.
- Assess and complete checklist for possible fibrinolytic treatment.
- Optimally, door to fibrinolytic treatment is less than 30 minutes from first medical contact.
- Optimally, door to balloon (percutaneous coronary insertion) is less than 90 minutes from first medical contact.

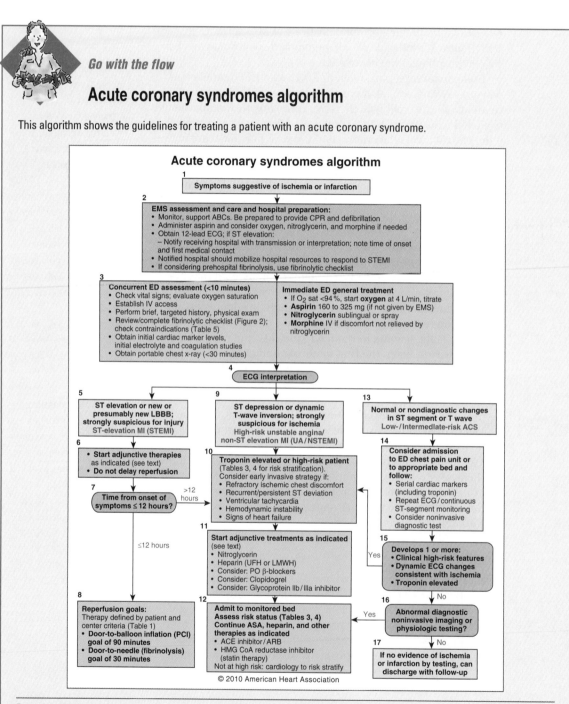

Go with the flow

Acute coronary syndromes algorithm

This algorithm shows the guidelines for treating a patient with an acute coronary syndrome.

Acute coronary syndromes algorithm

1
Symptoms suggestive of ischemia or infarction

2
EMS assessment and care and hospital preparation:
- Monitor, support ABCs. Be prepared to provide CPR and defibrillation
- Administer aspirin and consider oxygen, nitroglycerin, and morphine if needed
- Obtain 12-lead ECG; if ST elevation:
  – Notify receiving hospital with transmission or interpretation; note time of onset and first medical contact
- Notified hospital should mobilize hospital resources to respond to STEMI
- If considering prehospital fibrinolysis, use fibrinolytic checklist

3
Concurrent ED assessment (<10 minutes)
- Check vital signs; evaluate oxygen saturation
- Establish IV access
- Perform brief, targeted history, physical exam
- Review/complete fibrinolytic checklist (Figure 2); check contraindications (Table 5)
- Obtain initial cardiac marker levels, initial electrolyte and coagulation studies
- Obtain portable chest x-ray (<30 minutes)

Immediate ED general treatment
- If O_2 sat <94%, start **oxygen** at 4 L/min, titrate
- **Aspirin** 160 to 325 mg (if not given by EMS)
- **Nitroglycerin** sublingual or spray
- **Morphine** IV if discomfort not relieved by nitroglycerin

4
ECG interpretation

5
ST elevation or new or presumably new LBBB; strongly suspicious for injury
ST-elevation MI (STEMI)

6
- **Start adjunctive therapies** as indicated (see text)
- **Do not delay reperfusion**

7
Time from onset of symptoms ≤ 12 hours?
>12 hours
≤12 hours

8
Reperfusion goals:
Therapy defined by patient and center criteria (Table 1)
- **Door-to-balloon inflation (PCI) goal of 90 minutes**
- **Door-to-needle (fibrinolysis) goal of 30 minutes**

9
ST depression or dynamic T-wave inversion; strongly suspicious for ischemia
High-risk unstable angina/non-ST elevation MI (UA/NSTEMI)

10
Troponin elevated or high-risk patient (Tables 3, 4 for risk stratification). Consider early invasive strategy if:
- Refractory ischemic chest discomfort
- Recurrent/persistent ST deviation
- Ventricular tachycardia
- Hemodynamic instability
- Signs of heart failure

11
Start adjunctive treatments as indicated (see text)
- Nitroglycerin
- Heparin (UFH or LMWH)
- Consider: PO β-blockers
- Consider: Clopidogrel
- Consider: Glycoprotein IIb/IIIa inhibitor

12
Admit to monitored bed
Assess risk status (Tables 3, 4)
Continue ASA, heparin, and other therapies as indicated
- ACE inhibitor/ARB
- HMG CoA reductase inhibitor (statin therapy)
Not at high risk: cardiology to risk stratify

13
Normal or nondiagnostic changes in ST segment or T wave
Low-/Intermediate-risk ACS

14
Consider admission to ED chest pain unit or to appropriate bed and follow:
- Serial cardiac markers (including troponin)
- Repeat ECG/continuous ST-segment monitoring
- Consider noninvasive diagnostic test

15
Develops 1 or more:
- Clinical high-risk features
- Dynamic ECG changes consistent with ischemia
- Troponin elevated
Yes
No

16
Abnormal diagnostic noninvasive imaging or physiologic testing?
Yes
No

17
If no evidence of ischemia or infarction by testing, can discharge with follow-up

© 2010 American Heart Association

as needed, to treat acute ischemia. Classify the patient as having ST-segment elevation or new left bundle-branch block (LBBB), ST-segment depression or dynamic T-wave inversion, or nondiagnostic or normal ECG.

Other actions include obtaining serial cardiac markers (including troponin), electrolyte levels, coagulation studies, repeat 12-lead ECG, chest X-ray and continuous ST-segment monitoring.

ST-segment elevation or new LBBB

Treat patients with an ST-segment elevation greater than or equal to 1 mm in two or more leads or with LBBB for acute MI (STEMI). More than 90% of patients who present with an ST-segment elevation greater than or equal to 1 mm will develop new Q waves and have positive serum cardiac markers.

Treatment options include:
• reperfusion therapy (with a goal of door to balloon [PCI] in 90 minutes and door to needle [fibrinolysis] in 30 minutes)
• beta-adrenergic blockers
• clopidogrel
• heparin (if you're using fibrin-specific thrombolytics).

ST-segment depression or dynamic T-wave inversion

Suspect ischemia with findings of ST depression greater than 1 mm, marked symmetrical T-wave inversion in multiple precordial leads, and dynamic ST-T changes with pain. Patients with ST depression indicating a posterior MI benefit most when a diagnosis of acute MI is confirmed. Keep in mind that repeating the ECG may be helpful for patients who have hyperacute T waves. Patients who display persistent symptoms and recurrent ischemia, diffuse or widespread ECG abnormalities, heart failure, and positive serum markers are considered at high risk for further heart damage.

Treatment options include:
• beta-adrenergic blockers
• clopidogrel
• heparin therapy
• glycoprotein IIb/IIIa inhibitors.

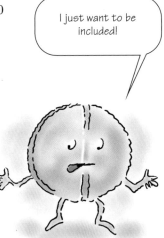

I just want to be included!

Normal or nondiagnostic ECG

A normal ECG won't show ST changes or arrhythmias. A non-diagnostic ECG may show an ST depression of 0.5 to 1 mm or a T-wave inversion or flattening in leads with dominant R waves. If further assessment is warranted, perform perfusion radionuclide imaging and stress echocardiography. Manage as high risk patients who have ECG changes, positive serum markers, or positive findings on any functional studies.

Treatment for the patient is individualized; however, you should include aspirin in all treatment plans.

Treatment

The 2010 AHA guidelines recommend that the order of treatment for every patient experiencing acute ischemia and MI is oxygen, aspirin, nitroglycerin, and morphine.

Oxygen

Administer oxygen to anyone experiencing chest discomfort who is dyspneic, has an oxygen saturation of less than 94%, or has signs of heart failure or shock. Deliver lower concentrations (less than 40%) of oxygen by nasal cannula and higher concentrations (over 40%) by mask. The type and amount of oxygen you need to administer is determined by the patient's oxygen saturation. Measure pulse oximetry, if possible, and maintain oxygen saturation at more than 90%.

Aspirin

Aspirin is considered a class I action in the treatment of a patient with MI. Give aspirin 160 to 325 mg by mouth as soon as possible. Chewed aspirin is absorbed the fastest and is preferred.

Nitroglycerin

Sublingual nitroglycerin is the initial treatment for a patient with chest pain that suggests ischemia. Nitrates are the preferred drug initially for the treatment of ischemic pain because they cause coronary dilation and allow for greater perfusion. They also decrease preload and afterload, reducing the heart's oxygen requirments. Don't give nitrates to patients with severe hypotension (less than 90 mm Hg systolic or 30 mm Hg or more below baseline), extreme bradycardia (heart rate less than 50 beats/ minute), tachycardia in the absence of heart failure, or right ventricular infarction.

Sublingually speaking

Give nitroglycerin 0.3 to 0.4 mg sublingually up to three times at 5-minute intervals as long as the patient's blood pressure is stable (usually systolic greater than 90 mm Hg). When nitroglycerin use will be prolonged, use the I.V. route because it allows for active titration.

Morphine

Morphine is indicated for central anxiety and is the drug of choice to relieve pain unresponsive to nitrates associated with acute MI. Use morphine carefully in patients with unstable angina non-STEMI because studies have shown that morphine causes more adverse effects in patients with these conditions. Give 2 to 4 mg initially by I.V. push with repeat doses of 2 to 8 mg every 5 to 10 minutes until the patient indicates pain relief. Pain affects heart rate, contractility, and systolic blood pressure, which adversely increases myocardial oxygen demand. Be sure to evaluate the patient's pain response and his vital signs. Remember to frequently monitor his respiratory rate, oxygen saturation, and blood pressure because morphine can cause respiratory depression and hypotension.

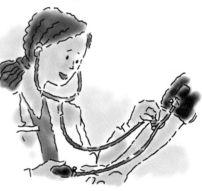

When you administer morphine or nitroglycerin, monitor blood pressure frequently because these drugs can cause hypotension.

Emergency department

If the patient with suspected ACS is brought to the ED, the CABD assessment and interventions continue. Obtain the patient's vital signs, oxygen saturation, brief and targeted history, 12-lead ECG results, I.V. access status, and assess whether he's a candidate for thrombolytic therapy or PCI. Remember to focus on rapid but accurate diagnosis.

Double duty

While assessment is underway, you may perform simultaneous treatment. This includes oxygen and medication administration. You can start adjunctive therapy while reperfusion strategies are being considered.

Adjunctive therapies include:
• beta-adrenergic blockers (decrease the workload of the heart)
• I.V. nitroglycerin (dilates coronary arteries, improves preload and afterload)
• clopidogrel to inhibit platelet aggregation

- heparin (indicated for patients receiving tissue plasminogen activator or reteplase [Retavase] and for patients who are candidates for percutaneous transluminal coronary angioplasty or surgical revascularization)
- angiotensin-converting enzyme inhibitors (block conversion of angiotensin; should be given within 24 hours of symptoms).
    Reperfusion strategies include:
- angiography
- PCI, which includes angioplasty with or without stents
- cardiothoracic bypass surgery
- fibrinolytic therapy.

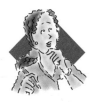

Quick quiz

1. When treating a patient in asystole, it's most important to:
    A. request a transcutaneous pacemaker.
    B. confirm the rhythm in a second lead.
    C. administer atropine 1 mg I.V. push.
    D. determine an underlying cause.

Answer: B. You must confirm the rhythm before proceeding to other steps because it's possible to have a false diagnosis of asystole. The most common cause of "false" asystole is operator error. Also be sure to assess the patient.

2. What's the initial treatment for a patient in VF?
    A. Lidocaine 1 mg/kg by I.V. push or I.O.
    B. Epinephrine 1 mg by I.V. push or I.O.
    C. Rapid defibrillation at 100 to 200 joules (biphasic energy)
    D. CPR for five minutes, followed by defibrillation at 360 joules

Answer: C. Rapid defibrillation of VF within minutes of collapse significantly increases the chances of a patient's survival to hospital discharge.

3. A patient is experiencing a regular wide-complex rhythm (0.12 second or more) of 250 beats/minute with diaphoresis, syncope, and decreased LOC. You should:
  A. defibrillate at 200 joules.
  B. administer lidocaine 1 mg by I.V. push.
  C. administer amiodarone 300 mg by I.V. push.
  D. perform synchronized cardioversion at 100 joules.

Answer: D. These symptoms describe an unstable patient. Perform immediate synchronized cardioversion using 100 joules. If synchronization is delayed, the patient's clinical condition continues to deteriorate, and he has no palpable pulse, perform defibrillation.

4. A patient is brought to the ED after a motor vehicle accident. He's unresponsive and EMS personnel are performing CPR. He has been intubated and has I.V. access. You place him on the monitor and his rhythm displays junctional tachycardia at a rate of 120 beats/minute. He has no discernible pulse. Which intervention is appropriate?
  A. Epinephrine 1 mg by I.V. push
  B. Sodium bicarbonate 1 mEq/kg by I.V. push
  C. Fluid bolus infusion
  D. Warming procedures

Answer: C. Your patient has a heart rhythm but no pulse. This is known as PEA. Hypovolemia is a possible cause of PEA and is the easiest to treat. You can rapidly infuse a fluid challenge while considering other causes.

5. Mr. H. is a patient in the intensive care unit after aortic aneurysm repair. He suddenly develops atrial fibrillation at a rate of 180 beats/minute. What medication should you consider using to convert the rhythm?
  A. Amiodarone
  B. Epinephrine
  C. Atropine
  D. Lidocaine

Answer: A. You can use amiodarone to convert atrial fibrillation for both the normal heart and the impaired heart.

Scoring

⭐⭐⭐ If you answered all five questions correctly, congratulations! Your score is a clear sign of your success.

⭐⭐ If you answered four questions correctly, good work! Your knowledge of algorithms is flowing nicely.

⭐ If you answered fewer than four questions correctly, it's no emergency! A quick review will point you to a perfect score next time.

9

ACLS in special situations

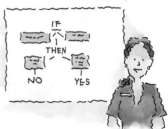

Just the facts

In this chapter, you'll learn:

◆ actions for treating patients experiencing acute stroke

◆ emergency care for pregnant women in cardiac arrest and patients in cardiac arrest caused by trauma

◆ special measures required for submersion or drowning, electric shock or lightning strike, and hypothermia

◆ emergency interventions to treat toxicologic emergencies, near-fatal asthma, and anaphylaxis.

A look at special situations

You may encounter situations in which it's difficult to apply the general guidelines presented in an algorithm. Such special situations require you to modify the general guidelines to increase your chance of successfully resuscitating the patient. These situations include acute stroke, pregnancy, trauma, submersion or drowning, electric shock or lightning strike, hypothermia, toxicologic emergencies, near-fatal asthma, and anaphylaxis. In addition, life-threatening electrolyte disturbances are frequently associated with cardiac arrest. Sereve electrolyte disturbances may be the cause of cardiac arrest or complicate resuscitation efforts during cardiac arrest from other causes. (See *Managing electrolyte disturbances associated with cardiac arrest*, pages 254 to 255.)

As with all emergencies, investigation into the background of the injury may be essential to treat the patient. For example, treatment measures for stroke are dependent on the amount of time that has elapsed since the onset of symptoms. Likewise, in toxicologic emergencies, knowledge of the specific drug or substance ingested helps to determine antidotal treatment.

> In special situations, you'll need to modify algorithm guidelines to provide the most effective care for your patient.

Managing electrolyte disturbances associated with cardiac arrest

Life-threatening electrolyte disturbances are often associated with cardiac arrest. In addition to standard advanced cardiac life support (ACLS) interventions, additional ACLS interventions may be necessary to improve the patient's cardiovascular stability during the cardiac arrest and hemodynamic recovery afterwards.

Electrolyte disturbance	Causes	Signs and symptoms
Severe hyperkalemia (serum potassium level > 6.5 mmol/L)	• Renal failure • Excess potassium administration • Drug therapy	• Flaccid paralysis • Paresthesia • Depressed reflexes • Respiratory problems
Severe hypokalemia (serum potassium level < 2.5 mmol/L)	• GI losses (severe vomiting, diarrhea, laxatives, GI tube drainage) • Renal losses (high-dose thiazide diuretics [furosemide] without potassium replacement) • Adrenal adenoma • Drug toxicities (chloroquine, risperidone, albuterol, terbutaline, digoxin, amphotericin B) • Epinephrine release during stress response (coronary ischemia)	• Muscle weakness • Hypoventilation • Respiratory arrest • Muscle cramps • Rhabdomyolysis • Myoglobinuria
Hypermagnesemia (serum magnesium level > 2.2 mEq/L)	• Renal failure • Toxicity due to magnesium replacement therapy • Magnesium laxative abuse	• Nausea and vomiting • Muscle weakness • Decreased deep tendon reflexes • Ataxia • Paralysis • Decreased level of consciousness (LOC) • Hypoventilation • Respiratory arrest • Hypotension • Cardiac arrest
Hypomagnesemia (serum magnesium level < 1.3 mEq/L)	• Thyroid hormone dysfunction • Diarrhea • Drug toxicities (cisplatin, diuretics, pentamidine, alcohol, amphotericin B, cyclosporine, proton pump inhibitors) • Malnutrition • Renal dysfunction (acute tubular necrosis, renal transplantation) • Bartter and Gitelman syndromes	• Anorexia • Generlized weaknesss • Positive Chvostek and Trousseau signs • Seizures • Decreased LOC

ECG changes	Possible additional ACLS interventions
• Peaked T waves • Long PR interval • Wide QRS complex • Merging of S and T waves • Flat or absent T waves • Idioventricular rhythm • Asystole	• Calcium chloride (10%) 5–10 mL (500 to 1,000 mg) I.V. over 2–5 minutes, or calcium gluconate (10%) 15–30 mL I.V. over 2–minutes • Sodium bicarbonate 50 mEq I.V. over 5 minutes • 25 g (50 mL of D50) glucose mixed with 10 units regular insulin and given I.V. over 15–30 minutes • Albuterol 10–20 mg nebulized over 15 minutes • Furosemide 40–80 mg I.V. • Kayexalate 15–50 g plus sorbitol P.O. or P.R. • Dialysis
• Decreased ST segment • Decreased amplitude of T waves with flattening • Increased amplitude of U wave • Atrial and junctional tachycardia • Sinus bradycardia • Atrioventricular block • Ventricular tachycardia (VT) • Ventricular fibrillation • Pulseless electrical activity • Asystole	• Treating hypomagnesemia if present • Estimating potassium deficit based upon underlying cause • Carefully monitoring electrolyte levels and replacing potassium by slow I.V. infusion
• Bradycardia • Prolonged PR interval • Wide QRS duration • Prolonged QT interval • Complete heart block	• Calcium chloride (10%) 5–10 mL I.V. over 2–5 minutes, or calcium gluconate (10%) 15–30 mL I.V. over 2–5 minutes
• Prolonged PR interval • Wide QRS complex • Peaked or flat T waves • Polymorphic VT (including torsades de pointes)	• Magnesium sulfate 1–2 g diluted in 10 mL D_5W I.V. or I.O.

Acute stroke

Acute stroke is a sudden impairment of cerebral circulation in one or more of the blood vessels supplying the brain. Stroke interrupts or diminishes oxygen supply and commonly causes serious damage or necrosis in brain tissues.

Playing the odds

About 85% of strokes are ischemic, resulting from thrombus formation in a blood vessel supplying the brain or from embolism (typically from the heart or carotid artery). Other strokes are hemorrhagic, resulting from the rupture of a cerebral artery or aneurysm.

The sooner, the better

The sooner normal blood flow is restored to the brain after a stroke, the better the patient's chance for recovery. A catch phrase that is commonly used is "time is brain." Therefore, prompt recognition and treatment of stroke can limit the extent of damage and significantly improve the patient's outcome. The National Institutes of Neurological Disorders and Stroke has established guidelines for the completion of tasks beginning from the minute the patient arrives in the emergency department (ED).

> Typically, you won't be able to immediately identify the cause of stroke; however, certain factors place the patient at greater risk for stroke.

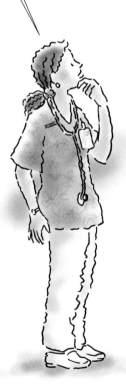

What causes it

Some strokes are caused by an arrhythmia (particularly atrial fibrillation) or a hypertensive crisis. In many cases, no precipitating event is identified. The risk of stroke is increased in patients with a history of:

- transient ischemic attacks (TIAs)
- atherosclerosis
- hypertension
- arrhythmias
- diabetes mellitus
- heart disease
- cigarette smoking
- hormonal contraceptive use
- personal or family history of stroke
- hypercoagulative state
- sickle cell disease
- carotid artery disease.

What to look for

Signs and symptoms of stroke vary with the artery affected (and, consequently, the portion of the brain it supplies), severity of damage, and extent of collateral circulation that develops to help the brain compensate for decreased blood supply.

Common signs and symptoms of stroke include the sudden onset of:
- hemiparesis on the affected side to unilateral or bilateral paralysis of the extremities
- unilateral sensory defect (such as numbness, tingling, or abnormal sensation), typically on the same side as the hemiparesis or hemiplegia
- slurred or indistinct speech or the inability to understand speech
- loss of half of the field of vision to the same side in both eyes, double vision, or transient vision loss in one eye (usually described as a shade coming down)
- mental status changes or loss of consciousness (particularly if associated with at least one of the above symptoms)
- severe headache (seen with hemorrhagic stroke).

How it's treated

For all patients with signs and symptoms of stroke:
- Maintain a patent airway and adequate oxygenation (oxygen saturation greater than 94%).
- Monitor for and treat hypoglycemia or marked hyperglycemia (serum glucose level of 185 mg/dL or less).
- Monitor blood pressure and manage it based on these considerations:
  – If the patient is a candidate for fibrinolytic therapy, keep his blood pressure below 185 mm Hg systolic or 110 mm Hg diastolic to minimize the risk of bleeding complications.
  – If the patient isn't a candidate for fibrinolytic therapy, treat only a severely elevated blood pressure (systolic blood pressure greater than 220 mm Hg, diastolic blood pressure greater than 120). Inducing lower perfusion pressures may increase ischemia and worsen the stroke.

Stroke Chain of Survial

As with the adult chain of survival for victims of cardiac arrest, remember the eight D's (links in the chain) to help minimize brain injury and maximize recovery.
- detection
- dispatch
- delivery
- door
- data
- decision
- drug
- disposition (See *Adult suspected stroke*, page 259.)

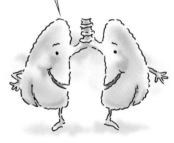

It's important to maintain a patent airway and adequate oxygenation when treating a patient with signs and symptoms of stroke.

The eight D's describe the essential steps in stroke treatment.
I think I really need to know this information!

Detection

Early detection of the signs and symptoms of stroke helps ensure the best outcome. A patient presenting with signs of stroke, such as difficulty talking or unresponsiveness, needs to be differentiated from other emergencies. For example, a patient with a low blood sugar may present with slurred speech or altered level of consciousness (LOC). A rapid blood sugar analysis can rule out hypoglycemia as a cause. If low blood sugar is the cause, rapid treatment should be initiated. Also, the quicker a patient suffering a stroke is evaluated and diagnosed, the faster he may qualify for certain treatments such as fibrinolytic therapy.

Dispatch

You must notify emergency medical service (EMS) personnel at the earliest signs of stroke to ensure a quick response. A patient with suspected stroke should receive the same priority as a patient experiencing an acute myocardial infarction (MI). The 911 dispatcher is trained to ask specific questions of the caller to determine what type of emergency is occurring and alert the EMS team as to how to respond.

Delivery

EMS responders will perform a quick assessment to rapidly confirm the signs and symptoms of stroke. You may use the National Institutes of Health (NIH) Stroke Scale or the Cincinnati Prehospital Stroke Scale (a simplified version of the NIH Stroke Scale). (See *NIH Stroke Scale*, pages 261 to 263. Also see *Cincinnati Prehospital Stroke Scale*, page 264.)

Primary priority

For a patient presenting with signs and symptoms of stroke, assess and manage his airway, breathing, and circulation, and intervene if necessary to provide cardiopulmonary support. Follow these steps:
- First, assess the patient for a head or neck injury because a fall may have accompanied the stroke. If indicated, apply a cervical collar and logroll the patient to prevent further injury. (Cervical spinal X-rays may be ordered in the ED.)
- Position the patient in the recovery position to prevent aspiration.
- Suction the airway as necessary to ensure patency because paralysis of the tongue, mouth, and throat commonly causes partial or complete airway obstruction, hampering the patient's ability to clear secretions. Aspiration is also possible.
- If the patient's breathing pattern is abnormal, you may need to insert an advanced airway. You may also need to provide

Go with the flow

Adult suspected stroke

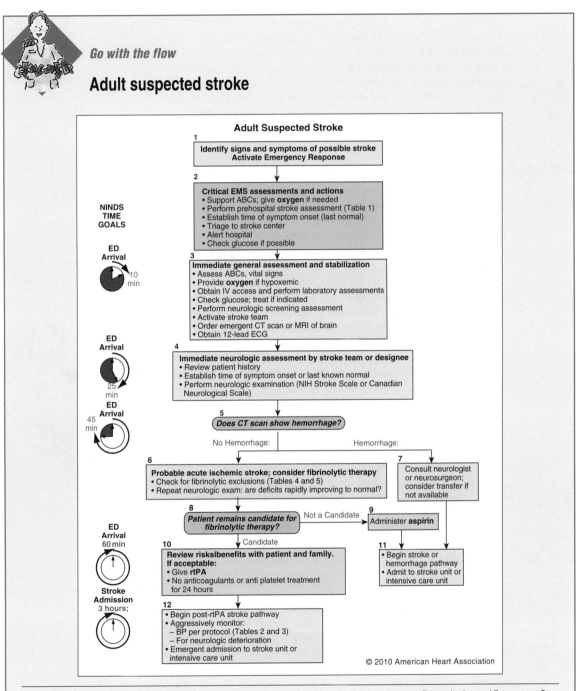

Adult Suspected Stroke

NINDS
TIME
GOALS

1
Identify signs and symptoms of possible stroke
Activate Emergency Response

2
Critical EMS assessments and actions
• Support ABCs; give **oxygen** if needed
• Perform prehospital stroke assessment (Table 1)
• Establish time of symptom onset (last normal)
• Triage to stroke center
• Alert hospital
• Check glucose if possible

ED
Arrival
10 min

3
Immediate general assessment and stabilization
• Assess ABCs, vital signs
• Provide **oxygen** if hypoxemic
• Obtain IV access and perform laboratory assessments
• Check glucose; treat if indicated
• Perform neurologic screening assessment
• Activate stroke team
• Order emergent CT scan or MRI of brain
• Obtain 12-lead ECG

ED
Arrival
25 min

4
Immediate neurologic assessment by stroke team or designee
• Review patient history
• Establish time of symptom onset or last known normal
• Perform neurologic examination (NIH Stroke Scale or Canadian Neurological Scale)

ED
Arrival
45 min

5
Does CT scan show hemorrhage?

No Hemorrhage:

Hemorrhage:

6
Probable acute ischemic stroke; consider fibrinolytic therapy
• Check for fibrinolytic exclusions (Tables 4 and 5)
• Repeat neurologic exam: are deficits rapidly improving to normal?

7
Consult neurologist or neurosurgeon; consider transfer if not available

8
Patient remains candidate for fibrinolytic therapy?

Not a Candidate

9
Administer **aspirin**

ED
Arrival
60 min

Candidate

10
Review risks/benefits with patient and family. If acceptable:
• Give **rtPA**
• No anticoagulants or anti platelet treatment for 24 hours

11
• Begin stroke or hemorrhage pathway
• Admit to stroke unit or intensive care unit

Stroke
Admission
3 hours;

12
• Begin post-rtPA stroke pathway
• Aggressively monitor:
 – BP per protocol (Tables 2 and 3)
 – For neurologic deterioration
• Emergent admission to stroke unit or intensive care unit

© 2010 American Heart Association

ventilatory assistance through a bag-mask device. (Breathing patterns are typically normal except when the patient is comatose.) Administer oxygen to keep oxygen saturation at greater than 94%.

• Apply a portable cardiac monitor. (Cardiac arrest is uncommon except in cases of intracranial hemorrhage; however, you may detect underlying cardiac arrhythmias on the monitor. If cardiac arrest occurs, begin cardiopulmonary resuscitation [CPR].)

• Check the patient's blood glucose level, but don't delay transport for further assessment.

Critical interval

After completing the initial assessment, attempt to establish the time of the patient's onset of symptoms. The interval between the onset of symptoms and the initiation of treatment is critical. If no one is able to identify when the patient's symptoms began, the onset of symptoms is defined as the last time the patient was observed to be normal.

The patient should be transported to a stroke-prepared hospital, primary stroke center, or comprehensive stroke center. Studies show that patients admitted to dedicated stroke units have a greater chance of improved functional outcomes. Facilities with established stroke programs have protocols that may establish a diagnosis of stroke more quickly than a facility without one. Remember that communicating with the receiving facility while the patient is en route is critical to ensuring prompt action in the ED when the patient arrives.

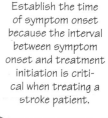

Establish the time of symptom onset because the interval between symptom onset and treatment initiation is critical when treating a stroke patient.

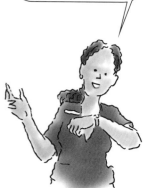

Door

As soon as the patient comes through the door of the ED (within 10 minutes), rapid assessment and evaluation of baseline vital signs should begin. The patient should be evaluated to determine if he's a candidate for fibrinolytic therapy. At this time, complete the secondary assessment. Follow these steps:

• Reassess the patient's airway and breathing.

• If the patient is breathing adequately without assistance, administer oxygen to keep his saturation at greater than 94%.

• Reassess circulation, assess blood pressure, and evaluate cardiac rhythm.

• Make sure that I.V. access has been established.

• Obtain appropriate laboratory studies (including blood glucose level, CBC, and cogqulation studies) and a 12-lead electrocardiogram (ECG). (Don't delay the computed tomography [CT] scan to obtain the ECG.)

• Assess the patient's neurologic status to determine the extent of his deficits using a standardized tool such as the NIH Stroke Scale. (For a patient with a subarachnoid hemorrhage, you may use the Hunt and

(Text continues on page 263)

NIH Stroke Scale

You can use a neurologic flow sheet, such as the National Institutes of Health (NIH) Stroke Scale, to record frequent neurologic assessments. For each item, choose the score that reflects what the patient can actually do at the time of the assessment. Add the scores for each item and record the total. The higher the score, the more severe the neurologic deficits.

Category	Description	Score	Date/time 3/3/12 1100	2 hours post treatment
1a. Level of consciousness (LOC)	Alert	0	1	
	Drowsy	1		
	Obtunded	2		
	Unresponsive	3		
1b. LOC questions (Ask patient what month it is and his age.)	Answers both correctly	0	0	
	Answers one correctly	1		
	Incorrect	2		
1c. LOC commands (Have patient open/close his eyes, make a fist, and then let go.)	Obeys both correctly	0	1	
	Obeys one correctly	1		
	Incorrect	2		
2. Best gaze (Eyes open; have patient follow your finger or face.)	Normal	0	0	
	Partial gaze palsy	1		
	Forced deviation	2		
3. Visual (Introduce visual stimulus/ threat to patient's visual field quadrants.)	No vision loss	0	1	
	Partial hemianopsia	1		
	Complete hemianopsia	2		
	Bilateral hemianopsia	3		
4. Facial palsy (Have patient show his teeth, raise his eyebrows, and squeeze his eyes shut.)	Normal	0	2	
	Minor	1		
	Partial	2		
	Complete	3		
5a. Motor arm—left (Elevate extremity to 90 degrees and score drift/ movement.)	Normal, no drift	0	4	
	Drift	1		
	Some effort against gravity	2		
	No effort against gravity	3		
	No movement	4		
	Not tested (amputation, joint fusion)(explain)	UN		

(continued)

NIH Stroke Scale (continued)

Category	Description	Score	Date/time 3/3/12 1100	2 hours post treatment
5b. Motor arm—right (Elevate extremity to 90 degrees and score drift/ movement.)	Normal, no drift Drift Some effort against gravity No effort against gravity No movement Not tested (amputation, joint fusion) (explain)	0 1 2 3 4 UN	0	
6a. Motor leg—left (Elevate extremity to 30 degrees and score drift/ movement.)	Normal, no drift Drift Some effort against gravity No effort against gravity No movement Not tested (amputation, joint fusion) (explain)	0 1 2 3 4 UN	4	
6b. Motor leg—right (Elevate extremity to 30 degrees and score drift/ movement.)	Normal, no drift Drift Some effort against gravity No effort against gravity No movement Not tested (amputation, joint fusion) (explain)	0 1 2 3 4 UN	0	
7. Limb ataxia (Perform finger-nose, heel down shin testing.)	Absent Present in one limb Present in two limbs Not tested (amputation, joint fusion) (explain)	0 1 2 UN	1	
8. Sensory (Pinprick patient's face, arm, trunk, and leg—compare side to side.)	Normal Partial loss Severe loss	0 1 2	0	
9. Best language (Have patient name items, describe a picture, and read sentences.)	No aphasia Mild to moderate aphasia Severe aphasia Mute	0 1 2 3	1	
10. Dysarthria	Normal articulation Mild to moderate dysarthria	0 1	1	

NIH Stroke Scale *(continued)*

Category	Description	Score	Date/time 3/3/12 1100	2 hours post treatment
(Have patient repeat listed words—evaluate speech clarity.)	Near to intelligible or worse Intubated or other physical barrier (explain)	2 UN		
11. Extinction and inattention (Use information from previous testing to identify neglect or double simultaneous stimuli testing.)	No abnormality Partial Profound	0 1 2	0	
		Total	16	

Individual administering scale: *Helen Horeson, RN*

Source: National Institute of Neurologic Disorders and Stroke. *NIH Stroke Scale.* Available at *www.ninds.nih.gov.*

Hess Scale to evaluate stroke severity. This scale may also help predict the patient's risk of complications and chance of survival.)
• Obtain a CT scan without contrast medium within 25 minutes of the patient's arrival in the ED. (The results should be available within 45 minutes of patient arrival to determine whether a subarachnoid hemorrhage is present.)
• Institute continuous cardiac monitoring.

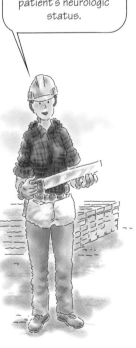

Be sure to use a standardized tool when assessing the patient's neurologic status.

Just to be sure

During the first few hours after an ischemic stroke, the CT scan may not show signs of ischemia. Those with a subarachnoid hemorrhage will have a normal CT scan only about 5% of the time. If you suspect a subarachnoid hemorrhage despite a normal CT scan, a lumbar puncture should be performed. Fibrinolytic therapy is contraindicated in patients who have experienced a subarachnoid hemorrhage.

Data

Data, such as your assessment, patient history, vital signs, and CT scan results, help the neurosurgical team determine the best treatment plan for the patient. If the patient has signs of brain hemorrhage and a neurosurgical team isn't available, consider transferring the patient to another facility that can offer him the appropriate neurologic support.

Cincinnati Prehospital Stroke Scale

The Cincinnati Prehospital Stroke Scale is a simplified scale for evaluating patients with suspected stroke derived from the National Institutes of Health Stroke Scale. Use this scale to evaluate facial palsy, arm weakness, and speech abnormalities. An abnormality in any one of the categories below indicates that the probability of stroke is 72%.

Facial droop

Tell the patient to show his teeth or smile. If he hasn't had a stroke, both sides of his face will move equally. If he has had a stroke, one side of his face won't move as well as the other side.

Normal response

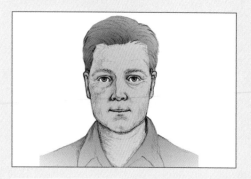

Facial droop on right side of face

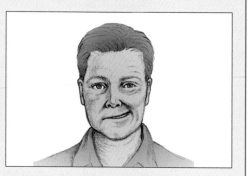

Arm drift

Tell the patient to close her eyes and hold both arms straight out in front of her for 20 seconds. If she hasn't had a stroke, her arms won't move or, if they do move, they'll move the same amount. If the patient has had a stroke, one arm won't move or one arm will drift down compared with the other arm.

Normal response

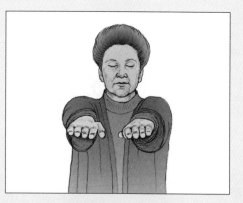

One-sided motor weakness in right arm

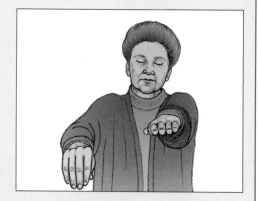

Abnormal speech

Have the patient say, "You can't teach an old dog new tricks." If he hasn't had a stroke, he'll use correct words and his speech won't be slurred. If he has had a stroke, he may use the wrong words, slur the words, or be unable to speak at all.

Decision

The type of treatment you provide is based on the assessment parameters and the patient's situation and type of injury.
• Fibrinolytic therapy is indicated for acute ischemic stroke if it can be initiated within the first 3 hours of symptom onset.
• Emergency angiography may be necessary if the patient has a subarachnoid hemorrhage.
• If an aneurysm is present, treatment may include aneurysm clipping, coiling, or exclusion; administering nimodipine; and correcting hyponatremia and water loss (if diabetes insipidus develops).
• If intracerebral hemorrhage is present, treatment may include preventing continued bleeding, managing intracranial pressure (ICP) and, possibly, neurosurgical decompression.

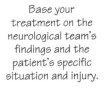

Base your treatment on the neurological team's findings and the patient's specific situation and injury.

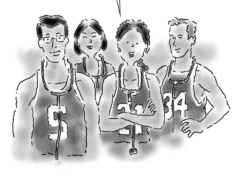

Drug

Initiate appropriate medical treatment within 60 minutes of the patient's arrival in the ED. Fibrinolytics are the drug therapy of choice, but the patient must meet certain criteria to be considered for this type of treatment. (See *Who's suited for fibrinolytic therapy?* page 266.)

Maybe, maybe not

Hypertension is commonly seen in stroke patients as a result of stress from the stroke and usually resolves without treatment. Avoid using typical treatments for hypertension because hypotension may result, which can impair cerebral perfusion.

Elevated blood pressure after a stroke isn't a hypertensive emergency unless the patient has other medical conditions. The occurrence of acute MI, severe left ventricular dysfunction, aortic dissection, or hypertensive encephalopathy indicates a need to maintain more normal blood pressure.

Push or drip? It's all good!

Appropriate antihypertensives for the stroke patient who's a candidate for fibrinolytic therapy include labetalol (Trandate) or nicardipine (Cardene).
• Administer labetalol 10 to 20 mg by I.V. push over 1 to 2 minutes; may repeat once.
• Start nicardipine infusion at 5 mg/hour and titrate by 2.5 mg/hour every 5 to 15 minutes (maximum, 15 mg/hour).

Disposition

Patients should be admitted to a specialized stroke unit or critical-care unit quickly (within 3 hours of arrival is recommended).

Who's suited for fibrinolytic therapy?

Not every stroke patient is a candidate for fibrinolytic therapy. Each patient must be evaluated to see whether he meets the established criteria.

Criteria that must be present
- Acute ischemic stroke associated with significant neurologic deficit
- Onset of symptoms less than 3 hours before treatment begins
- Age 18 or older

Criteria that must *not* be present
- Evidence of intracranial hemorrhage during pretreatment evaluation
- Signs and symptoms of subarachnoid hemorrhage during pretreatment evaluation
- Blood glucose level less than 50 mg/dL
- Intracranial neoplasm, arteriovenous malformation, or aneurysm
- History of intracranial hemorrhage
- History of recent (within 3 months) intracranial or intraspinal surgery, serious head trauma, or previous stroke
- Active bleeding
- Noncompressible arterial puncture within past week
- Known bleeding diathesis, involving but not limited to:
  - current use of oral anticoagulants, such as warfarin, or International Normalized Ratio greater than 1.5 or prothrombin time greater than 15 seconds
  - receipt of heparin within 48 hours before the onset of stroke and having a partial thromboplastin time greater than the upper normal limit
  - platelet count less than 100,000/µL
- Uncontrolled hypertension at time of treatment greater than (185 mm Hg or diastolic greater than 110 mm Hg)
- Computed tomography scan shows multilobar infarction

Criteria that shouldn't be present
- Seizure at stroke onset with post-seizure neurological impairments
- GI or urinary tract hemorrhage within 21 days
- Major surgery or trauma within 14 days
- Acute myocardial infarction within 3 months
- Only minor or rapidly improving signs and symptoms of stroke

> The health care team must evaluate the patient to determine whether he's a candidate for fibrinolytic therapy.

Studies show that care delivered in a stroke unit is higher quality than in general medical units and the positive effects of that care can persist for years.

What to consider

- If the patient has a fever, use acetaminophen (Tylenol) or other cooling measures to reduce hyperthermia.

- If seizures occur, administer anticonvulsants
- If you suspect cerebral edema (clinically significant in only 10% to 20% of stroke patients), you must maintain ICP sufficient for adequate cerebral perfusion but low enough to avoid brain herniation. Treatments may include:
  - elevating the head of the bed 20 to 30 degrees
  - modestly restricting fluids
  - providing oxygenation and ventilation support to avoid hypoxemia and hypoventilation and inducing hyperventilation
  - initiating hyperosmolar therapy by giving mannitol (Osmitrol) to lower ICP; effects usually occur about 20 minutes after administration

Cardiac arrest during pregnancy

Cardiovascular and respiratory systems are altered significantly during pregnancy. As a result, a pregnant woman is more susceptible to the effects of cardiovascular and respiratory difficulties. MI is the most common cause of maternal death from cardiac disease.

When treating a pregnant patient, remember that circulating blood volume, cardiac output, heart rate, oxygen consumption, and minute ventilation increase during pregnancy while systemic and pulmonary vascular resistance, pulmonary functional residual capacity, and colloid oncotic pressure decrease.

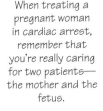

When treating a pregnant woman in cardiac arrest, remember that you're really caring for two patients— the mother and the fetus.

Treatment for two

Keep in mind that you need to consider optimal care for the mother and the fetus when managing cardiac arrest in a pregnant woman. If the mother isn't doing well, the fetus will also be affected. The key to resuscitation of the fetus is resuscitation of the mother because the two are inseparable in this situation.

What causes it

Cardiac arrest in a pregnant woman is typically caused by precipitating events that may be indirectly attributed to the physiologic changes that occur during pregnancy.
These include:

- bleeding/disseminated intravascular coagulation
- pulmonary embolism
- cardiac disease (MI, aortic dissection, cardiomyopathy)
- trauma
- hypertension (preeclampsia, eclampsia)
- amniotic fluid embolism

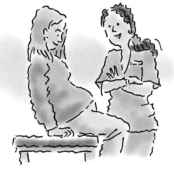

- placenta abruptio, previa
- complications of tocolytic therapy, such as arrhythmias, MI, or heart failure
- anesthetic complications, including spinal shock
- uterine atony
- sepsis.

What to look for

Signs of cardiac arrest in a pregnant patient don't differ from those in another patient. They include:
- loss of consciousness
- inadequate breathing
- absence of a pulse.

How it's treated

Treatment of a pregnant patient during advanced cardiac life support (ACLS) involves assessment of the patient, with some adjustments based on the size of the fetus.

Position supposition

First, stay aware of the patient's position. When a pregnant woman is in a supine position, the pressure of the uterus on abdominal blood vessels (particularly the inferior vena cava) can inhibit venous return and filling of the abdominal aorta. This can produce hypotension and decreased cardiac output, which may result in signs of shock. For this reason, a pregnant patient requires displacement of the uterus to the left when placed in a supine position. To accomplish this, use one of the following methods:
- Place a foam wedge, the backs of overturned chairs, pillows, blankets, or other supporting material under the patient's right torso (optimally, her torso should be angled 30 to 45 degrees from the floor).
- Position your knees and thighs under the patient's right hip and back to tilt her torso to the left.
- Manually displace the uterus to the left while resuscitation efforts proceed.

Circulation

You may need to perform chest compressions slightly higher on the sternum (slightly above the center) of a patient in advanced pregnancy to accommodate the shifting of abdominal contents toward the patient's head. You will need proper hand position to achieve a pulse.

When replacing fluid volume, remember that there's a normal increase in blood volume of up to 50% during pregnancy.

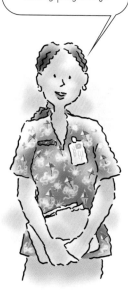

When replacing fluid volume, remember that there's a normal increase in blood volume of up to 50% during pregnancy.

In addition, you must monitor blood supply to the neonate to maintain stability. Establish I.V. access above the diaphragm.

Airway

Secure the airway early in the resuscitation effort. Airway management of a pregnant patient is more difficult than with a nonpregnant patient. There is also an increased risk of pregnancy-related complications in airway management.

Breathing

Be aware that the gravid uterus pushes up on the diaphragm and may decrease ventilatory volume, which makes providing positive-pressure ventilation difficult. As in any resuscitation, make sure that there's adequate rise to the chest when providing ventilations. It is especially important in pregnancy to provide good ventilations with 100% oxygen and bag-mask before intubation.

Defibrillation

Defibrillation requirements are unchanged when resuscitating a pregnant patient. Shocks haven't been found to transfer a significant current to the developing fetus. If internal or external fetal monitors are in use, it's a good idea to remove them before defibrillating.

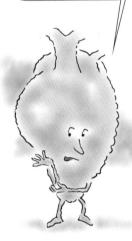

Defibrillation is OK for a pregnant patient because shocks don't transfer significant current to the fetus.

Differential diagnosis

In certain situations, an emergency cesarean delivery may be indicated. This may increase the chance of survival for the mother and fetus when performed within 5 minutes of the cardiac arrest because blood supply to the fetus becomes rapidly hypoxic and acidotic. Points to consider when making this decision include:
• the patient's response to appropriate basic life support (BLS) and ACLS care
• the presence of an inevitably fatal injury or condition in the patient
• the possible benefit of a cesarean delivery to the mother (Removing the fetus and the placenta benefits the mother even if the fetus is too small to compress the inferior vena cava.)
• gestational age and viability of the fetus
• time that has elapsed between collapse of the mother and possible removal of the fetus
• availability of personnel able to perform a cesarean delivery and to support the mother and neonate after the procedure.

If a cesarean delivery has been performed, provide supportive measures to the mother and neonate, as indicated, to promote their chance of survival.

What to consider

• If persistent arrest is due to an immediately reversible problem (such as excessive anesthesia or analgesia or bronchospasm), cesarean delivery isn't indicated.

• If standard BLS and ACLS measures fail and there's a chance that the fetus is viable, consider immediate perimortem cesarean delivery.

Cardiac arrest as a result of trauma

The treatment of a trauma patient with cardiac or respiratory arrest is complex. Your prime consideration should be the patient's need for rapid transport to a facility capable of managing his condition rather than performing multiple resuscitation attempts.

> Ensuring rapid transport to a capable facility is your top priority when treating a trauma patient.

Traumatic times

If cardiac arrest is associated with uncontrolled internal hemorrhage or pericardial tamponade, immediate surgical intervention in a capable facility is required. In some situations, the number of critical patients may exceed the capability of ACLS providers and the EMS team. If this occurs, trauma patients without a pulse should be considered lower in priority for care during the triage process.

What causes it

Some of the potential causes of cardiac or respiratory arrest in a trauma patient include:

• tension pneumothorax; ruptured diaphragm, or pericardial tamponade that causes significant compromise to cardiac output

• exsanguination or internal bleeding with subsequent hypovolemia and inadequate oxygen delivery

• central neurologic injury that causes cardiovascular collapse

• severe hypothermia that complicates injuries occurring in a cold environment or during an avalanche.

• hypoxia from airway obstruction, severely lacerated or crushed trachea or bronchi, large open pneumothorax, or neurologic injury

• severe direct injury to vital organs, such as the heart, and to such structures as the aorta or pulmonary artery

• underlying medical problems that led to the injury such as cardiac arrest precipitating a motor vehicle accident.

• Blunt trauma to the anterior chest wall can cause cardiac contusion with ECG changes and rhythm disturbances. If the blow occurs during repolarization, ventricular fibrillation (VF) can result (commotio cordis).

What to look for

The signs and symptoms of cardiac arrest may occur suddenly or insidiously, depending on the mechanism of injury and the patient's age and medical history. If the trauma involves multiple injuries, be sure to look past them to assess for circulation, airway, and breathing.

Signs of cardiac arrest in a trauma patient don't differ from those in another patient. They include:

- loss of consciousness
- inadequate breathing
- absence of a pulse.

How it's treated

First, if the patient is trapped, extricate him immediately using standard precautions. As a health care provider, if you suspect cervical injury, remember to immobilize the patient's neck before extrication and transport. Immobilization is usually accomplished by using lateral neck supports and strapping the patient securely to a backboard to assist in transport. You should also apply a firm cervical collar, which has been appropriately sized for the patient. These actions minimize neck and spinal cord injury while caring for, moving, and transporting the patient.

Next, perform the primary and secondary CABD assessments. Keep in mind that several special considerations exist when treating a trauma patient. (See *Assessment of the trauma patient*, page 273.) Most emergency interventions for the trauma patient will be performed by a practitioner with special training.

Circulation

Provide chest compressions, as needed, to maintain the patient's cardiac output. Apply firm, direct pressure with dry dressing material to control external hemorrhage. A patient with uncontrollable hemorrhage should be transported immediately to a hospital for surgical intervention.

Trauma to the thoracic cage increases the risk that chest compressions may cause tension pneumothorax. If compressions are necessary, synchronize them with ventilations to minimize damaging the patient's already traumatized lungs.

Airway

Remember that you must immobilize the spine when performing BLS procedures on a patient with suspected head or neck trauma or with multisystem trauma. This can make providing the required patient care challenging. If possible, have another rescuer support

the patient's neck during airway procedures. Follow these steps to ensure a patent airway:
• Open the airway using the jaw-thrust maneuver (preferred over the head-tilt, chin-lift maneuver).
• Use the finger sweep maneuver or suction to clear the airway of secretions, including blood and vomitus.
• If intubation is needed to obtain or maintain an adequate airway, perform orotracheal intubation (preferred over nasotracheal intubation). (Remember to confirm proper tube placement initially and with any movement or transfer of the patient, if unable to initiate continuous waveform capnography.)
• If intubation is unsuccessful or if the patient has experienced massive facial injury and edema, perform cricothyrotomy.

I'm best given in high concentrations. If I'm not, I get kind of cranky.

Breathing

If ventilation is required, immobilize and maintain the patient's cervical spine. Always provide ventilation with high concentrations of oxygen, even if the patient's oxygenation appears adequate. When using a bag-mask device, remember to deliver breaths slowly to reduce the chance of gastric distention and regurgitation, which can easily lead to aspiration.

Pitfall potential

Follow these steps if you suspect the presence of conditions that are interfering with the patient's ability to breathe on his own:
• Assess for open pneumothorax and seal the pleural cavity if present. (If ventilation attempts don't cause the patient's chest to expand despite repeated attempts to open the airway using the jaw-thrust maneuver, suspect tension pneumothorax or hemothorax.)
• If the patient has suffered chest injury, check for asymmetry of breath sounds or resistance to ventilation, which may indicate tension pneumothorax. (If tension pneumothorax is present, immediately perform needle decompression, followed by the insertion of a chest tube to help expand the patient's lungs.)
• If significant flail chest is present, intubate the patient and provide positive-pressure ventilation because he'll be unable to maintain adequate oxygenation.
• If penetrating trauma occurred to the patient's left chest and is associated with signs of decreased cardiac output or tamponade (jugular vein distention, hypotension, and muffled heart tones), suspect penetrating cardiac injury. (If penetrating cardiac injury is present, perform emergency open thoracotomy, which allows direct cardiac massage as well as management of thoracic hemorrhage and cardiac tamponade. Aortic cross-clamping can also be performed during this procedure.)

Memory jogger

To help remember what information to obtain during your assessment of the trauma patient, use the acronym **SAMPLE:**

Signs and symptoms

Allergies

Medications

Past medical history

Last meal

Events leading to injury.

Assessment of the trauma patient

This chart shows what to look for and what to do during the assessment of the trauma patient.

Parameter	Assessment	Interventions
Circulation	• Pulse and blood pressure • Bleeding or hemorrhage • Capillary refill, color of skin and mucous membranes • Cardiac rhythm	• Perform cardiopulmonary resuscitation, administer medications, and perform defibrillation or synchronized cardioversion. • Control hemorrhaging with direct pressure or pneumatic devices. • Establish I.V. access and provide fluid therapy, such as isotonic fluids and blood. • Treat life-threatening conditions such as cardiac tamponade.
Airway	• Airway patency • Position of trachea (midline or deviation)	• Position the patient and make sure that his neck is midline and stabilized, and then perform the jaw-thrust maneuver. • Use airway adjuncts, such as an oral or a nasal airway, an endotracheal tube, an esophageal-tracheal Combi-tube, or cricothyrotomy. • Suction as needed. • Remove foreign bodies that may obstruct the airway.
Breathing	• Respirations (rate, depth, effort) • Breath sounds • Chest wall movement and chest injury	• Administer 100% oxygen using a bag-mask device. • Treat life-threatening conditions, such as pneumothorax or tension pneumothorax.
Disability	• Neurologic assessment, including level of consciousness, pupils, and motor and sensory function	• Institute cervical spine immobilization until X-rays confirm the absence of cervical spine injury.
Exposure to environment	• Injuries and environmental exposure (extreme cold or heat)	• Institute appropriate therapy (warming therapy for hypothermia or cooling therapy for hyperthermia).

• If blunt trauma occurred to the patient and is associated with extreme tachycardia, arrhythmias, and ST-T wave changes, suspect blunt cardiac injury, which can result in significant arrhythmias or impairment in function. (Confirm this diagnosis with an ECG or radionuclide angiography.)

Turn up the volume

Successful resuscitation usually depends on restoring adequate circulating blood volume; however, don't let establishing I.V.

access, fluid resuscitation, or administering medications delay transport of the patient to a trauma facility. Initiate these measures at the scene only if extrication of the patient is prolonged. In all other cases, these actions can be initiated en route to a trauma facility. Keep in mind that aggressive volume replacement may be necessary to obtain adequate perfusion pressures.

Control bleeding as quickly as possible. If external pressure doesn't stop internal bleeding or if you suspect penetrating cardiac injury, surgical exploration is required. Hemorrhage may require blood replacement.

Explore the possibilities

Surgical exploration is also indicated in trauma patients in the following situations:
• hemodynamic instability despite volume resuscitation
• excessive thoracic drainage (greater than 300 mL/hour for 3 hours or total drainage of 1.5 to 2 L)
• significant hemothorax on X-ray
• cardiac trauma
• gunshot wound to the abdomen
• penetrating injury to the torso
• positive diagnostic peritoneal lavage
• significant solid organ or bowel injury.

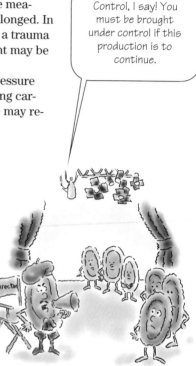

Control, I say! You must be brought under control if this production is to continue.

Defibrillation

If indicated, use defibrillation for VF and pulseless ventricular tachycardia (VT).

Differential diagnosis

It's essential that you identify and treat the underlying causes of arrhythmias. Cardiac monitoring may reveal pulseless electrical activity (PEA), bradycardia, VF, or VT. Although epinephrine is typically administered to treat these arrhythmias, it may be ineffective if severe hypovolemia is present and left uncorrected.

Treating PEA requires treating the causes. You may need to reverse hypovolemia, hypothermia, cardiac tamponade, or tension pneumothorax. Bradycardic rhythms are commonly due to severe hypovolemia or hypoxemia or cardiopulmonary failure.

What to consider

• Trauma from a head injury or shock can produce loss of consciousness.
• Spinal cord injuries can result in a conscious patient with neurologic deficits. Monitor the patient's responsiveness closely

because deterioration can result from neurologic compromise or cardiorespiratory failure.

• A gastric tube may be indicated to decompress the stomach; however, if the patient has severe maxillofacial injury, a nasogastric tube is contraindicated because it can migrate intracranially. (In this case, an oral gastric tube is indicated.)

• The patient may experience heat loss if his clothing is removed to determine the extent of injuries or if blood or other fluids evaporate. Keep the patient warm, if possible, because hypothermia promotes coagulopathy and subsequent bleeding.

> Keep the trauma patient warm to prevent hypothermia.

Submersion or drowning

You can classify a patient who's been involved in a water accident according to the type of incident.

• Water rescue: An event in which a patient is alert, experiences distress while swimming, and receives help. Generally, this patient isn't transported to the hospital for further evaluation unless injured.

• Submersion: An event in which a patient requires support in the field and is transported to a facility for observation and treatment.

• Drowning: An event that results in respiratory arrest when a patient is submerged in a liquid medium, usually water. Death may occur at the scene or within 24 hours of the event. (Up to the time of the drowning-related death, the patient is considered a submersion patient.)

Duration determination

When treating a patient who has been submerged, you should first try to determine the duration of the submersion, along with the duration and severity of the resultant hypoxia. Hypoxia can cause multisystem complications, such as hypoxic encephalopathy and acute respiratory distress syndrome as well as increased pulmonary capillary permeability, which results in pulmonary edema. The patient may also develop hypothermia if he's been submerged in cold water.

> A water rescue usually doesn't require ACLS measures unless the patient is injured.

Even if you can't determine the duration of submersion, promptly initiate resuscitation efforts to restore the patient's oxygenation, ventilation, and perfusion unless you note obvious evidence of death, such as rigor mortis, dependent lividity, or putrefaction. Submersion patients who require resuscitation should be transported to the hospital and evaluated.

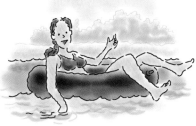

What causes it

Submersion or drowning may occur in such situations as:
• unattended toddler in a bathtub or around water
• residential swimming
• injury after diving
• swimming while under the influence of alcohol or drugs
• child abuse
• boating accident
• underlying disease process, such as diabetes, seizure disorder, MI, anxiety, or panic disorder
• suicide attempt
• scuba diving accident.

What to look for

The degree of injury caused by a water incident varies depending on the amount of time that the patient was submerged and his age and medical history. For example, an elderly patient with a history of lung disease may suffer from water submersion quicker than a healthy adolescent.

Additional considerations include injury occurring before sub-mersion and the temperature of the water. For example, cervical injury that occurs while diving may cause drowning due to spinal injury. The risk of hypothermia develops in water temperatures less than 25° F (–3.9° C), which is the temperature of most natural water in the United States. Also, physical exertion increases the body's heat loss up to 50% faster, thereby allowing hypothermia to set in more quickly.

How it's treated

First, retrieve the patient from the water as quickly as possible while maintaining the safety of the rescuers. Arrange to transport him to a hospital for further evaluation and treatment, even if he has responded to resuscitation efforts. Attempt to determine the cause of submersion and length of time under water. Although the 2010 American Heart Association (AHA) guidelines for CPR now begin with chest compressions, they recommend that you use the traditional ABC approach for drowning victims because the cause for the arrest is hypoxia. Begin cycles of CPR with two rescue breaths.

Airway

The 2010 AHA guidelines state that research findings show routine cervical spine immobilization isn't necessary for a submersion patient except in cases when trauma is likely (diving, water slide, signs of injury or alcohol intoxication). If a potential spinal cord injury is suspected, maintain the patient's head and neck in a neutral position while in the water and immobilize the cervical and thoracic spine before removing the patient from the water.

Breathing

Initiate rescue breathing as soon as possible. Remember, you don't need to clear the patient's airway of water before beginning rescue breathing. In most cases, the volume aspirated is small and quickly absorbed by the lung tissue. After you've intubated the patient, deliver positive-pressure ventilation with a bag-mask device. Continue oxygen administration during transport. Keep in mind that it may take several hours for pulmonary injury to manifest.

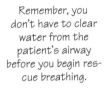

Remember, you don't have to clear water from the patient's airway before you begin rescue breathing.

Circulation

After you've established rescue breathing, assess the patient for a pulse and initiate compressions, if indicated. Assess pulse rate for a maximum of 10 seconds. If you are unable to detect a pulse, begin compressions. The pulse of a near-drowning patient may be difficult to palpate because of peripheral vasoconstriction. Don't attempt compressions while the patient is still in the water unless special equipment (such as a transport board) is available to support his back and rescuers have been specifically trained to use such equipment.

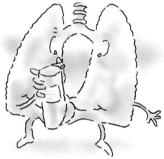

Defibrillation

Use defibrillation if a shockable rhythm is identified. Follow electrical safety precautions, remove the patient from the water, and quickly dry his chest before defibrillation. If the patient has a core temperature of 86° F (30° C) or less (severe hypothermia), follow standard BLS and ACLS algorithms, including defibrillation, while using rewarming techniques.

Differential diagnosis

The cause of submersion or drowning should be considered during rescue attempts. If the patient is in VF or has suffered a spinal injury, you should attempt to simultaneously treat that emergency along with providing respiratory resuscitation and treating hypothermia.

What to consider

• Don't attempt deep-water breathing techniques unless you're specifically trained in their use.

- Be aware that nearly all drowning patients will experience some degree of hypothermia as a result of the submersion and from evaporation during resuscitation.
- Despite aggressive care, patients presenting with significant neurologic hypoxia aren't typically affected by attempts to improve outcome.

Electric shock or lightning strike

Electric shock or lightning strike can cause many injuries with varying degrees of severity accompanied by cardiac or respiratory arrest. Initiate ACLS measures immediately if rescuer safety is assured. Although it isn't possible to readily predict a patient's prognosis, those without preexisting cardiopulmonary disease, especially the young, have a good potential for survival when immediate support is provided.

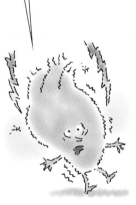

Electric shock or lightning strike can cause cardiac arrest.

What causes it

Although most electric shocks to children occur in the home, most of the incidents involving adults occur in the workplace. Lightning strikes typically occur when the victim is outdoors during a thunderstrom. Many factors determine the type and severity of injury, including:
- magnitude of energy received
- voltage
- duration of contact (contact with alternating current can cause skeletal muscle contractions that "lock" the patient to the source, leading to prolonged exposure)
- resistance to current flow
- path of current flow.

What to look for

Primary respiratory arrest following electric shock or lightning strike can occur due to:
- inhibition of the patient's respiratory center function as the result of electric current passing through the brain
- tetanic contraction of the patient's respiratory muscles during the passing of the electric current
- continued paralysis of the patient's respiratory muscles up to several minutes after the electric current has ended.

Lightning strikes may also affect the patient's cardiovascular and neurologic systems. Cardiac arrest may take the form of VF, asystole, or VT, which may deteriorate to VF. Myocardial injury may occur as a direct effect of the current and from coronary artery spasm. Neurologic injuries may result directly from effects on the patient's brain or secondarily from complications of cardiac arrest and hypoxia.

The current may produce such problems as:
- hemorrhages in the brain
- edema
- small-vessel injury
- neuronal injury
- hypoxic encephalopathy (from cardiac arrest)
- myelin damage to the peripheral nervous system.

Shot to the heart

Lightning strikes cause an instantaneous, massive direct current countershock. Depolarization occurs to the entire myocardium resulting in VF cardiac arrest. In many cases, cardiac cell automaticity restores organized cardiac activity. Excessive catecholamine release or autonomic nervous system stimulation can result in:
- hypertension
- tachycardia
- nonspecific ECG changes (including a prolonged QT interval and T-wave inversion)
- myocardial necrosis.

How it's treated

First, be certain that the electrical current has been turned off or removed before touching a patient who has been shocked. (A victim of lightning strike isn't electrified.) As a health care provider, if you suspect head or neck trauma, maintain the patient's head in a neutral position and immobilize his spine. Spinal injuries can occur with electric shock due to tetanic contraction of skeletal muscles.

Safety first

If rescuers must remain with the patient near live current, only those specially trained to perform in this circumstance should do so. Remember to maintain the safety of rescuers at all times.

If the patient is caught in an unsafe environment, such as high on a telephone pole, he must be brought to safety before treatment. After you've ensured the patient's safety, initiate vigorous resuscitative measures during the CABD assessment.

Circulation

If you don't detect signs of circulation, initiate chest compressions as soon as possible. Hypovolemic shock can occur from significant tissue destruction and fluid

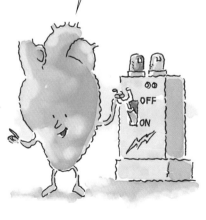

Before touching a patient who has been shocked, make sure that the electric current is turned off or removed.

loss due to increased capillary permeability. Administer adequate I.V. fluids to support circulating blood volume and to produce diuresis. This will promote excretion of myoglobin and potassium, which are by-products of extensive tissue damage. Edema may occur locally at the site of the patient's injuries. Remove jewelry and other constrictive objects to promote circulation.

Airway

Secure a patent airway if the patient can't maintain one naturally. It's important to intubate the patient early because significant tissue swelling and edema may develop, especially if facial burns are present. Insert an endotracheal (ET) tube before signs of airway obstruction become severe. If you suspect head or neck injury, use the jaw-thrust maneuver (preferred over the head-tilt, chin-lift maneuver). Keep in mind that electric burns on the face, mouth, or anterior neck can result in a compromised airway.

Breathing

Initiate rescue breathing if the patient doesn't spontaneously breathe on his own. Provide ventilatory support and supplemental oxygenation.

Defibrillation

If pulseless VT or VF is present, defibrillate to convert the rhythm.

Differential diagnosis

After you treat the patient's injuries, you should evaluate and address the precipitating event such as faulty wiring.

What to consider

• Electrothermal burns and underlying tissue injury may need surgical treatment. Transport the patient to a capable facility as soon as possible for a thorough evaluation of his injuries.
• In addition to potential spinal injuries, the patient may suffer muscular strains or fractures due to the tetanic response of his skeletal muscles.
• The patient may experience thermal damage from smoldering clothing, shoes, and belts. Remove these items to prevent further injury.

Hypothermia

Patients with severe hypothermia may appear to be clinically dead, with pulses and respiratory efforts difficult to detect and marked depression of brain function. Don't withhold

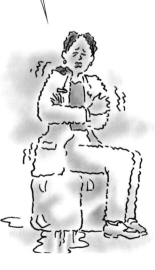

Initiate lifesaving procedures for the patient with hypothermia unless he has lethal injuries or his body is frozen.

lifesaving procedures unless the patient has obvious lethal injuries or his body is frozen to the point that chest compressions are impossible.

What causes it

Hypothermia occurs from exposure to cold temperatures. Unintentional hypothermia may be associated with poverty, mental illness, or the use of drugs and alcohol. Hypothermia may also be a secondary occurrence, such as in the case of a trauma or cardiopulmonary arrest patient found in a cold environment. It may also result from exposure to avalanches during winter recreational activities. It's a common occurrence in a submersion or drowning patient.

What to look for

Hypothermia has a physiologic effect on vital organs. Severe hypothermia results in:
- depression of cerebral blood flow
- diminished oxygen requirements
- reduced cardiac output
- decreased arterial pressure.

Keep in mind that hypothermia may have a protective effect on the brain and vital organs to some extent in cardiac arrest. If the patient cools rapidly, organ ischemia may be reduced because of decreased oxygen consumption.

> Severe hypothermia affects vital organs by causing cerebral blood flow depression, decreased oxygen requirements, and reduced cardiac output.

How it's treated

Some patients with hypothermia maintain a perfusing rhythm and only require rewarming. If the patient has maintained a perfusing rhythm:
- Remove wet clothing, insulate his body, and protect him from wind.
- Transport him to the hospital, carefully avoiding rough movement that may precipitate VF.
- Monitor his core temperature and cardiac rhythm. (You may need to use needle electrodes if adhesive electrodes won't function on very cold skin.)
- Gently provide additional supportive measures, such as intubation, as needed while continuing to monitor cardiac rhythm.

Now we're really warming up!

Institute rewarming for a patient with a core temperature lower than 93° F (33.9° C). If appropriate equipment is available, rescuers in the field should assess core temperature (tympanic or rectal) because rewarming techniques vary based on the severity of hypothermia. Rewarming techniques include passive, active external, and active internal.

In passive rewarming, the patient is placed in a warm room and wrapped in blankets. Manage a conscious patient with mild or moderate hypothermia with passive and active rewarming procedures.

In active external rewarming, heating devices, such as forced hot air, warm bath water, warm packs, or warming blankets, are carefully employed.

Use active internal rewarming for patients with severe hypothermia. Follow these steps:
- Administer humidified oxygen that has been warmed to 108° to 115° F (42.2° to 46.1° C).
- Centrally administer I.V. fluids warmed to 110° F (43.3° C) at 150 to 200 mL/hour.
- Perform peritoneal lavage with potassium-free fluid, 2 L at a time, that has been warmed to 110° F.
- Perform pleural lavage with warm normal saline solution instilled into the patient's chest tube.
- Use extracorporeal blood warming with partial bypass, if available.

Other patients may experience cardiopulmonary arrest and require resuscitation as well as rewarming. If the patient experiences cardiopulmonary arrest, institute standard ACLS procedures.

Circulation

Assess for a pulse for no longer than 10 seconds because peripheral vasoconstriction and bradycardia may make the patient's pulse difficult to detect. If he has profound bradycardia or no detectable pulse, initiate chest compressions immediately and connect the patient to a cardiac monitor as soon as possible to evaluate his rhythm.

An extended cold spell

Patients who are hypothermic for 45 minutes or longer have additional concerns that you'll need to address:
- Administer fluid to counteract the expansion of the vascular space that occurs during vasodilation in rewarming procedures.
- Monitor the patient's heart rate and hemodynamic level because of increased fluid requirements and his response to rewarming techniques.
- Monitor the patient's serum potassium level carefully because significant hyperkalemia may develop. Manage a high serum potassium level with I.V. calcium chloride, sodium bicarbonate, glucose, and insulin or use a sodium polystyrene sulfonate

> A patient's fluid requirements increase if he's hypothermic for 45 minutes or longer.

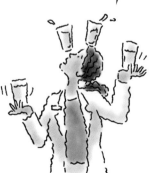

(Kayexalate) enema. (More aggressive treatments include dialysis or exchange transfusion.)

Airway

Make sure that the patient with hypothermia has a patient airway. There should be a visible rise and fall of his chest. If this isn't apparent, use the head-tilt, chin-lift maneuver to open the patient's airway. Intubate the patient if neccessary to provide ventilatory support.

Breathing

After securing a patent airway, assess the patient for breathing. If the patient isn't breathing, initiate rescue breathing immediately and provide warmed humidified oxygen (108° to 115° F) when possible.

Defibrillation

As soon as a defibrillator is available, assess the patient's cardiac rhythm. Attempt defibrillation if pulseless VT or VF is present.

Differential diagnosis

Address underlying disorders and coinciding conditions while treating hypothermia. These situations may include drug overdose, alcohol use, and associated trauma.

> Ahh, this is the life! I get to enjoy the warmth and humidity, and the patient with hypothermia benefits. Talk about a win-win situation!

What to consider

- In the past, ACLS modification in hypothermia suggested withholding or increasing the interval between drug doses because metabolism is reduced when core temperatures are low. Current research is unclear regarding administering or withholding medications. However, using vasopressors may improve the chance of return of spontaneous circulation, especially if rewarming techniques are also being used. It's reasonable to give vasopressors during cardiac arrest according to the standard ACLS algorithm.
- In severe hypothermia, bradycardia may be physiologic and the heart may not respond to artificial pacing. (Pacing isn't indicated unless bradycardia persists after rewarming.)

Toxicologic emergencies

Although exposure to poisons is common, poisoning rarely causes cardiac arrest. If you suspect poisoning is the cause of the patient's cardiac arrest, base your treatment on the specific poison involved. Obtain a careful history from available family members or friends as to which substance was ingested to provide faster treatment.

Remember that a toxicologic emergency can occur from ingestion of many things besides medication. Other substances that may cause a toxicologic emergency include:

- illicit drugs
- household cleaners
- alcohol
- plants
- dangerous gas or fumes.

What causes it

Poisoning can be accidental or intentional. In all cases, it's important to know the drug or substance involved, the approximate amount ingested, and the time that's elapsed since ingestion. For example, if an ingestion error of opioids occurs, respiratory depression may result before cardiac arrest. Also, certain gases, such as carbon monoxide, may cause a toxicologic emergency and resuscitation may be necessary.

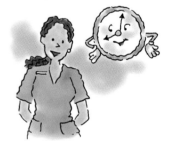

In all poisoning cases, it's helpful to know what was ingested and how much time has elapsed since ingestion.

What to look for

The symptoms of poisoning vary with the substance that the patient has ingested. (See *Substances that can cause toxicity.*) General symptoms include:

- hypoventilation
- bradycardia
- tachycardia
- altered LOC
- hypotension or hypertension
- hypothermia or hyperthermia
- tachypnea
- breath odor
- nystagmus
- miosis
- mydriasis.

How it's treated

Keep in mind that standard protocols for critically poisoned patients may not result in optimal outcomes. A scene survey may add valuable information as to appropriate treatment. However, in all toxicologic emergencies, follow ACLS procedures.

Substances that can cause toxicity

Overuse or overdose of a variety of substances can cause life-threatening toxicity. Signs and symptoms of toxicity vary according to the substance ingested.

Substances that cause hypoventilation
- Anesthetics
- Carbon monoxide
- Clonidine
- Cyanide
- Ethanol
- Opioids
- Sedative-hypnotics

Substances that cause bradycardia
- Beta-adrenergic blockers
- Calcium channel blockers
- Clonidine
- Digoxin (Lanoxin)
- Mushrooms
- Opioids
- Organophosphates
- Sedative-hypnotics

Substances that cause tachycardia
- Amphetamines
- Anticholinergic agents
- Antihistamines
- Atropine
- Caffeine
- Cocaine
- Cyanide
- Ethanol
- Nicotine
- Salicylates
- Sympathomimetics
- Theophylline
- Tricyclic antidepressants

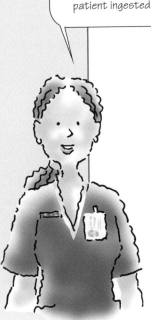

Many substances can cause toxicity; however, symptoms vary depending on which substance the patient ingested.

Circulation

Support and maintain circulation. Assess the patient's heart rhythm and palpate for a pulse. Toxicologic ingestion may cause PEA. When treating a patient who has ingested a potentially lethal amount of drug or toxin presenting within 1 hour of ingestion, administer activated charcoal. If a comatose patient requires charcoal, you must intubate him before beginning the charcoal administration to avoid aspiration. (In addition, try to remove and reverse the toxic agent, if applicable.)

Antidote anyone?

Consider specific therapies to reverse the effects of the drug or toxin ingested. (See *Combating drug toxicity*, pages 288 and 289.) Remember that some agents have antidotes. References that may provide specific antidotal information include:
- poison control
- poison index
- toxicologist.

Airway

Assess the patient's airway frequently. If he has an altered LOC, there's an increased risk of airway occlusion caused by the tongue.

Breathing

Frequently assess adequacy of breathing because the poisoned patient's status can deteriorate quickly, depending on the type and amount of drug ingested. This is especially necessary in the case of opioid overdose.

Defibrillation

Perform defibrillation if the patient with a toxicologic emergency deteriorates to VF or pulseless VT.

Differential diagnosis

After ensuring adequate circulation, determine further treatment based on the type of drug taken or the effects of the drug on the patient. Also, consider specific therapies based on the cardiopulmonary effect of the poisoning agent.

Torsades de pointes

Torsades de pointes can occur with exposure to many drugs. Treatment includes correcting contributing factors, such as hypoxemia and electrolyte abnormalities.

Electrical overdrive pacing (100 to 120 beats/minute) or pharmacologic overdrive pacing with isoproterenol (Isuprel) may also be effective when treating torsades de pointes as a result of drug overdose or poisoning.

What to consider

- Consult a medical toxicologist or certified regional poison information center for unusual poisoning cases. Receiving specific information quickly will help you treat the patient as effectively and efficiently as possible.
- Activated charcoal administration is recommended for patients who present within 1 hour of ingestion.
- Prolonged resuscitation attempts are warranted in poisoned patients. (If attempts are unsuccessful, organ donation may still be an option.)
- Avoid high-dose epinephrine in cases of sympathomimetic poisoning.
- The usual criteria for brain death aren't valid during acute toxic encephalopathy and can be used only after drug levels are no longer toxic.

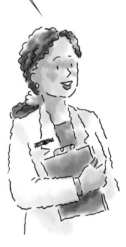

To treat torsades de pointes caused by drug toxicity, consider overdrive pacing.

Near-fatal asthma

Severe exacerbation of asthma, with signs and symptoms developing in less than $2^{1}/_{2}$ hours, can lead to sudden death. Commonly, death occurs due to asphyxia from severe bronchospasm and mucus plugging.

The patient's outcome may be affected by:
- whether he has true active asthma or another severe condition
- preexisting conditions, such as cardiac disease, pulmonary disease, acute allergic bronchospasm or anaphylaxis, and pulmonary embolism or vasculitis (Churg-Strauss syndrome)
- medications or illicit drug use (Beta-adrenergic blockers, cocaine, and opioids can cause bronchospasm.)
- discontinuation of long-term corticosteroid therapy, which may result in adrenal insufficiency and other problems.

What causes it

Cardiac arrest can result from hypoxia-induced cardiac arrhythmias and tension pneumothorax. Positive pressure generated in the patient's lungs as a result of air trapping can also induce cardiac arrest.

Combating drug toxicity

Drug classes produce varying signs of toxicity that require different treatment measures. This table shows the signs of toxicity for various drug classes and their treatment options.

Drug class	Signs of toxicity	Treatment options
Beta-adrenergic blockers atenolol (Tenormin) propranolol (Inderal)	• Bradycardia • Cardiac arrest • Impaired conduction • Hypotension, shock	• Administer glucagon high-dose insulin, or calcium I.V. • Apply an external pacemaker, insert a temporary pacemaker, or use intra-aortic baloon counterpropulsion, ventricular assist devices, extracorporeal membrane oxygenation.
Calcium channel blockers diltiazem (Cardizem) nifedipine (Procardia) verapamil (Calan)	• Bradycardia • Cardiac arrest • Impaired conduction • Shock	• Infuse calcium I.V. • Apply an external pacemaker or insert a temporary pacemaker.
Cardiac glycosides digoxin (Lanoxin) foxglove oleander	• Bradycardia, atrioventricular (AV) block • Ventricular arrhythmias • Hyperkalemia, hypomagnesmia • Cardiac arrest • Shock	• Administer ovine digoxin immune Fab (Digibind). • Infuse magnesium I.V. for hypomagnesemia. • Apply an external pacemaker or insert a temporary pacemaker. • Adminster glucose and insulin for life-threatening hyperkalemia.
Cholinergics carbamates organophosphates nerve agents	• Bradycardia • Cardiac arrest • Impaired conduction • Shock • Supraventricular and ventricular arrhythmias	• Administer atropine. • Administer pralidoxime (Protopam).
Opioids heroin fentanyl (Sublimaze) methadone (Dolophine) oxycodone (OxyContin)	• Bradycardia • Hypotension • Slow, shallow respirations	• Administer naloxone.

(continued)

Combating drug toxicity *(continued)*

Drug class	Signs of toxicity	Treatment options
Sympathomimetics amphetamines cocaine methamphetamine	• Acute coronary syndrome • Cardiac arrest • Hypertensive crisis • Impaired conduction • Shock • Supraventricular and ventricular arrhythmias • Tachycardia	• Administer an alpha-adrenergic blocker. • Administer benzodiazepines. • Administer sodium bicarbonate.
Tricyclic antidepressants amitriptyline desipramine (Norpramin) nortriptyline	• Bradycardia • Cardiac arrest • Impaired conduction, AV block • Shock • Tachycardia • Ventricular arrhythmias, torsades de pointes	• Consider sodium bicarbonate. • Administer a mixed alpha-beta agonist or an alpha agonist. • Administer vasopressors. • Administer lidocaine. (Procainamide is contraindicated.)

What to look for

An asthma attack may begin dramatically, with the simultaneous onset of many symptoms, or insidiously, with gradually increasing shortness of breath. An asthma attack typically includes progressively worsening shortness of breath, cough, wheezing, and chest tightness or some combination of these signs or symptoms. Cyanosis, confusion, and lethargy indicate the onset of respiratory failure.

How it's treated

Aggressively treat the severe asthmatic crisis before it deteriorates to full cardiac or respiratory arrest. Administer oxygen to all patients and arrange to transport the patient to a health care facility as soon as possible.

Medicate and evaluate

Medications for the treatment of acute asthma include:
• beta-agonists such as nebulized albuterol (Proventil)—Give 2.5 to 5 mg every 15 to 20 minutes intermittently or give continuous nebulization of 10 to 15 mg/hour.

> Uh-oh...During an asthma attack, worsening symptoms can lead to respiratory failure... I think I need my inhaler!

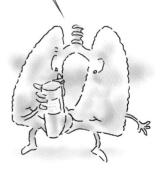

• epinephrine (if the patient doesn't respond to albuterol or if the situation is life-threatening)—Give 0.01 mg/kg of a 1:1,000 solution divided into three doses subcutaneously at 20-minute intervals.

• corticosteroids—Give initial dose of methylprednisolone (Medrol) 125 mg I.V. after administering oxygen and initiating beta-agonist therapies.

• nebulized anticholinergics such as ipratropium (Atrovent)—Because these drugs have an onset of 20 minutes, give 0.5 mg in combination with albuterol, which acts immediately.

In addition, magnesium sulfate can improve respiratory function when used in combination with nebulized albuterol and methylprednisolone. For severe refractory asthma in adults, give magnesium sulfate 2 g I.V. over 20 minutes.

Airway

Because asthma affects airway patency, focus ACLS efforts on maitaining a patent airway. The patient with asthma may have difficulty maintaining an adequate airway secondary to bronchospasm and mucus plugging. Oral suctioning may be necessary to open the airway. If you can't maintain a patent airway, ET intubation may be necessary.

Breathing

Administer oxygen to achieve a partial pressure of arterial oxygen greater than or equal to 92 mm Hg. Keep in mind that an elevated partial pressure of arterial carbon dioxide doesn't indicate the severity of the asthmatic episode. Always treat the patient according to his clinical symptoms.

It's all positive

Bilevel positive airway pressure can help reduce the work of breathing and help delay or prevent the need for intubation. You may also give heliox (a mixture of 70% helium and 30% oxygen) to delay intubation while other medications are taking effect. Heliox decreases the work of breathing by decreasing the resistance of air flow to the bronchial branches by 28% to 48%.

To intubate or not to intubate

In an asthmatic crisis, intubate the patient, using rapid-sequence intubation, if you note:

• a decline in LOC

• profuse diaphoresis

> Intubate the patient in an asthmatic crisis if you note a decline in LOC or if he shows signs of hypoxemia.

- poor muscle tone (a clinical sign of hypercarbia)
- severe agitation, confusion, and fighting against the oxygen mask (clinical signs of hypoxemia).

Circulation

Hypoxia resulting from a severe asthma attack may result in cardiac arrhythmias and cardiac arrest. Assess the patient experiencing an asthma attack for adequate perfusion and circulation. Monitor the patient's cardiac rhythm and vital signs.

Defibrillation

Perform defibrillation if pulseless VT or VF occurs. These arrhythmias may result from a hypoxic state.

Differential diagnosis

Attempt to identify the trigger for an acute asthma attack. Possible asthma triggers include:
- infection
- exercise
- cold weather
- tobacco smoke
- air pollution
- allergens
- chemical odors.

What to consider

- Attempt to identify asthma triggers so that the patient can avoid these triggers, if possible.
- Treating an asthma attack early can help avoid progressive respiratory distress that may compromise the patient's airway and ventilation.
- An asthma action plan should be developed for patients that directs them when to use asthma medications and when to seek medical treatment.

Anaphylaxis

Anaphylaxis is a hypersensitivity reaction triggered by allergens, such as food, medications, insect venom, or latex. Anaphylaxis is life-threatening because it causes rapid airway constriction. The time it takes for treatment to be initiated is extremely important to ensure a positive patient outcome. Initial exposure to the allergen may not cause a reaction. Typically, it's the reexposure to an antigen that causes the reaction.

What causes it

The most common causes of anaphylaxis are:
• insect stings (especially bees, wasps, yellow jackets, and fire ants)
• drugs (such as antibiotics and aspirin)
• contrast media that contain iodine
• foods (such as peanuts, shellfish, eggs, or dairy products)
• latex, which is contained in a large amount of medical supplies.

What to look for

The sooner a reaction occurs after exposure to an antigen, the more likely it is to be severe. Signs and symptoms of anaphylaxis include:
• agitation, feeling faint
• hypotension, tachycardia
• bronchospasm, upper and lower airway edema
• cardiovascular collapse due to vasodilation and increased capillary permeability
• urticaria, rhinitis, pruritis
• abdominal pain, vomiting, and diarrhea
• sense of impending doom.

How it's treated

Depending on the reaction, the patient with anaphylaxis may exhibit various signs and symptoms, which can vary in intensity and severity over time. In the case of an insect sting, scrape away any insect parts at the site of a sting (don't squeeze a venom sac that's intact). Then apply ice to the area to slow absorption. Arrange to transport the patient to a health care facility as soon as possible.

A special kind of pen

You may give epinephrine to treat shock, airway swelling, or difficulty breathing. If the patient is aware of his allergy, he may carry an EpiPen that should be administered as quickly as possible. If there isn't an EpiPen

> Now, wait a minute. You mean to tell me that the EpiPen is shaped like a pen but it delivers epinephrine instead of ink? What an amazing invention!

available, administer 0.2 to 0.5 mg (1:1,000) of epinephrine I.M. and repeat after 5 to 15 minutes if you don't note improvement in the patient's condition. You should also administer epinephrine (1:10,000) 0.05 to 0.1 mg I.V. over 5 minutes in profound, immediately life-threatening situations. A continuous I.V. infusion at 5 to 15 mcg/minute may be necessary.

Medication advantage

In addition, you may consider giving the following medications to treat an anaphylactic reaction:
• antihistamines such as diphenhydramine (Benadryl)—Give 10 to 50 mg slowly I.V. or I.M.
• inhaled albuterol (Proventil) (if bronchospasm is significant)— If the patient is hypotensive, give epinephrine before inhaled albuterol to prevent a drop in blood pressure.
• corticosteroids—Give a high dose slowly I.V. or I.M. for a severe attack, especially in an asthmatic patient; the effect won't be evident for 4 to 6 hours.
• inhaled ipratropium (Atrovent)—helpful for patients taking beta-adrenergic blockers.

For patients experiencing anaphylaxis, modify the standard ACLS treatments of circulation, airway, and breathing. Focus intially on maintaining a patent airway.

Airway

Observe the patient closely during drug therapy. A typical anaphylactic reaction includes swelling of the tongue and throat, followed by difficulty breathing. Be sure to monitor airway patency if you suspect an allergic reaction. Early and rapid intubation is critical if hoarseness, lingual edema, and posterior or oropharyngeal swelling occur because the patient is at high risk for respiratory compromise. Also, intubate a patient if airway swelling is present and he doesn't rapidly respond to pharmacologic interventions. Use caution when giving paralytic agents to ease intubation because these drugs deprive the patient of the ability to attempt spontaneous breathing. Manually ventilate the patient with a bag-valve mask device until spontaneous breathing returns.

Breathing

Deliver 100 % oxygen, as appropriate. Support is essential to maintain oxygen delivery and circulation until the effects of anaphylaxis have resolved. Monitor pulse oximetry to make sure that adequate oxygenation is occurring.

How to use an anaphylaxis kit

An anaphylaxis kit contains everything the patient needs to treat an allergic reaction:
• prefilled syringe containing two doses of epinephrine
• alcohol swabs
• antihistamine tablets.

Instruct the patient to notify the practitioner immediately if anaphylaxis occurs (or to ask someone else to call) and to use the anaphylaxis kit as outlined here.

Getting ready
• Take the prefilled syringe from the kit and remove the needle cap. Hold the syringe with the needle pointing up. Expel air from the syringe by pushing in the plunger until it stops.
• Next, clean about 4″ (10 cm) of the skin on your arm or thigh with an alcohol swab. (If you're right-handed, clean your left arm or thigh; if you're left-handed, clean your right arm or thigh.)

Injecting the epinephrine
• Rotate the plunger one-quarter turn to the right so that it's aligned with the slot. Insert the entire needle—like a dart—into the skin.
• Push down on the plunger until it stops. It will inject 0.3 mL of the drug. Withdraw the needle. (*Note:* This dosage is for a patient older than age 12. Epinephrine use in an infant or a child age 12 or younger must be directed by a practitioner.)

Taking the antihistamine tablets
• Chew and swallow the antihistamine tablets. (A child age 12 or younger should follow the directions supplied by the practitioner or provided in the kit.)

Following up
• Apply ice packs, if available, to the sting site (if appropriate).
• Avoid exertion.
• Keep warm.
• See a practitioner or go to the emergency department immediately.
• Give yourself a second injection by following the directions in the kit if you don't notice an improvement within 10 minutes. (If the syringe has a preset second dose, don't depress the plunger until you're ready to give the second injection.)

Special instructions
• Keep the kit handy for emergency treatment at all times.
• Ask the pharmacist for storage guidelines.
• Periodically check the epinephrine in the preloaded syringe. A pinkish brown solution must be replaced.
• Note the kit's expiration date and replace it before that date.
• Instruct other family members on proper use of the kit in case they would be required to administer the medication.

Deterioration descriptors

Deterioration of the patient is evident with:
- stridor
- severe dysphonia or aphonia
- laryngeal edema
- massive lingual swelling
- face and neck swelling
- hypoxemia.

These symptoms can occur anywhere from 3 minutes to 3 hours after exposure to an allergen.

Consider the alternative

Alternative methods of oxygenation and ventilation include:
- fiber-optic tracheal intubation
- digital tracheal intervention (using the rescuer's fingers and a smaller [less than 7-mm diameter] ET tube)
- needle cricothyrotomy followed by transtracheal ventilation
- cricothyrotomy for the patient with massive neck swelling.

Use caution when attempting tracheal intubation or cricothyrotomy because these measures can result in increased laryngeal edema, bleeding, and further narrowing of the glottic opening.

Circulation

If the patient is unresponsive, be sure to check for a pulse. If there's no pulse, initiate CPR and follow the ACLS protocol for cardiac arrest.

Administer 2 to 4 L of an isotonic crystalloid solution, such as normal saline solution, and high-dose epinephrine to rapidly expand fluid volume. Continue to administer isotonic crystalloid I.V. solutions for hypotension that doesn't respond promptly to epinephrine. Rapidly infuse I.V. solutions from 1 to 2 L up to 4 L to maintain circulatory support.

Defibrillation

The patient experiencing anaphylaxis may deteriorate to hypoxia, resulting in myocardial ischemia and arrhythmias. Follow the cardiac arrest algorithm and defibrillate if appropriate.

Differential diagnosis

While treating the patient, you should identify and investigate the underlying cause of anaphylaxis. Be sure to check the patient for medical alert information, usually in the form of a bracelet or necklace, that may identify allergy information. If no allergen is identified after investigating patient exposures, he may have idiopathic anaphylaxis.

What to consider

• Observe the patient for up to 24 hours because signs and symptoms of anaphylaxis may recur in 1 to 8 hours despite effective initial treatment.
• If the practitioner orders an anaphylaxis kit for the patient on discharge, teach the patient about its contents. (See *How to use an anaphylaxis kit*, page 294.)

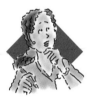

Quick quiz

1. The risk of stroke is increased in patients with a history of:
   A. atherosclerosis.
   B. multiple sclerosis.
   C. rheumatic arthritis.
   D. hypotension.

Answer: A. The patient with a history of atherosclerosis is at increased risk for stroke. Other risk factors include hypertension, cardiac arrhythmias, diabetes, smoking, history of TIAs, and family history of stroke.

2. A pregnant patient experiencing a cardiac arrest requires:
   A. displacement of her uterus to the left when in a supine position.
   B. placement on her right side.
   C. raising her head 30 to 45 degrees.
   D. being kept in a supine position during chest compressions.

Answer: A. The large uterus presses on vital blood vessels and needs displacement to the left when a pregnant patient is in the supine position. The patient may also be slightly tilted to her left to assist with this measure.

3.   When treating a patient for submersion or drowning after a diving accident:
   A.   clear the patient's airway of water before initiating rescue breathing.
   B.   initiate the primary CABD survey while the patient is still in the water.
   C.   consider the patient to have a spinal cord injury.
   D.   administer abdominal thrusts.

Answer: C. Consider the submersion or drowning patient to have a head or neck injury unless proven otherwise. Use the jaw-thrust maneuver to open the patient's airway instead of the head-tilt, chin-lift maneuver. You should also apply a cervical collar as soon as possible.

4.   Primary respiratory arrest after electric shock can occur from:
   A.   paralysis of respiratory muscles during shock.
   B.   pneumothorax from injury.
   C.   contraction of respiratory muscles.
   D.   VF.

Answer: C. Tetanic contraction of respiratory muscles occurs during the passage of the electric current and can result in respiratory arrest.

5.   After receiving the second dose of an antibiotic, the patient develops hoarseness and lingual edema. Immediate actions should include:
   A.   defibrillation.
   B.   administration of epinephrine.
   C.   infusion of blood products.
   D.   administration of high-dose corticosteroids.

Answer: B. The patient who develops hoarseness and lingual edema after receiving a medication, especially antibiotics, may be experiencing an anaphylactic reaction. Your priority in this situation is to protect the airway. Administer epinephrine immediately and support the patient with an isotonic crystalloid solution such as normal saline solution.

Scoring

☆☆☆ If you answered all five questions correctly, way to go! Your knowledge of ACLS is special.

☆☆ If you answered four questions correctly, great effort! Your understanding of what to do in an emergency is emerging.

☆ If you answered fewer than four questions correctly, try again! A quick review will make you a "specialist" in no time.

Megacode review

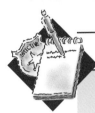

Just the facts

In this chapter, you'll learn:

♦ the role of the team leader during the Megacode

♦ the role of the team members performing airway management, cardiopulmonary resuscitation, and emergency medication administration

♦ appropriate actions to take during emergency situations.

A look at the Megacode

The Megacode station in an advanced cardiac life support (ACLS) class provides a rehearsal to help team members organize their roles when involved in a real code situation. A case study approach is used to present a realistic picture of what occurs during a code. Each student takes a turn at each of the four roles:
• team leader
• team member in charge of airway management
• team member in charge of cardiopulmonary resuscitation (CPR)
• team member in charge of I.V. access and drug administration.

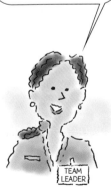

As a team leader, it's your responsibility to direct the activities of other members and delegate actions based on your assessment of the situation.

TEAM LEADER

Team member roles

During the Megacode, the team leader serves as the director of care activities and delegates responsibilities to the other team members accordingly. The team leader assesses and manages circulation, airway, breathing, and defibrillation. Other components of the team leader role include:
• monitoring the quality of CPR being performed
• long-term objectives such as controlling rescuers and bystanders on the scene

- investigating the existence of advance directives
- deciding when to stop resuscitation
- incorporating family needs and concerns during and after the resuscitation process
- providing opportunities to conduct an objective critique of the resuscitation event.

There's no "I" in team

Remember, the team leader needs to be open to suggestions from other team members because many different activities occur simultaneously during a Megacode. For example, the team member administering drugs may notice that 3 minutes have passed since the last dose of epinephrine was given or the team member who intubated the patient may realize that breath sounds haven't been checked. Team members who respond to code situations frequently can quickly and smoothly work through algorithms because they need infrequent prompting from the team leader to perform appropriately to achieve a positive outcome.

Algorithms

Within the Megacode, algorithms serve as guides to patient care, pointing the team in a unified direction. However, don't use an algorithm as a replacement for your team's assessment skills. Remember that research findings may alter the current recommendations, so team members must keep up-to-date and be aware of changes in standards of practice.

Megacode testing

At Megacode testing stations, the ACLS instructor will give you a brief patient scenario. These stations typically include any equipment the situation demands. Before testing day, you'll be given the opportunity to practice with the equipment.

Some instructors try to set up scenarios that apply to the student's likely work situation. For example, if the student is a critical care nurse, the patient situation may take place in an intensive care setting. If the student is employed in a free-standing surgical center, the situation may occur there.

Raise your hand

When presented with the patient situation, you may find that you need additional information to take an action or make a

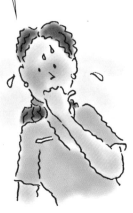

Try not to be nervous. Your instructor is there to guide you, not to deliberately throw you off track.

sound decision. Don't be afraid to ask for that information. If you ordered an arterial blood gas analysis, you might need to ask if the results have arrived. This information is helpful if you need to make adjustments in oxygenation.

In turn, the instructor may ask you for information that's appropriate to the situation. For example, she may ask you if an alternative medication could be given or remind you that an I.V. line hasn't been started (or that the team is trying to insert a line). The instructor won't be trying to trick you, but she will be trying to determine if you're thinking along the correct route or simply guessing. A seasoned instructor can differentiate an unprepared student from a nervous one and will provide guidance to redirect you back to the algorithm.

Line up!

It may be helpful to line up the equipment as you intend to use it or in an order you find most comfortable. You may also use the equipment to remind yourself about what has occurred during the testing scenario. For example, you might place epinephrine nearer to the patient's I.V. site as a reminder that one dose has been given.

Sample Megacode scenarios

Here are three simulations to help you prepare for the Megacode section of the ACLS examination. Remember to only look at each scenario from the perspective of one team member at a time because trying to think about every single responsibility may prove overwhelming.

Scenario #1

INSTRUCTOR: A patient arrives in your emergency department (ED) complaining of palpitations and mild dizziness. She's visibly anxious and crying. Her vital signs are: blood pressure, 98/50 mm Hg; heart rate, 210 beats/minute; and respiratory rate, 24 breaths/minute. You attach a pulse oximeter and her oxygen saturation is 90%. You attach her to the monitor, which shows this rhythm:

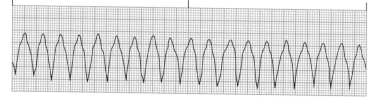

TEAM LEADER: The rhythm on the monitor appears to be ventricular tachycardia (VT). I would perform a CABD assessment and administer oxygen 4L/minute by nasal cannula.

INSTRUCTOR: The CABD assessment indicates that the patient is conscious and breathing with a palpable pulse. The patient's airway is natural and her breathing is adequate. Oxygen is in place by nasal cannula. An I.V. line has been started and a 12-lead electrocardiogram (ECG) is performed. A diagnosis of stable VT is made.

TEAM LEADER: I would direct a team member to administer adenosine 6 mg IV as quickly as possible, followed by a 20-mL saline flush.

INSTRUCTOR: There is no change in rhythm.

TEAM LEADER: I would direct a team member to give adenosine 12 mg as quickly as posssible followed by a 20-mL saline flush.

INSTRUCTOR: That's correct. There is no change in rhythm. The patient's blood pressure is 70/20 mm Hg and she has become more restless. She's arousable but can't answer questions.

TEAM LEADER: I would check the carotid pulse.

INSTRUCTOR: The patient's carotid pulse is present with this rhythm.

TEAM LEADER: Does this defibrillator deliver monophasic or biphasic energy?

INSTRUCTOR: It's a biphasic device.

TEAM LEADER: I would direct a team member to place the defibrillator's gel pads or "hands off" pads on the patient's chest. I would announce "all clear" and "remove oxygen source from patient" and visually confirm that team members are clear of the patient and the oxygen is turned off. I would select the synchronize mode on the defibrillator and perform synchronized cardioversion at 100 joules.

INSTRUCTOR: The patient converts to this rhythm after cardioversion:

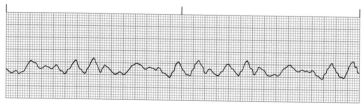

TEAM LEADER: I would check the carotid pulse.

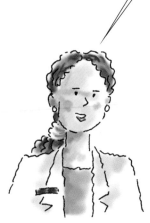

> You need to initiate the primary assessment to ascertain circulation, airway, and breathing.

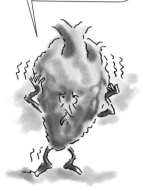

> Cardioversion is indicated because the patient is becoming unstable. Remember, synchronization is critical in a rhythm with a pulse.

INSTRUCTOR: The patient's carotid pulse is checked and is absent.

TEAM LEADER: I would then turn off the synchronize mode on the defibrillator, visually verify and announce "all clear" and "remove oxygen source from patient," and defibrillate the patient at 200 joules.

INSTRUCTOR: The patient's carotid pulse is absent with no change in rhythm.

TEAM LEADER: I would direct team members to perform CPR, beginning with chest compressions. I would monitor the quality of the compressions and the bag-mask ventilations. I would have the team intubate the patient in less than 10 seconds or insert a supraglottic advanced airway based on their skill level, and administer epinephrine 1 mg by I.V. push. CPR shouldn't be interrupted to place a supraglottic advanced airway.

INSTRUCTOR: An endotracheal (ET) tube is placed and confirmed with five-point chest auscultation and secondary confirmation and monitoring using waveform capnography is begun. Epinephrine is administered and CPR is in progress.

TEAM LEADER: I would announce "all clear" and "remove oxygen source from patient," and then defibrillate the patient at 200 joules after 2 minutes of CPR. I would then have to team immediately resume chest compressions, making sure team members switch performing compressions every 2 minutes. I would administer amiodarone 300 mg by rapid I.V. infusion diluted in 20 to 30 mL of dextrose 5% in water (D_5W).

INSTRUCTOR: Amiodarone is administered.

TEAM LEADER: I would visually verify and announce "all clear" and "remove oxygen source from patient" and then defibrillate the patient again at 200 joules after 2 minutes of CPR.

INSTRUCTOR: The patient is defibrillated.

TEAM LEADER: I would resume CPR for 2 minutes and then check the carotid pulse and rhythm on the monitor.

INSTRUCTOR: There's no change in the patient's pulse or cardiac rhythm.

TEAM LEADER: I would direct team members to continue CPR and, if it has been 3 to 5 minutes since 1 mg of epinephrine was given, I would administer vasopressin 40 units by I.V. push.

INSTRUCTOR: Vasopressin is administered.

> When defibrillating this patient, you don't need to apply synchronization. The key is to look at the defibrillator to determine whether the "synch" command is on or off and make sure you know what the patient's condition requires.

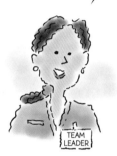

TEAM LEADER

TEAM LEADER: I would announce "all clear" and "remove oxygen source from patient" and then defibrillate the patient again at 200 joules.

INSTRUCTOR: The patient is defibrillated.

TEAM LEADER: After 2 minutes of CPR, I would check the carotid pulse and rhythm on the monitor.

INSTRUCTOR: The patient has this rhythm on the monitor:

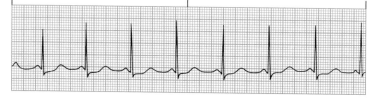

TEAM LEADER: I would check the carotid pulse again.

INSTRUCTOR: The patient has a pulse and the rhythm on the monitor is normal sinus rhythm.

TEAM LEADER: I would direct a team member to begin a continuous infusion of amiodarone at 1 mg/minute.

INSTRUCTOR: The amiodarone infusion is initiated.

TEAM LEADER: I would perform CABD assessment and then admit the patient to the intensive care unit (ICU).

INSTRUCTOR: The patient has return of spontaneous circulation but remains unconscious. What post-arrest treatment might be considered?

TEAM LEADER: The patient should be evaluated for possible therapeutic hypothermia if available and possible percutaneous coronary intervention if indicated.

Note: This scenario followed the algorithm for adult tachycardia (with pulse) and adult cardiac arrest.

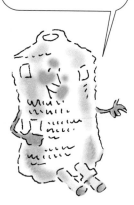

Remember, if the patient's rhythm is successfully converted, an antiarrhythmic may be given by continuous infusion.

Scenario #2

INSTRUCTOR: A 75-year-old woman is admitted to the coronary care unit with the diagnosis of acute myocardial infarction (MI). She denies chest pain or shortness of breath. Her vital signs are: blood pressure, 100/70 mm Hg; heart rate, 210 beats/minute; respiratory rate, 20 breaths/minute; and temperature 98.6° F (37°C). Pulse oximetry is 94%. After returning to bed from the bathroom, her monitor shows this rhythm:

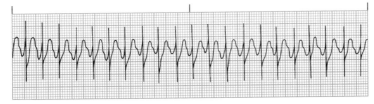

TEAM LEADER: The rhythm on the monitor appears to be a narrow complex tachycardia. I would perform a CABD assessment.

INSTRUCTOR: The assessment indicates that the patient is conscious and breathing adequately with a palpable pulse. Pulse oximetry is 88%.

TEAM LEADER: I would administer oxygen via nasal cannula at 4 L. If there's no I.V. access, I would direct someone to secure an I.V. line. If I.V. access is already present, I would make sure that it's patent.

INSTRUCTOR: Oxygen is on at 4 L. Pulse oximetry is 98%. I.V. access is already established and functioning.

TEAM LEADER: I would instruct someone to administer adenosine (Adenocard) 6 mg by rapid I.V. push, followed by a 20-mL flush of normal saline solution and then elevate the extremity. I would watch the cardiac monitor closely for any change.

INSTRUCTOR: The patient's rhythm is unchanged.

TEAM LEADER: I would direct someone to administer adenosine 12 mg by rapid I.V. push, followed by a normal saline solution flush, and then elevate the extremity. I would watch the monitor for any change in rhythm.

INSTRUCTOR: The patient's rhythm changes to this:

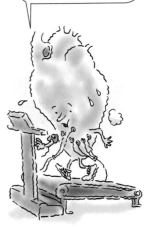

Order oxygen administration for a patient with cardiac injury or disease to help meet the increased oxygen demands caused by an increased heart rate.

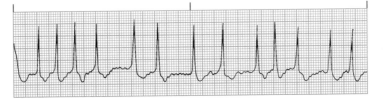

TEAM LEADER: The rhythm on the monitor appears to be rapid rate atrial fibrillation.

INSTRUCTOR: The rhythm returns to what it was initially (regular narrow-complex tachycardia), only the patient's heart rate has increased to 240 beats/minute; blood pressure, 75/40 mm Hg; and respiratory rate, 28 breaths/minute. The patient is complaining of chest pain and shortness of breath. She then becomes unresponsive.

TEAM LEADER: I would have someone check for a carotid pulse.

INSTRUCTOR: The patient has a carotid pulse.

TEAM LEADER: I would direct a team member to place the defibrillator's gel pads or "hands off" pads on the patient's chest. I would select the synchronize mode on the defibrillator, announce "all clear" and "remove oxygen source from patient," and visually confirm that these actions are done. I would then perform a synchronized cardioversion at 50 joules.

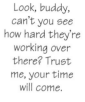

Hey! Let me through! I want to know what's taking so long.

Look, buddy, can't you see how hard they're working over there? Trust me, your time will come.

INSTRUCTOR: The rhythm converts again to this:

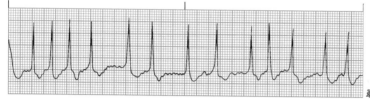

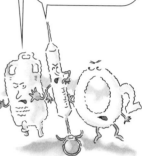

TEAM LEADER: I would check the patient's vital signs.

INSTRUCTOR: The patient's blood pressure is 90/50 mm Hg and her heart rate is 130 beats/minute. Her respiratory rate is 20 breaths/minute. Pulse oximetry is 96%. The rhythm on the monitor is rapid atrial fibrillation. She's waking up.

TEAM LEADER: I would order diltiazem (Cardizem) 15 mg (0.25 mg/kg) I.V. over 2 minutes for initial rate control and consult the cardiologist. I would have the team continue to observe the patient in the ICU. A 12-lead ECG should be obtained.
Note: This scenario followed the algorithm for tachycardia with a pulse.

When someone complains of chest pain, the possibility of an MI is the priority until ruled out. In this situation, rescuers must determine whether the chest pain started before or after the accident.

Scenario #3

INSTRUCTOR: A 66-year-old man is involved in a motor vehicle accident in which his vehicle hit a telephone pole. He complains of pain in his chest, and he's pale and diaphoretic. A bystander at the scene calls 911. While waiting for help, the patient becomes unconscious, isn't breathing, and has no pulse. Bystanders initiate CPR.

The first person to arrive is a police officer. He has an automated external defibrillator and applies the patches. The machine analyzes the patient's rhythm and instructs the officer to push the SHOCK button. One shock is delivered and the patient has a carotid pulse and spontaneous breathing but remains unconscious.

The paramedics arrive. The patient is now conscious and complaining of chest pain. It's noted that the steering wheel is bent. The paramedics call into the dispatcher and begin the CABD assessment: circulation and breathing adequate, airway secured and differential diagnosis made. The patient is conscious and his airway is patent. A cervical collar is applied. Oxygen is delivered at 4 L/minute by nasal cannula.

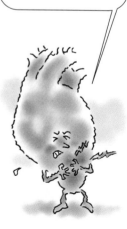

I.V. access is obtained and a 12-lead ECG is performed. The patient is transported to the ED. He arrives in your ED and is attached to a monitor. He has normal saline solution infusing I.V. and oxygen is being administered at 4 L/minute. The patient rates his chest pain as 5 on a scale of 0 to 10, with 0 being no pain and 10 being the worst pain imaginable. A 12-lead ECG is repeated.

The patient's wife arrives in the ED. The paramedics report that the chest pain started after the accident occurred and that the patient hit the steering wheel with enough force to bend it. The patient's vital signs are: blood pressure, 126/82 mm Hg; heart rate, 84 beats/minute; and respiratory rate, 22 breaths/minute. His monitor strip shows the following rhythm:

> The trauma patient needs rapid assessment to identify life-threatening conditions that may impede his airway, oxygenation, ventilation, or circulation.

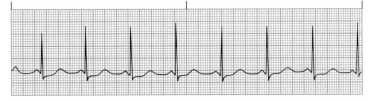

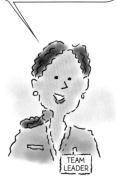

INSTRUCTOR: The patient's 12-lead ECG shows no ST-segment elevation. Now, all eyes turn to you for direction. Please describe your next action as team leader.

TEAM LEADER: I would quickly assess the patient for injury related to the accident as well as obtain a medical history.

INSTRUCTOR: The patient's medical history is benign and he isn't on any medications; however, he suddenly complains of difficulty breathing and then becomes unconscious.

TEAM LEADER: I would direct a team member to assess for breathing and check for a pulse. I would also check the monitor for a rhythm.

INSTRUCTOR: The patient isn't breathing and he has no palpable pulse. The monitor continues to show normal sinus rhythm.

TEAM LEADER: I would assess that the patient is in pulseless electrical activity (PEA). Then I would direct team members to begin CPR starting with chest compressions, and continue for five cycles. I would continually monitor the quality of the CPR. I would direct the team to intubate the patient or insert a supraglottic airway based on the skill level of the team. I.V. access is already established, so I would order I.V. fluids to be run wide open and epinephrine 1 mg to be administered by I.V. push. Then I would assess for a reversible cause of PEA.

INSTRUCTOR: Intubation is complete and tube placement is confirmed by the end-tidal carbon dioxide level and continuous waveform capnography and five-point chest auscultation. The patient

> I.V. fluids run wide open may help reverse hypovolemia, which is the most common cause of PEA.

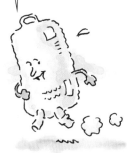

is receiving 100% oxygen with assisted ventilation. The tube is secured. Pulse oximetry is 97%.

TEAM LEADER: I would check for a pulse.

INSTRUCTOR: The patient has no pulse.

TEAM LEADER: I would direct team members to continue CPR. I would assess breath sounds bilaterally.

INSTRUCTOR: The patient has equal bilateral breath sounds.

TEAM LEADER: I would then order pericardiocentesis to relieve cardiac tamponade.

INSTRUCTOR: Pericardiocentesis is complete; 20 mL of blood was obtained.

TEAM LEADER: I would check for a pulse while checking the rhythm on the monitor.

INSTRUCTOR: You check the monitor and this rhythm appears on the screen:

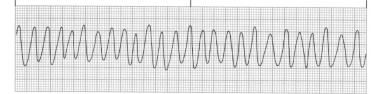

TEAM LEADER: I would ask for a pulse check.

INSTRUCTOR: The patient has no pulse.

TEAM LEADER: I would instruct a team member to place the defibrillator's gel pads or "hands off" pads on the patient's chest. I would place the defibrillator paddles appropriately and announce "all clear" and "remove oxygen source from patient," while looking around to confirm that all team members are clear of the patient. I would then defibrillate the patient at 360 joules because the defibrillator is monophasic and then resume CPR for 2 minutes. I would then check the monitor again for rhythm assessment. If there was still no change, I would defibrillate again at 360 joules.

INSTRUCTOR: The patient has no change in rhythm.

TEAM LEADER: I would ask for a carotid pulse check.

INSTRUCTOR: The patient has no carotid pulse and ventricular fibrillation (VF) continues. Team members are performing high-quality CPR.

TEAM LEADER: I would tell a team member to administer 1 mg of epinephrine by I.V. push.

INSTRUCTOR: Epinephrine is administered I.V. according to protocol.

> Even though the CABD assessment has been done before, it's performed again, taking into account any treatment of the patient.

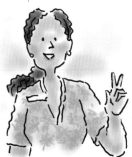

TEAM LEADER: I would direct the team to continue CPR.

INSTRUCTOR: Team members are still performing CPR. The patient has a femoral pulse with chest compressions.

TEAM LEADER: After 2 minutes of CPR, I would check the monitor again to assess rhythm. If there was still no change, I would defibrillate the patient at 360 joules. I would announce "all clear" and "remove oxygen source from patient" again and visually confirm that all team members are clear of the patient.

INSTRUCTOR: The patient is defibrillated according to protocol. The monitor still shows VF.

TEAM LEADER: I would continue CPR and ensure that team members are rotating every 2 minutes.

INSTRUCTOR: There's no carotid pulse; the cardiac monitor is unchanged.

TEAM LEADER: I would tell a team member to administer amiodarone 300 mg by rapid I.V. infusion diluted in 20 to 30 mL of D_5W.

INSTRUCTOR: An amiodarone infusion is initiated.

TEAM LEADER: I would direct the team to continue CPR.

INSTRUCTOR: CPR continues for 2 minutes.

TEAM LEADER: I would check the monitor again to assess rhythm. If there was still no change, I would defibrillate the patient again at 360 joules after 2 minutes of CPR. I would announce "all clear" and "remove oxygen source from patient" again and visually confirm that all team members are clear of the patient.

INSTRUCTOR: The patient is defibrillated according to protocol. The monitor is unchanged after defibrillation.

TEAM LEADER: I would confirm cardiac rhythm on the monitor and check the patient's carotid pulse and continue CPR.

INSTRUCTOR: The carotid pulse is checked and there's none present.

TEAM LEADER: I would direct a team member to administer vasopressin 40 units by I.V. push.

INSTRUCTOR: Vasopressin is administered according to protocol.

TEAM LEADER: I would continue CPR for 2 minutes and then defibrillate the patient again at 360 joules.

INSTRUCTOR: CPR has continued for 2 minutes.

TEAM LEADER: I would announce "all clear" and "remove oxygen source from patient" again and visually confirm that all team members are clear of the patient.

> The course of treatment is drug-defibrillate-drug-defibrillate. When the patient isn't being defibrillated, the team leader should ensure that high-quality CPR continues in the interim.

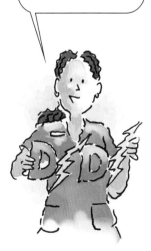

INSTRUCTOR: The patient is defibrillated according to protocol and the monitor shows this rhythm:

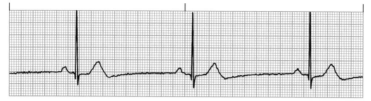

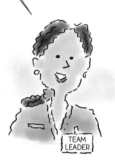

Remember, you can always ask for information during the Megacode.

TEAM LEADER: I see that the monitor shows a change in rhythm, and I check the carotid pulse.

INSTRUCTOR: There's a carotid pulse.

TEAM LEADER: It appears to be sinus bradycardia. I would reassess using the CABD assessment.

INSTRUCTOR: The rest of the assessment is unchanged and the patient remains unconscious.

TEAM LEADER: I would direct a team member to start an amiodarone infusion at 1 mg/minute and have a transcutaneous pacemaker on standby because of the slow heart rate.

INSTRUCTOR: A transcutaneous pacemaker is kept at the bedside.

TEAM LEADER: I would ask a team member for the patient's vital signs (blood pressure, pulse, respirations).

INSTRUCTOR: The patient's blood pressure is 70/20 mm Hg, heart rate, 35 beats/minute; and respiratory rate, 12 breaths/minute with a bag-valve mask device.

TEAM LEADER: I would instruct the team to apply the pacing pads and set the pacer at a rate of 60 beats/minute.

INSTRUCTOR: The following cardiac rhythm is seen on the monitor after transcutaneous pacing is started:

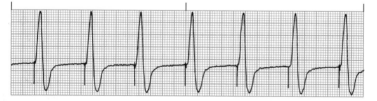

TEAM LEADER: The monitor shows a ventricular paced rhythm with capture. I would check the carotid pulse.

INSTRUCTOR: A pulse is present with this rhythm.

TEAM LEADER: I would direct the team to run an I.V. infusion of 500 mL of normal saline solution over a few minutes, and I would recheck the patient's blood pressure.

INSTRUCTOR: An I.V. infusion of 500 mL of normal saline solution has infused. The patient's blood pressure is unchanged and his heart rate is 80 beats/minute.

TEAM LEADER: I would direct a team member to continue the normal saline solution infusion at 100 mL/hour and begin a dopamine (Intropin) infusion at 5 mcg/kg/minute, titrated to maintain a systolic blood pressure of 90 mm Hg. I would then direct the team to reassess the patient's vital signs.

INSTRUCTOR: The dopamine infusion is started. Systolic blood pressure is maintained at 90 mm Hg with initiation of the infusion.

TEAM LEADER: I would then complete the trauma assessment. When that's finished, I would transfer the patient to the ICU.
Note: This scenario followed the algorithm for pulseless arrest and bradycardia.

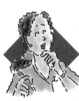

Quick quiz

1. An important step before performing defibrillation is:
    A. calling "all clear" and "remove oxygen source from patient."
    B. setting the defibrillator to 50 joules.
    C. increasing the oxygen flow rate.
    D   setting the defibrillator to synchronize mode.

Answer: A. To defibrillate, you first need to program the defibrillator to 360 joules (for a monophasic machine). You then need to charge the defibrillator. Before discharging the shock, disconnect any oxygen source and call "all clear" and "remove oxygen source from patient" to prevent a fire from the oxygen-enriched environment. Visually ascertain that no one is in contact with the patient before delivering the shock.

2. The team leader is responsible for:
    A. directing the other team members to deliver care following appropriate ACLS algorithms.
    B. delivering medications to the patient as ordered.
    C. recording team member activites and patient response during resuscitation.
    D. checking all equipment before use.

Answer: A. It's the team leader's responsibility to direct the activities of other team members and delegate actions based on her assessment of the situation.

3. What is the most reliable method for confirming and monitoring ET tube placement?

    A. Continuous cardiac output monitoring
    B. Continuous waveform capnography
    C Pulse oximetry
    D. Measuring resistance with a bag-mask device

Answer: B. Continuous waveform capnography is the most reliable method of confirming and monitoring correct placement of ET tubes.

4. Which step is important to perform when there's a change in cardiac rhythm on the monitor?

    A. Check the oxygen setting.
    B. Check for a carotid pulse.
    C. Check the patient's electrolytes.
    D. Check the patient's cardiac enzymes.

Answer: B. When there's a change in cardiac rhythm, check the patient for a palpable pulse.

5. When should synchronized cardioversion be switched to defibrillation?

    A. When asystole occurs.
    B. When atrial fibrillation occurs.
    C. When VF occurs.
    D. Synchronized cardioversion never needs to be switched to defibrillation.

Answer: C. Synchronized cardioversion should be switched to defibrillation if the patient's cardiac rhythm deteriorates to VF.

Scoring

☆☆☆ If you answered all five questions correctly, impressive! You have a "mega" command of the Megacode.

☆☆ If you answered four questions correctly, not bad! You'll make a fine team leader.

☆ If you answered fewer than four questions correctly, don't sweat it! After a quick review, you'll be a Megacode megastar in no time.

Appendices and index

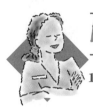

Practice makes perfect

1. After an ET tube is inserted, you should:
   A. deliver ventilations in sync with chest compressions.
   B. deliver ventilations at a rate of 20 to 30/minute.
   C. immediately secure the tube to the patient to prevent movement of the tube.
   D. deliver ventilations asynchronously with chest compressions at a rate of 8 to 10 ventilations/minute.

2. What's a feature of a pocket face mask?
   A. Low-resistance one-way valve
   B. Two-way valve
   C. Reusable filter
   D. Made of transparent, rigid plastic

3. After you insert an esophageal-tracheal tube and attach a bag-mask device to the first (esophageal) lumen, you note that the patient's chest isn't rising and falling, and you hear sounds over the epigastrium. The next step is to:
   A. attach the bag-mask device to the second (endotracheal) lumen and ventilate.
   B. inflate both cuffs to prevent the escape of oxygen.
   C. pull up on the tube so that the printed ring is 2″ (5 cm) above the teeth.
   D. deflate both cuffs to allow emptying of the epigastric area.

4. When you're assisting with pericardiocentesis, it's most important to notify the practitioner if:
   A. the patient develops dyspnea.
   B. blood enters the syringe.
   C. jugular vein distention develops.
   D. arrhythmias are noted.

5. Emergency treatment of tension pneumothorax includes:
   A. needle thoracostomy.
   B. pericardiocentesis.
   C. emergency thoracotomy.
   D. intubation.

6. Death occurs from tension pneumothorax due to:
   A. compression of the organs in the thoracic cavity.
   B. massive hemorrhage into the pleural space.
   C. increased venous return.
   D. collapse of the lungs.

7. What's the most common initial rhythm in sudden cardiac arrest?
   A. VT
   B. Atrial fibrillation with rapid ventricular response
   C. Bradycardia
   D. VF

8. What's an indication for cardiac pacing?
   A. Hemodynamically unstable bradycardia
   B. Asystole
   C. Sinus arrhythmia
   D. PACs

9. When an adult is found unresponsive, which action should you take first?
   A. Defibrillate the patient.
   B. Activate the EMS.
   C. Open the patient's airway.
   D. Begin CPR.

10. The P wave represents:
    A. atrial repolarization.
    B. atrial depolarization.
    C. ventricular depolarization.
    D. ventricular repolarization.

11. Which ECG component gives you information about impulse conduction from the atria to the ventricles?
    A. P wave
    B. PR interval
    C. ST segment
    D. QRS complex

12. The period when myocardial cells are vulnerable to extra stimuli begins with the:
    A. end of the P wave.
    B. start of the R wave.
    C. peak of the T wave.
    D. peak of the QRS complex.

13. For a patient with symptomatic sinus bradycardia, appropriate nursing interventions include establishing I.V. access to administer which agent?
    A. Atropine
    B. An anticoagulant
    C. A calcium channel blocker
    D. A thrombolytic

14. Treatment for symptomatic high-grade AV block includes:
A. beta-adrenergic blockers.
B. ventilatory support.
C. pacemaker insertion.
D. fluid administration.

15. Which scenario indicates the need for administration of amiodarone 300 mg by I.V. push?
A. Pulseless VT
B. Symptomatic supraventricular tachycardia
C. Symptomatic bradycardia
D. Asystole

16. In atrial flutter, the key consideration in determining treatment is:
A. atrial rate.
B. ventricular rate.
C. configuration of the flutter waves.
D. configuration of the fibrillatory waves.

17. Carotid sinus massage is used to:
A. prevent the continual development of PACs.
B. increase the ventricular rate in AV block.
C. convert paroxysmal atrial tachycardia to sinus rhythm.
D. treat VT.

18. The inherent rate for the AV junction is:
A. 20 to 40 beats/minute.
B. 40 to 60 beats/minute.
C. 60 to 80 beats/minute.
D. 80 to 100 beats/minute.

19. During an ACLS situation, which of the following is a responsibility of the team leader?
A. Contacting the patient's family
B. Obtaining arterial blood gas values
C. Monitoring the quality of CPR being performed
D. Signing the death certificate

20. After you deliver a synchronized cardioversion shock to a patient with rapid SVT, his rhythm changes to VF. What's the treatment of choice for a patient with VF?
A. Defibrillation
B. Transesophageal pacing
C. Synchronized cardioversion at the same rate
D. Synchronized cardioversion at a higher rate

21. Which treatment should you give for a patient with third-degree AV block and a ventricular rate of 30 beats/minute?
- A. Lidocaine
- B. Dobutamine
- C. Transcutaneous pacing
- D. Diltiazem

22. Which drug would you give as an alternative to the first or second dose of epinephrine for a patient with VF or pulseless VT?
- A. Atropine
- B. Lidocaine
- C. Amiodarone
- D. Vasopressin

23. Which agent should you give first to a patient with anaphylaxis?
- A. A corticosteroid
- B. Epinephrine
- C. An antihistamine
- D. A histamine-2 blocker

24. Circulation, airway, breathing, and modifications for the patient with hypothermia include:
- A. assessing for breathing and pulse for 30 to 45 seconds.
- B. administering warming techniques immediately.
- C. withholding defibrillation until the patient is warmed.
- D. providing standard BLS and ACLS.

25. Aggressive care techniques and vigorous warming of the patient with hypothermia may result in:
- A. successful resuscitation of the patient.
- B. VF.
- C. aggravation of hypotension.
- D. no particular effect.

26. What action should you take as a hypothermic patient rewarms?
- A. Monitor serum electrolyte levels.
- B. Provide humidified oxygen.
- C. Assess for underlying conditions.
- D. Carefully monitor fluids to prevent hypertension.

27. Activated charcoal is recommended for:
- A. all patients who have ingested lethal amounts of drugs, regardless of time.
- B. overdose of antiarrhythmic agents.
- C. patients who present within 1 hour of ingestion.
- D. comatose patients.

28. What common arrhythmia can occur as a complication of such drugs as tricyclic antidepressants (TCAs) or procainamide?
   A. Tachycardia
   B. Bradycardia
   C. VF
   D. Torsades de pointes

29. Which first-line agent should be administered to treat torsades de pointes?
   A. Magnesium
   B. Calcium chloride
   C. Glucagon
   D. Epinephrine

30. Asthma can result in sudden death from:
   A. asphyxia from severe bronchospasm.
   B. hypoxia.
   C. diminished blood flow and blood pressure.
   D. unresolved preexisting problems.

31. Which sign indicates the need for ET intubation in a patient with asthma?
   A. Decreased Pa_{CO_2}
   B. Tachycardia
   C. Confusion
   D. Wheezing

32. A 74-year-old male presents to the emergency department with a cardiac rhythm determined to be stable, monomorphic, wide-complex tachycardia. Which of the following medications should the team leader consider administering at this time?
   A. Adenosine
   B. Atropine
   C. Vasopressin
   D. Epinephrine

33. A 72-year-old patient is experiencing the sudden onset of mental status change, including slurred speech and vision changes. You should immediately evaluate the patient for:
   A. anaphylaxis.
   B. unstable angina.
   C. stroke.
   D. MI.

34. Which tool is useful for an EMS responder to rapidly identify a patient with stroke?
   A. Glasgow coma scale
   B. Hunt and Hess prehospital scale
   C. Cincinnati prehospital stroke scale
   D. NIH stroke scale

35. Which antihypertensive agent should you give a patient who has experienced a stroke?

    A. Labetalol

    B. Nifedipine

    C. Mannitol

    D. Lorazepam

36. Which of the following is an appropriate treatment for the cardiac arrest patient with return of spontaneous circulation?

    A. Maintaining a temperature of at least 99° F (37° C) at all times

    B. Providing therapeutic hypothermia

    C. Discussing placement in a long-term care facility

    D. Administering an atropine drip

37. What should you consider when defibrillating a pregnant patient?

    A. Initially, half the amount of joules should be administered.

    B. Defibrillation is contraindicated in pregnant patients due to the developing fetus.

    C. The fetus should be removed by emergency cesarean delivery before defibrillation.

    D. Defibrillation requirements are unchanged for a pregnant patient.

38. Physiologic considerations of the pregnant patient in cardiac arrest include:

    A. decreased cardiac output and a normal heart rate.

    B. increased systemic and pulmonary vascular resistance.

    C. increased blood volume and oxygen consumption.

    D. increased pulmonary functional capacity.

39. What intervention is a priority when treating a trauma patient who has decreased responsiveness, facial trauma, and possible spinal cord injury?

    A. Application of a cervical collar

    B. Assessment of neurologic status

    C. Removal of blood from the patient's mouth and use of the jaw-thrust maneuver to open the airway

    D. Determination of oxygen saturation

40. Ventricular arrhythmias in a patient with blunt chest trauma may be due to which of the following?

    A. myocardial contusion.

    B. tension pneumothorax.

    C. hypovolemia.

    D. neurologic changes.

41. What's the priority treatment for a submersion victim?
A. Perform synchronized cardioversion.
B. Administer vasopressin.
C. Defibrillate at 360 joules.
D. Initiate rescue breathing.

42. Cardiac pacing may be initiated for which of the following conditions?
A. Pulseless electrical activity
B. Asystole
C. Hemodynamically unstable bradycardia
D. Ventricular tachycardia

43. How should you treat PEA?
A. Immediately defibrillate the patient.
B. Administer amiodarone.
C. Treat the underlying causes.
D. Use an external pacemaker.

44. What should you see on the ECG of a patient with acute coronary syndrome before you consider administering thrombolytics?
A. ST-segment elevation
B. ST-segment depression
C. T-wave inversion
D. Right bundle-branch block

45. Acidosis in the patient with cardiac arrest is:
A. unrelated to metabolic factors.
B. due to inadequate ventilation.
C. treated immediately with bicarbonate.
D. treated with fluids.

46. How many joules should you initially deliver to a patient in VF when using a monophasic defibrillator?
A. 100 joules
B. 200 joules
C. 300 joules
D. 360 joules

47. A dopamine infusion administered at 20 mcg/kg/minute will result in:
A. constriction of the peripheral vessels.
B. decreased cardiac output.
C. dilation of the great vessels.
D. renal arterial vasodilation.

48. While performing synchronized cardioversion on a patient with symptomatic tachycardia, you note that the patient's cardiac rhythm changes to VF. The defibrillator fails to deliver a shock of 200 joules. Which of the following is the most likely cause?
    A. The defibrillator can only be used once per session.
    B. The defibrillator is in SYNC mode.
    C. The defibrillator monitor didn't recognize the VF rhythm.
    D. The defibrillator has malfunctioned.

49. Which of the following is the AHA-recommended method for confirming and monitoring ET tube placement?
    A. Serial arterial blood gas sampling
    B. Daily chest X-ray
    C. Assessment of breath sounds every 15 minutes
    D. Continuous quantitative waveform capnography

50. Asystole can sometimes be mistaken for which type of arrhythmia?
    A. Idioventricular rhythm
    B. Pulseless VT
    C. Fine VF
    D. Complete heart block

Answers

1. D. You should give ventilations asynchronously with chest compressions at 8 to 10 ventilations/minute. Secure the tube after positive confirmation and monitor placement with continuous waveform capnography.

2. A. The pocket face mask is a barrier device with a low-resistance one-way valve that diverts the patient's exhaled gas. It's made of transparent, moldable plastic that allows visualization so that emesis can be detected. It has a disposable filter that prevents contact between the rescuer and the patient's secretions.

3. A. In this situation, your next step would be to attach the bag-mask device to the second lumen, which has endotracheal placement, and ventilate the patient. You should note chest expansion with bag-mask ventilations.

4. D. During pericardiocentesis, arrhythmias may occur if the needle touches the myocardium. Echocardiography or cardiac ultrasound may be used to definitely identify the location of the needle.

5. A. Immediate needle thoracostomy is indicated for a patient with tension pneumothorax to allow air to escape and organs to return to their original position.

6. A. In tension pneumothorax, organs in the thoracic cavity are compressed, resulting in decreased ventricular filling and decreased cardiac output. Death will occur if this condition isn't treated.

7. D. The most common rhythm seen in sudden cardiac arrest is VF. The only effective treatment is defibrillation.

8. A. Bradycardia that causes hemodynamic changes, such as hypotension and shock, may require cardiac pacing.

9. B. You should immediately activate the EMS after discovering an unresponsive person. Next, initiate chest compressions at a rate of at least 100/minute at a depth of 2 inches.

10. B. The P wave is a reflection of the impulse spreading across the atria, causing depolarization.

11. B. The PR interval measures the interval between atrial depolarization and ventricular depolarization. A normal PR interval is 0.12 to 0.20 second.

12. C. The peak of the T wave represents the beginning of the relative, not the absolute, refractory period when the cells are vulnerable to stimuli.

13. A. Atropine is the standard treatment for symptomatic sinus bradycardia.

14. C. A pacemaker is commonly used to maintain a steady heart rate in patients with symptomatic AV block.

15. A. You may administer amiodarone 300 mg by I.V. push for pulseless VT that isn't responsive to multiple shocks. For recurrent VT, consider administrating an additional dose of 150 mg I.V. and starting an infusion at 1 mg/minute.

16. B. If the ventricular rate is too fast or too slow, the patient's cardiac output will be compromised. A rapid ventricular rate may require immediate cardioversion.

17. C. Carotid sinus massage triggers atrial standstill by inhibiting the firing of the SA node and slowing AV conduction. This allows the SA node to reestablish itself as the primary pacemaker.

18. B. The normal, or inherent, rate for the AV junction is 40 to 60 beats/minute.

19. C. The responsibilities of the team leader include monitoring the quality of CPR being performed as well as assessing the outcome of the actions.

20. A. A patient with VF is in cardiac arrest and requires defibrillation.

21. C. Transcutaneous pacing is a temporary way to increase the patient's heart rate and improve cardiac output.

22. D. After giving epinephrine to treat a patient with VF or pulseless VT, you may administer vasopressin. Vasopressin is a powerful vasoconstrictor when used at high doses.

23. B. Epinephrine is the drug of choice for the patient in anaphylactic shock. You should also give oxygen at a high flow rate.

24. D. Circulatory function can be difficult to assess in a patient with severe hypothermia; however, BLS and ACLS treatment shouldn't be delayed. Once no pulse is confirmed for no more than 10 seconds, CPR compressions should be initiated immediately and the ACLS guidelines followed.

25. B. The patient with hypothermia is susceptible to VF. Be careful to avoid aggressive rewarming.

26. A. When rewarming a patient with hypothermia, hyperkalemia may develop due to metabolic changes. Monitor serum electrolyte levels and treat deficiencies promptly.

27. C. Activated charcoal is indicated for patients who have ingested a potentially lethal amount of drug or toxin and present within 1 hour of ingestion.

28. D. Torsades de pointes can occur with exposure to many drugs, including TCAs and antiarrhythmics, such as procainamide and disopyramide.

29. A. Magnesium (1 to 2 g I.V.) is usually effective in converting torsades de pointes, even if the patient's magnesium level is normal.

30. A. Asphyxia caused by bronchospasm and mucus plugging—both common complications—can lead to sudden death in the asthma patient.

31. C. Confusion is an early clinical sign of respiratory failure and hypoxia that requires ET intubation. Other signs of hypoxia include obtundation, profuse diaphoresis, poor muscle tone, and severe agitation.

32. A. Adenosine is now recommended as an initial treatment of stable, regular, monomorphic wide-complex tachycardia.

33. C. The patient is experiencing the early signs of stroke. Immediate evaluation and treatment will improve his outcome.

34. C. The Cincinnati Prehospital Stroke Scale checks for facial droop, arm weakness, and speech abnormality and can rapidly identify patients with stroke.

35. A. You should administer labetalol for patients with elevated blood pressure caused by acute ischemic stroke. The recommended initial dosage is 10 to 20 mg I.V. for 1 to 2 minutes.

36. B. Post–cardiac arrest care includes therapeutic hypothermia, along with percutaneous coronary interventions, electroencephalogram, and cardiopulmonary and neurologic support.

37. D. Defibrillation hasn't been shown to harm a developing fetus; therefore, you would defibrillate a pregnant patient in the standard manner.

38. C. The pregnant patient will have increases in blood volume, oxygen consumption, cardiac output, and heart rate.

39. C. Ensuring a patent airway and assessing for breathing is essential. When opening the patient's airway, remember to have another rescuer immobilize the patient's spine until you can apply immobilization equipment.

40. A. Blunt chest trauma causes myocardial contusion, which may result in tachycardia and arrhythmias as well as ST-T wave changes.

41. D. After removing the submersion victim from the water and immobilizing his spine, initiate rescue breathing immediately. Then initiate compressions, if indicated, and defibrillate if you identify a shockable rhythm. Support the patient's oxygenation, ventilation, and perfusion until he can be transported to a facility.

42. C. Bradycardia that causes hemodynamic changes, such as chest pain, hypotension, and altered mental status, may require cardiac pacing.

43. C. You must treat the underlying causes of PEA, including hypovolemia, hypothermia, cardiac tamponade, and tension pneumothorax. Cardiac pacing is no longer recommended with PEA.

44. A. You may give thrombolytics when the patient's 12-lead ECG indicates ST-segment elevation or new left bundle-branch block.

45. B. Acidosis in the patient with cardiac arrest may be caused by respiratory factors, such as inadequate ventilation, and metabolic factors, such as high potassium. It can be initially corrected with adequate perfusion and ventilation.

46. D. When defibrillating a patient in VF using a monophasic defibrillator, you should use 360 joules initially. Deliver one shock and then immediately resume CPR for five cycles or 2 minutes.

47. A. Dopamine administered at the rate of 20/mcg/kg/minute will result in peripheral arterial vasoconstriction.

48. B. When performing synchronized cardioversion, if the patient's rhythm changes to VF, you need to switch off the synchronize mode. Cardioversion delivers an electric charge to the myocardium at the peak of the R wave because synchronizing the electrical charge with the R wave ensures that the current won't be delivered on the vulnerable T wave and disrupt repolarization. VF is irregular and doesn't have an R wave with which to synchronize; therefore, the defibrillator won't deliver a shock.

49. D. Continuous quantitative waveform capnography is recommended by the AHA for confirming and monitoring correct ET tube placement based on end-tidal volume carbon dioxide values.

50. C. In some cases, VF masquerades as asystole; however, the more common cause of a false report of asystole is operator error. Always verify asystole in two leads.

BLS guidelines for health care provider: CPR (adult)

Check for unresponsiveness	Gently tap the victim on the shoulder, carefully shake the patient, and shout "Are you OK?" Check for no breathing or no normal breathing.
Yell for help—activate emergency medical service	Immediately yell for help; call 911. Get an automated external defibrillator (AED) if possible. If a second rescuer is available, send him to get help and an AED.
Position	Place the patient in a supine position on a hard, flat surface, if possible, but don't delay initiating chest compressions.
Check pulse	Palpate the carotid pulse for no more than 10 seconds.
Pulse definitely present	Give one breath every 5 to 6 seconds and recheck the pulse every 2 minutes.
Pulse not found	Begin chest compressions by placing the heel of one hand in the center of the chest with the heel of the second hand atop the first so your hands overlap.
Depth of compressions	Compress the chest at least 2 inches (5 cm) with each compression. Allow complete recoil after each compression.
Rate of compressions	Give 30 chest compressions at a rate of at least 100/minute followed by two breaths. If an advanced airway is in place, discontinue "cycles" of compressions. Give continuous chest compressions.
Open airway	Use the head-tilt, chin-lift maneuver unless it's contraindicated by trauma. If you suspect trauma, use the jaw-thrust maneuver.
Provide ventilations	For two-rescuer cardiopulmonary resuscitation (CPR), with no advanced airway in place, provide two breaths after every 30 compressions, with the compressor pausing to allow delivery of breaths. With an advanced airway, provide one breath every 6 to 8 seconds, with no pause by the compressor.
Pulse check	Palpate the carotid pulse every 2 minutes or after five cycles of compressions, for no longer than 10 seconds. Minimize interruptions in compressions.
AED/defibrillator	Check rhythm and defibrillate shockable rhythm. Resume CPR immediately for 2 minutes, then check pulse.
Compressor rotation	Switch compressor/ventilator roles at a minimum of every 2 minutes to prevent fatigue and deterioration in quality of compressions. Switching roles should take less than 5 seconds.

BLS guidelines: obstructed airway management (adult)

Choking—conscious adult

Symptoms

- Grabbing throat with hand
- Inability to speak
- Weak, ineffective coughing
- High-pitched sounds while inhaling

Interventions

1. Ask the person, "Are you choking? Can you speak?" Assess for airway obstruction. Don't intervene if the person is coughing forcefully and can speak; a strong cough can dislodge the object. Quickly activate emergency medical services if the patient is having difficulty breathing.

2. Stand behind the person and wrap your arms around her waist. (If the person is pregnant or obese, wrap your hands around the chest.)

3. Make a fist with one hand and place the thumb side of your fist just above the person's navel and well below the sternum.

4. Grasp your fist with your other hand.

5. Perform quick, upward and inward thrusts with your fist. (If the person is pregnant or obese, use chest thrusts.)

6. Continue thrusts until the object is dislodged or the person loses consciousness.

7. If the person loses consciousness, activate the emergency response system and provide cardiopulmonary resuscitation. (Each time you open the airway to deliver rescue breaths, look in the person's mouth and remove any object you see. Never perform a blind finger sweep.)

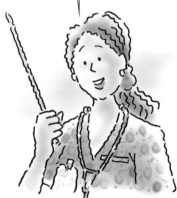

Continue thrusts until the object is dislodged or the person loses consciousness

Guide to common antiarrhythmic drugs

Antiarrhythmic drugs are categorized into four main classes based on their electrophysiologic actions and how they affect the action potential. The mechanism of action of antiarrhythmic drugs can vary, and some drugs exhibit properties common to more than one class. Several drugs don't fall into any of the classes and are, therefore, listed as miscellaneous antiarrhythmics.

Drugs	Indications	Special considerations
Class IA antiarrhythmics Disopyramide phosphate, procainamide hydrochloride, quinidine	• Ventricular tachycardia (VT) • Atrial fibrillation with rapid rate in Wolff-Parkinson-White syndrome • Paroxysmal atrial tachycardia • Monomorphic wide-complex tachycardia	• Check the patient's apical pulse rate before starting therapy. If you note extremes in pulse rate, withhold the dose and notify the prescriber. • Monitor for electrocardiogram (ECG) changes (widening QRS complexes, prolonged QT interval).
Class IB antiarrhythmics Lidocaine, mexiletine, tocainide	• VT • Ventricular fibrillation (VF)	• IB antiarrhythmics may potentiate the effects of other anti-arrhythmics. • Use an infusion pump to administer I.V. infusions.
Class IC antiarrhythmics Flecainide, moricizine, propafenone	• VT • VF • Supraventricular arrhythmias • Atrial fibrillation • Atrial flutter	• Correct electrolyte imbalances before administration. • Monitor the patient's ECG before and after dosage adjustments. • Monitor for ECG changes (widening QRS complexes, prolonged QT interval) and new atrioventricular block (AV) blocks.
Class II antiarrhythmics Acebutolol, atenolol, esmolol, propranolol	• Atrial flutter • Atrial fibrillation • Paroxysmal atrial tachycardia	• Monitor the patient's apical heart rate and blood pressure. • Abruptly stopping these drugs can exacerbate angina and precipitate myocardial infarction. • Monitor for ECG changes (prolonged PR interval). • Use cautiously in patients with asthma.
Class III antiarrhythmics Amiodarone, dofetilide, ibutilide, sotalol	• VF, pulseless VT • Atrial arrhythmias	• Monitor the patient's blood pressure and heart rate and rhythm for changes. • Amiodarone increases the risk of digoxin toxicity in patients taking digoxin. • Monitor for signs of pulmonary toxicity (dyspnea, nonproductive cough, and pleuritic chest pain) in patients taking amiodarone. • Monitor for ECG changes (prolonged QT interval) in patients taking dofetilide, ibutilide, and sotalol.

(continued)

Drugs	Indications	Special considerations
Class IV antiarrhythmics Diltiazem, verapamil	• Supraventricular arrhythmias • Atrial fibrillation and atrial flutter	• Carefully monitor the patient's blood pressure and heart rate and rhythm when initiating therapy or increasing the dosage. • Calcium supplements may reduce effectiveness.

Miscellaneous antiarrhythmics

Adenosine	• Paroxysmal supraventricular tachycardia • Regular, monomorphic wide-complex tachycardia	• Adenosine must be administered over 1 to 2 seconds, followed by a 20-mL flush of normal saline solution. • Record rhythm strip during drug administration.
Atropine	• Symptomatic sinus bradycardia, AV block	• Monitor the patient's heart rate and rhythm. • Use cautiously in patient's with myocardial ischemia; not recommended for third-degree AV block or type II AV block. • In adult patients, avoid doses less than 0.5 mg because of the risk of paradoxical slowing of the heart rate.
Epinephrine	• VF, pulseless VT, asystole, PEA • Symptomatic bradycardia (after atropine administration)	• Carefully monitor the patient's blood pressure and heart rate and rhythm. • Don't mix I.V. dose with alkaline solutions. • Give the drug into a large vein to prevent irritation or extravasation at site.
Vasopressin	• VF nonresponsive to shock	• Carefully monitor the patient's blood pressure and heart rate and rhythm.

Post–cardiac arrest care

The goals of immediate post–cardiac arrest care after the return of spontaneous circulation (ROSC) include optimizing tissue perfusion, restoring metabolic homeostasis and supporting organ function, implementing goal-directed critical care, identifying and treating the causes of arrest, and objectively assessing the prognosis for recovery. Targeted treatment during the postresuscitation period increases the likelihood that the patient will survive neurologically intact. This care should be multidisciplinary, structured, and delivered in a consistent manner. The American Heart Association recommends that post–cardiac arrest victims be transported to facilities capable of providing this level of care.

Objectives for care after ROSC	Immediate interventions	Rationale
Optimize ventilation and oxygenation	• Maintain oxygen saturation at 94% or greater. Consider advanced airway. Avoid hyperventilation. • Optimize mechanical ventilation and titrate oxygen to the lowest level necessary to maintain oxygen saturation at 94% or more. • Use waveform capnography to monitor and achieve target carbon dioxide levels (35 to 40 mm Hg). • Use continuous pulse oximetry to monitor oxygen saturation.	• Interventions confirm that the airway is secure and help detect causes or complications of cardiac arrest (such as hypoxia, pneumonia, and pulmonary edema), minimize acute lung injury, and prevent oxygen toxicity.
Optimize hemodynamics	• Monitor blood pressure frequently by cuff or direct arterial line. • Administer I.V. or I.O. fluid bolus of 1 to 2 L of normal saline or lactated Ringer's solution. • Initiate vasopressor infusion, such as epinephrine, norepinephrine, or dopamine, to keep systolic blood pressure at 90 mm Hg or greater or mean arterial pressure at 65 or greater.	• These measures maintain adequate tissue perfusion.
Optimize cardiac function	• Implement continuous cardiac monitoring. • Obtain and monitor troponin levels. • Obtain 12-lead electrocardiogram to detect ischemia (ST-segment elevation or new left bundle-branch block). • Consider early cardiac catheterization if indicated. • Consider coronary reperfusion procedure (percutaneous coronary intervention [PCI]) or fibrinolytic therapy for ST-elevation myocardial infarction (MI) or acute MI. • Treat arrhythmias as needed. • Obtain echocardiogram. • Administer antiplatelet therapy and heparin if indicated.	• Continuous monitoring and laboratory and diagnostic studies help identify cardiac structure abnormalities, acute coronary syndrome, myocardial ischemia, MI, arrhythmias, and QT-interval abnormalities. • Prompt PCI or fibrinolysis provides prompt revascularization of cardiac vessels, reduces ischemia, and helps preserve cardiac function.

Objectives for care after ROSC	Immediate interventions	Rationale
Optimize cardiac function *(continued)*	• Administer vasoactive drugs (e.g., epinephrine, dopamine, and dobutamine) if needed. • Consider mechanical augmentation (intra-aortic balloon pump therapy) if needed.	• Vasoactive drugs and mechanical augmentation can help support cardiac output.
Identify, treat, and prevent causes of arrest: hypovolemia, hypoxia, hydrogen ion (acidosis), hypokalemia, hyperkalemia, tension pneumothorax, cardiac tamponade, toxins, thrombosis (coronary or pulmonary).	• Obtain appropriate laboratory studies (such as serum electrolyte, magnesium, and calcium levels; arterial blood gas analysis; CBC with differential; glucose level; renal and liver function tests; coagulation profile; and toxicologic screens). • Correct electrolyte imbalances. • Obtain chest X-ray, computed tomography (CT) scan and other diagnostic tests to identify tension pneumothorax and pulmonary embolism. • Correct hypothermia with warming techniques. • Consider fibrinolytic therapy to treat pulmonary embolism.	• Identifying the underlying cause of cardiac arrest will help direct postresuscitation care—from administering appropriate medications, fluids, and antidotes to performing diagnostic tests and procedures to help stabilize organ function, prevent complications, and improve survival.
Protect, optimize, and assess prognosis for neurologic recovery	• If patient isn't following commands, consider therapeutic hypothermia (TH). Follow facility policy and procedure for treatment. • Treat post–cardiac arrest hyperthermia with antipyretics and cooling techniques as indicated. • Promptly obtain an electroencephalogram (EEG) to diagnose seizure activity. Use continuous EEG monitoring for comatose patients to detect seizure activity. • Administer anticonvulsants to control seizures. • Treat pain, anxiety, agitation, and shivering (due to hypothermia) with sedatives, analgesics, opioids, and intermittent or continuous sedation as needed. • Obtain nonenhanced head CT scan to detect intracranial disease (tumor, stroke). • Avoid hypotonic fluid replacement.	• TH is a recommended therapy for comatose adult survivors of cardiac arrest with ROSC, and patients should be transported to an inpatient critical-care facility capable of providing this care. This therapy aims to protect the brain and other organs by cooling the body (for at least 12 hours), which slows metabolism and reduces oxygen demand and consumption. (There are multiple methods for inducing hypothermia.) • Post–cardiac arrest hyperthermia may result from activation of inflammatory cytokines and impair brain recovery. • EEG may be helpful to predict outcomes in comatose survivors of cardiac arrest. • Prolonged seizures can cause brain injury • Pain, anxiety, and shivering increase release of catecholamines, resulting in increased oxygen demand and increased intracranial pressure. • Hypotonic fluids can increase cerebral edema.

Glossary

aberrant conduction: the abnormal pathway of an impulse traveling through the heart's conduction system

adrenergics: medications used to restore heart rate and rhythm and blood pressure during resuscitation of the patient

afterload: resistance that the left ventricle must work against to pump blood through the aorta

amplitude: the height of a waveform

analgesics: medications used primarily to help alleviate pain and promote relaxation

anaphylaxis: severe allergic reaction to a foreign substance

angiotensin-converting enzyme inhibitors: medications used to reduce mortality and improve left ventricular function in post-acute myocardial infarction (MI) patients, prevent adverse left ventricular remodeling, delay progression of heart failure, and decrease sudden death and recurrent MI

antiarrhythmics: medications used to treat, suppress, or prevent three major mechanisms of arrhythmias: increased automaticity, decreased conductivity, and reentry

antiplatelet drugs: medications used to block the final common pathway of platelet aggregation and thrombus formation

arrhythmia: a disturbance of normal cardiac rhythm due to abnormal origin, discharge, or conduction of electrical impulses

artifact: waveform interference in an electrocardiogram tracing that results from patient movement or poorly placed or malfunctioning equipment

asthma: chronic disorder in which airways are hyperresponsive

asystole: the total absence of ventricular activity

atrial fibrillation: chaotic, asynchronous, electrical activity in atrial tissue that stems from impulses firing in reentry pathways at a rate of 400 to 600 times/minute, causing the atria to quiver instead of contract

atrial flutter: a cardiac rhythm characterized by an atrial rate of 250 to 400 beats/minute that originates in a single atrial focus, resulting from reentry and, possibly, increased automaticity

atrial kick: the amount of blood pumped into ventricles as a result of atrial contraction; contributes about 30% of total cardiac output

atrioventricular node: the node situated low in the septal wall of the right atrium that slows the impulse conduction between the atria and ventricles, providing time for the contracting atria to fill the ventricles with blood before the lower chambers contract

automaticity: the ability of a cardiac cell to initiate an impulse on its own

bigeminy: a premature beat occurring every other beat that alternates with normal complexes

biphasic: a complex containing both an upward and a downward deflection; usually seen when the electrical current is perpendicular to the observed lead

bundle-branch block: the slowing or blocking of an impulse as it travels through one of the bundle branches

capture: successful pacing of the heart, represented on an electrocardiogram by a pacemaker spike followed by a P wave or QRS complex

cardiac output: the amount of blood ejected from the left ventricle in 1 minute (the normal value is 4 to 8 L/minute)

cardioversion: the restoration of normal rhythm by synchronized electric shock or drug therapy

carotid sinus massage: manual pressure applied to the carotid sinus to slow the heart rate

compensatory pause: the period following a premature contraction during which the heart regulates itself, allowing the sino-atrial node to resume normal conduction

conduction: the transmission of electrical impulses through the myocardium

conductivity: the ability of one cardiac cell to transmit an electrical impulse to another cell

contractility: the ability of a cardiac cell to contract after receiving an impulse

couplet: a pair of premature beats that occur together

defibrillation: the termination of ventricular fibrillation by electrical shock

deflection: the direction of a waveform, based on the direction of a current

depolarization: the response of a myocardial cell to an electrical impulse that causes movement of ions across the cell membrane, which triggers myocardial contraction

diastole: the phase of the cardiac cycle during which both atria (atrial diastole) or both ventricles (ventricular diastole) are at rest and filling with blood

ectopic beat: a contraction that occurs as a result of an impulse generated from a site other than the sinoatrial node

electrocardiogram complex: waveform representing the electrical events of one cardiac cycle, consisting of five main waveforms (labeled P, Q, R, S, and T), a sixth waveform (labeled U) that occurs under certain conditions, the PR and QT intervals, and the ST segment

endotracheal intubation: oral or nasal insertion of a flexible tube through the larynx into the trachea to control the airway and mechanically ventilate the patient

enhanced automaticity: a condition in which pacemaker cells increase the firing rate above their inherent rate

excitability: the ability of a cardiac cell to respond to an electrical stimulus

first-degree atrioventricular (AV) block: a cardiac rhythm that occurs when impulses from the atria are consistently delayed during conduction through the AV node

hypoxemia: oxygen deficit in arterial blood (lower than 80 mm Hg)

hypoxia: reduction of oxygen in body tissues to below normal levels

intrinsic: naturally occurring electrical stimulus from within the heart's conduction system

inverted: a negative or downward deflection on an electrocardiogram

junctional tachycardia: three or more premature junctional contractions occurring in a row, caused by an irritable focus from the atrioventricular junction that enhances automaticity and overrides the sinoatrial node to function as the heart's pacemaker, which depolarizes the atria by means of retrograde conduction (usually the rate measures between 100 and 200 beats/minute)

lead: perspective of the electrical activity in a particular area of the heart through the placement of electrodes on the chest wall

monomorphic: a form of ventricular tachycardia in which the QRS complexes have a uniform appearance from beat to beat

multifocal atrial tachycardia: a cardiac rhythm that results from an extremely rapid firing of multifocal ectopic sites

multiform or multifocal: a type of premature contraction that has differing QRS configurations as a result of originating from different irritable sites in the atria or ventricles

nonrebreather mask: type of oxygen delivery system involving a one-way inspiratory valve, which opens on inhalation and directs oxygen from a reservoir bag into the mask, allowing the patient to breathe air only from the bag

nonsustained ventricular tachycardia: ventricular tachycardia that lasts less than 30 seconds

normal sinus rhythm: the standard against which all other rhythms are compared; an impulse that starts in the sinus node and progresses to the ventricles through a normal conduction pathway—from the sinus node to the atria and atrioventricular node, through the bundle of His, to the bundle branches, and on to the Purkinje fibers

oropharyngeal airway: curved rubber or plastic device inserted into the mouth to the posterior pharynx to establish or maintain a patent airway

pacemaker: a group of cells that generates impulses to the heart muscle or a battery-powered device that delivers an electrical stimulus to the heart to cause myocardial depolarization

paroxysmal: an episode of an arrhythmia that starts and stops suddenly

pneumothorax: collapse of part or all of the lung due to air in the pleural space

polymorphic: a type of ventricular tachycardia in which the QRS complexes change from beat to beat

preload: a stretching force exerted on the ventricular muscle by the blood it contains at the end of diastole

proarrhythmia: a rhythm disturbance caused or made worse by drugs or other therapy

pulmonary edema: a life-threatening condition in which an abnormal amount of fluid accumulates in the lungs

pulmonary embolism: sudden obstruction of a pulmonary artery by foreign substances or a blood clot

pulseless electrical activity: a cardiac rhythm in which isolated electrical activity occurs sporadically without evidence of effective myocardial contraction; commonly caused by a clinical condition that can be reversed when identified quickly and treated appropriately

pulse oximetry: relatively simple, noninvasive procedure used to monitor arterial oxygen saturation

quadrigeminy: a premature beat occurring every fourth beat that alternates with three normal complexes

reentry mechanism: the failure of a cardiac impulse to follow the normal conduction pathway; instead, it follows a circular path

refractory: a type of arrhythmia that doesn't respond to usual treatment measures

refractory period: a brief period during which excitability in a myocardial cell is depressed

repolarization: the recovery of myocardial cells after depolarization during which the cell membrane returns to its resting potential

rhythm strip: the length of electrocardiogram (ECG) paper that shows multiple ECG complexes representing a picture of the heart's electrical activity in a specific lead

second-degree atrioventricular (AV) block (type I, Wenckebach or Mobitz I): a cardiac rhythm that occurs when diseased tissues in the AV node delay conduction of impulses to the ventricles; each impulse from the sinotrial node is delayed slightly longer than the previous impulse with a pattern of progressive prolongation of the PR interval, eventually leading to a dropped beat when the impulse isn't conducted to the ventricles; the pattern then repeats after the dropped beat

second-degree atrioventricular block (type II): a cardiac rhythm produced by a conduction disturbance in the His-Purkinje fibers, causing an intermittent conduction delay or block (the PR and R-R intervals remain constant before the dropped beat)

sinoatrial (SA) node: the node located on the endocardial surface of the right atrium near the superior vena cava, which serves as the heart's normal pacemaker by firing an impulse throughout the right and left atria, resulting in atrial contraction (under normal conditions, the SA node generates an impulse 60 to 100 times/minute)

sinus bradycardia: a cardiac rhythm in which the sinus rate is below 60 beats/minute and all impulses come from the sinoatrial node

sinus tachycardia: an acceleration of the firing of the sinoatrial node beyond its normal discharge rate, resulting in a heart rate of 100 to 150 beats/minute (rates greater than 150 beats/minute may indicate an ectopic focus)

status asthmaticus: emergency, life-threatening situation resulting from an acute asthma attack that goes untreated or in which the person doesn't respond to drug therapy after 24 hours

Stokes-Adams attack: a sudden episode of light-headedness or loss of consciousness caused by an abrupt slowing or stopping of the heartbeat

sustained ventricular tachycardia: a type of ventricular tachycardia that lasts longer than 30 seconds

systole: the phase of the cardiac cycle during which both atria (atrial systole) or both ventricles (ventricular systole) are contracting

tension pneumothorax: air trapped within the pleural space that can be fatal without prompt treatment

third-degree atrioventricular block: a cardiac rhythm in which all supraventricular impulses are prevented from reaching the ventricles; the atria and ventricles beat independently of each other

torsades de pointes: a polymorphic ventricular tachycardia characterized by a prolonged QT interval and QRS polarity that seem to spiral around the isoelectric line

trigeminy: a premature beat occurring every third beat that alternates with two normal complexes

triplet: three premature beats occurring together

uniform or unifocal: a type of premature ventricular contraction that has the same or similar QRS configuration and originates from the same irritable site in the ventricle

vagal stimulation: the pharmacologic or manual stimulation of the vagus nerve to slow the heart rate

Valsalva's maneuver: a technique of forceful expiration against the closed glottis that's used to slow the heart rate

ventilation: gas distribution into and out of the pulmonary airways

ventricular fibrillation: a chaotic pattern of electrical activity in the ventricles in which electrical impulses arise from many different foci, producing no effective muscular contraction and no cardiac output

Venturi mask: type of oxygen delivery system that allows for the mixture of a specific volume of air and oxygen to deliver a highly accurate oxygen concentration

Wolff-Parkinson-White syndrome: abnormality of cardiac rhythm that occurs when an anomalous atrial bypass tract (bundle of Kent) develops outside the atrioventricular junction, connecting the atria and ventricles and causing impulses to be conducted to either the atria or ventricles

Selected references

Albers, G. W., Amarenco, P., J. Easton, D., Sacco, R. L., & Teal, P. (2008). Antithrombotic and thrombolytic therapy for ischemic stroke: American College of Chest Physicians Evidence-Based Clinical Practice Guidelines (8th edition). *Chest, 133*(6), 630S–669S. doi:10.1378/chest.08-0720

American Heart Association. (2010). *Highlights of the 2010 American Heart Association Guidelines for CPR and ECC*. Retrieved from http://www.heart.org/idc/groups/heart-public/@wcm/@ecc/documents/downloadable/ucm_317350.pdf

American Heart Association. (2010). *2010 handbook of emergency cardiovascular care for healthcare providers*. Dallas, TX: Author.

ECG interpretation made incredibly easy (5th ed.). (2010). Philadelphia, PA: Lippincott Williams & Wilkins.

Emergency Nurses Association. (2010). *Sheehy's emergency nursing: Principles and practice* (6th ed.). St. Louis, MO: Mosby.

Lloyd, M. S., Heeke, B., Walter, P. F., & Langberg, J. J. (2008). Hands-on defibrillation: An analysis of electrical current flow through rescuers in direct contact with patients during biphasic external defibrillation. *Circulation, 117*(19), 2435–2436.

Marik, P. (2010). *Handbook of evidence-based critical care*. New York, NY: Springer.

Meaney, P., Nadkarni, V., Kern, K. B., Indik, J. H., Halperin, H. R., & Berg, R. A. (2010). Rhythms and outcomes of adult in-hospital cardiac arrest. *Critical Care Medicine, 38*(1), 101–108.

Middleton, P. (2009). Insertion techniques of the laryngeal mask airway: A literature review. *Journal of Perioperative Practice, 19*(1), 31–35.

Nettina, S. M. (2010). *Lippincott manual of nursing practice* (9th ed.). Philadelphia, PA: Lippincott Williams & Wilkins

Nursing 2012 drug handbook. (2011). Philadelphia, PA: Lippincott Williams & Wilkins.

Porth, C. (2010). *Essentials of pathophysiology concepts of altered health states* (3rd ed.). Philadelphia, PA: Lippincott Williams & Wilkins.

Sasson, C., Rogers, M. A., Dahl, J., & Kellerman, A. L. (2010). Predictors of survival from out-of-hospital cardiac arrest: A systematic review and meta-analysis. *Circulation: Cardiovascular Quality and Outcomes, 3*, 63–81.

Simmons, S. (2010). Taking the sting out of anaphylaxis. *Nursing Critical Care, 5*(3), 10–16.

2010 American Heart Association Guidelines for Cardiopulmonary Resuscitation and Emergency Cardiovascular Care. (2010, November 2). *Circulation, 122*(18, suppl 3).

Wiegand, D. J. (2011). *AACN procedure manual for critical care* (6th ed.). St. Louis, MO: Elsevier/Saunders.

Woods, S., Froelicher, E., Motzer, S., & Bridges, E. (2009). *Cardiac nursing* (6th ed.). Philadelphia, PA: Lippincott Williams & Wilkins.

Index